SUCCINCT CONCISE ANATOMY

for Dental Students with MCQs

Nagesh Khurana BDS MDS (Pursuing)
Department of Pedodontics and Preventive Dentistry
Modern Dental College and Research Centre
Indore, Madhya Pradesh, India

Aafreen Aftab BDS
People's Dental Academy
Bhopal, Madhya Pradesh, India

Forewords

MK Gupta
ND Shashikiran

JAYPEE

JAYPEE BROTHERS MEDICAL PUBLISHERS (P) LTD

New Delhi • London • Philadelphia • Panama

Jaypee Brothers Medical Publishers (P) Ltd.

Headquarters
Jaypee Brothers Medical Publishers (P) Ltd
4838/24, Ansari Road, Daryaganj
New Delhi 110 002, India
Phone: +91-11-43574357, Fax: +91-11-43574314
Email: jaypee@jaypeebrothers.com

Overseas Offices

J.P. Medical Ltd.
83, Victoria Street, London
SW1H 0HW (UK)
Phone: +44-2031708910
Fax: +02-03-0086180
Email: info@jpmedpub.com

Jaypee-Highlights Medical Publishers Inc.
City of Knowledge, Bld. 237, Clayton
Panama City, Panama
Phone: +507-301-0496
Fax: +507-301-0499
Email: cservice@jphmedical.com

Jaypee Medical Inc.
The Bourse
111, South Independence Mall East
Suite 835, Philadelphia, PA 19106, USA
Phone: + 267-519-9789
Email: joe.rusko@jaypeebrothers.com

Jaypee Brothers Medical Publishers (P) Ltd.
17/1-B Babar Road, Block-B, Shaymali
Mohammadpur, Dhaka-1207
Bangladesh
Mobile: +08801912003485
Email: jaypeedhaka@gmail.com

Jaypee Brothers Medical Publishers (P) Ltd.
Shorakhute, Kathmandu
Nepal
Phone: +00977-9841528578
Email: jaypee.nepal@gmail.com

Website: www.jaypeebrothers.com
Website: www.jaypeedigital.com

Inquiries for bulk sales may be solicited at: jaypee@jaypeebrothers.com

SUCCINCT Concise Anatomy For Dental Students with MCQs

First Edition: **2013**

ISBN : 978-93-5090-619-4

Printed at Rajkamal Electric Press, Plot No. 2, Phase-IV, Kundli, Haryana.

Dedicated to

Those who matter so much
Our Parents
Dr Aftab Mustaquim
Dr Shaheen Siddiqui
Dr Ved Prakash Khurana
Mrs Kanchan Khurana
And most especially and always
Our Teachers...

Inspired by

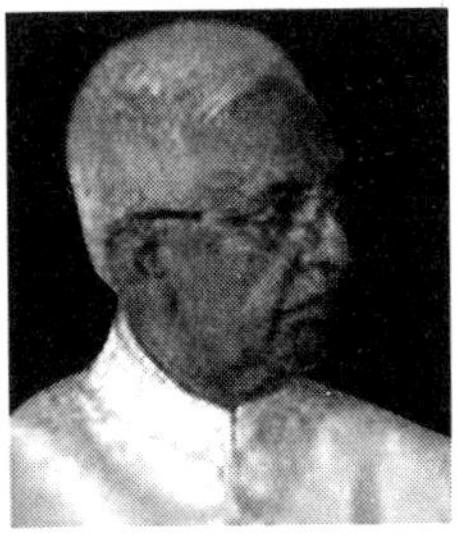

Late Dr Mahendra Pal Singh (Senior)
MBBS, MS (Anatomy)
Ex-Dean,
Gandhi Medical College, Bhopal, Madhya Pradesh, India
Professor and Head
Anatomy and Advisor
People's Group, Bhopal, Madhya Pradesh, India
Whose vision has always been a source of strength for us

Foreword

PEOPLE'S UNIVERSITY
(Established Under MP Act 17 of 2007)

PEOPLE'S DENTAL ACADEMY
AN ISO 9001: 2008 Certified Institute

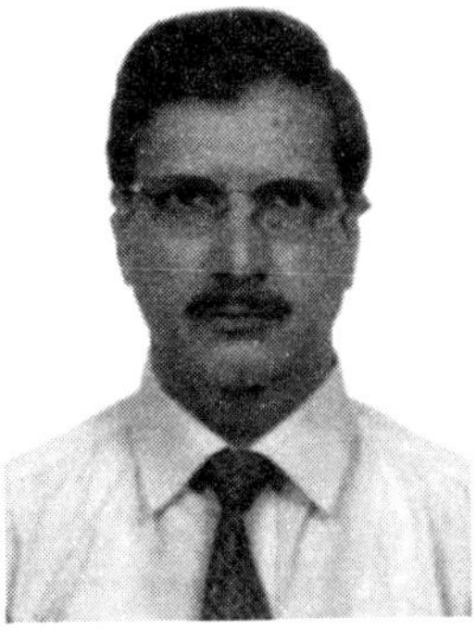

It gives me an immense pleasure to know that Dr Nagesh Khurana and Dr Aafreen Aftab are going to publish *SUCCINCT Concise Anatomy for Dental Students with MCQs.*

Anatomy is one of the basic sciences in dentistry, the thorough understanding of which can certainly bring out qualitative changes in our clinical approach towards amelioration of disease entity.

I have gone through the book and found it to be very informative and useful for undergraduate students. The texts have been presented in a very simple language, which is easy for the students to understand, assimilate and reproduce during examination.

My best wishes to Dr Khurana and Dr Aafreen for their humble beginning, sincere efforts and wishful contributions for the benefit of students.

MK Gupta
MDS FICD FPFA FIAOMS FICS (USA)
Dean
Professor and Head
Department of Oral and Maxillofacial Surgery
People's Dental Academy
Bhopal, Madhya Pradesh, India

Foreword

PEOPLE'S UNIVERSITY

(Established Under MP Act 17 of 2007)

PEOPLE'S DENTAL ACADEMY

AN ISO 9001: 2008 Certified Institute

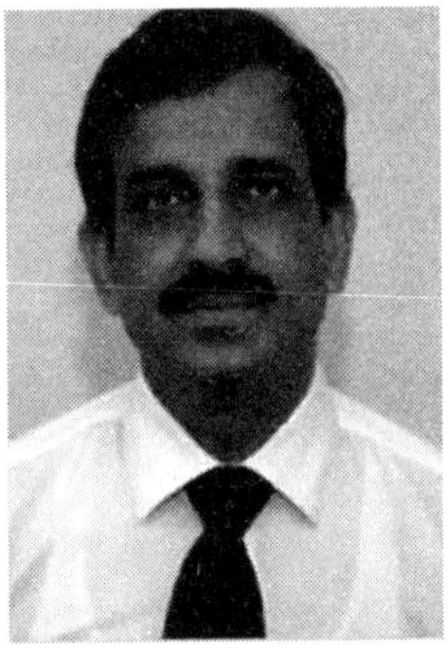

It gives me a great pleasure to write foreword for *SUCCINCT Concise Anatomy for Dental Students with MCQs* compiled by Dr Aafreen Aftab and Dr Nagesh Khurana.

This book is very concise and to the point with diagrammatic representation of various anatomic structures, which would be very beneficial for the 1st year BDS students. In addition, the contents of the book are well structured, and incorporates multiple choice questions, making it easy for the students.

The attention to minute details evident in the book reflects the meticulousness and efficiency of the authors. It is with a great pride, I wish authors all the very best for the success of this venture. I am sure that the book will guide students into gaining an insight from the vast field of anatomy.

ND Shashikiran MDS
Dean
Professor and Head
Department of Pedodontics and Preventive Dentistry
People's College of Dental Sciences
People's University
Bhopal, Madhya Pradesh, India

Preface

We hope that *SUCCINCT Concise Anatomy for Dental Students with MCQs* will become a helpful companion, especially for undergraduate and postgraduate medical and dental students as ready-reference.

This comprehensive compilation of Multiple Choice Questions and Previous Year Questions in easy-to-understand language has been in order to fulfill its purpose for pre-postgraduate and university examinations.

It is a privilege to achieve a dream come true to start this series on anatomy.

Nagesh Khurana
Aafreen Aftab

Acknowledgments

We adore and express deep sense of heartfelt indebtedness towards our parents and all family members.

We acknowledge with affection the constant support and motivation extended to us by Professor Jalees Siddiqui, Dr Kapil Khurana and Dr Nidhi Khurana. We also express profound gratitude to Dr Ashwini Deshpande for helping in proofreading and judicious suggestions. We are grateful to Dr Yogesh Sharma, for being a guiding light that was required for completing the arduous task.

We are grateful to our colleagues and senior staff members of People's Dental Academy (PDA), Bhopal, Madhya Pradesh, India, who were the spirit behind the idea of bringing out the book.

Our special thanks to:

1. Librarian, Mrs Krishna Verma and staff, PDA, Bhopal, Madhya Pradesh, India
2. Brothers and Sister—Yasir Aftab, Samreen Aftab and Musheer Mustaquim
3. Friends—Dr Prakash Singh, Dr Abhiruchi Saraf, Dr Nitish Dale, Dr Pushpraj Gaur and Dr Nalin Singhal
4. Students of People's Group—Shubham Sharma, Bhaskar Sharma (PDA) and Zain Saeed (PCDS), Dr Neetu Mishra, Department of Oral Pathology, Modern Dental College and Research Centre, Indore, Madhya Pradesh, India.
5. Mr Rajeev from Lyall Book Depot and Publishers, Bhopal, Madhya Pradesh, India.
6. Rajdeep Graphics, Bhopal for typing the script in the same way as we wanted
7. Shri Jitendar P Vij (Group Chairman), Mr Ankit Vij (Managing Director), Mr Tarun Duneja (Director-Publishing), Mr KK Raman (Production Manager) and Mr Subarata Adhikary (Commissioning Editor) of M/s Jaypee Brothers Medical Publishers Ltd, New Delhi, India, for publishing the book.

Contents

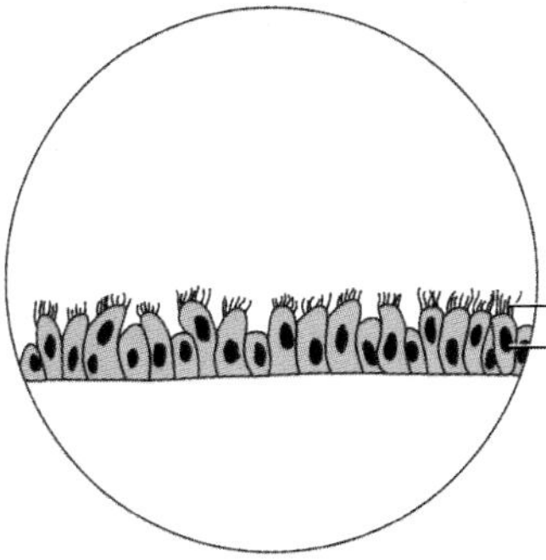
Cilia
Nucleus at different level

Fig. 30.1: Pseudostratified epithelium

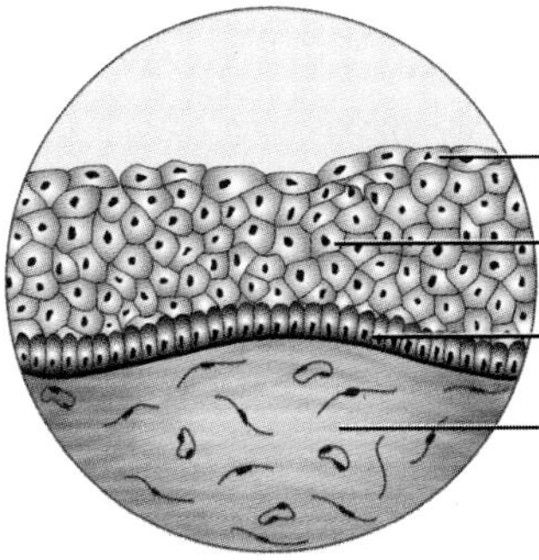
Umbrella shaped cell
Polygonal cell
Columnar basal cell
Connective tissue

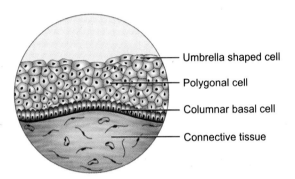

Fig. 30.2: Transitional epithelium

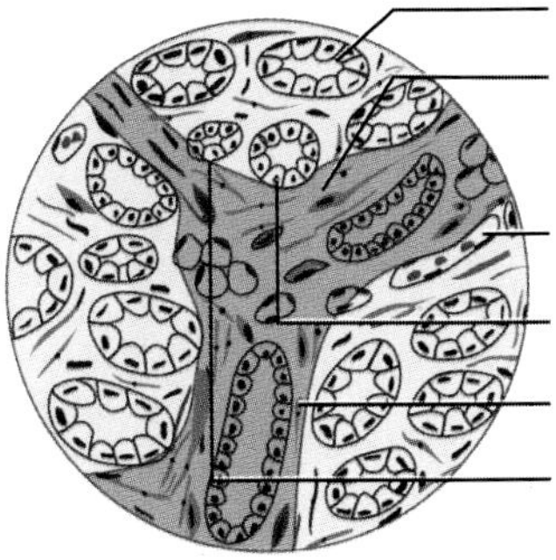
Mucous acini
Connective tissue septa dividing gland into lobes
Blood vessel
Intralobular duct
Interlobular duct
Intercalated duct

Fig. 30.3: Mucous salivary gland (Sublingual)

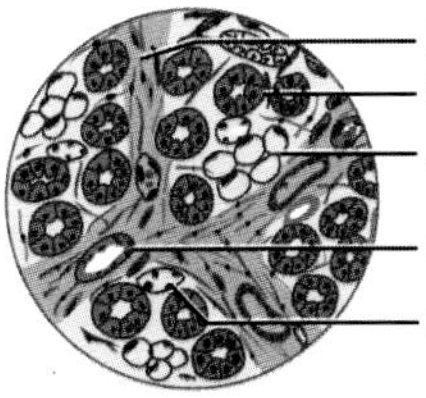
Interlobular connective tissue septa
Serous acini
Adipose tissue
Interlobular duct
Intralobular duct

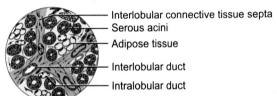

Fig. 30.4: Serous salivary gland (Parotid)

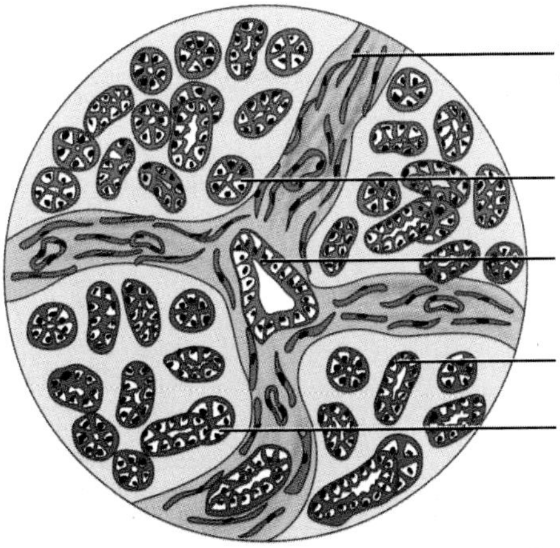
Connective tissue septa dividing gland into lobes
Mucous acini
Interlobular duct
Serous acini
Serous demilunes/demilune of gianuzzi

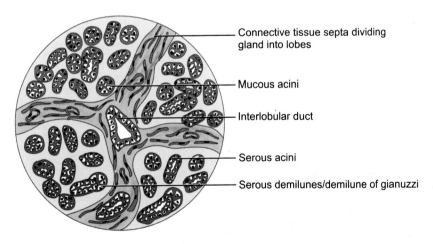

Fig. 30.5: Mixed salivary gland (Submandibular)

Plate 2

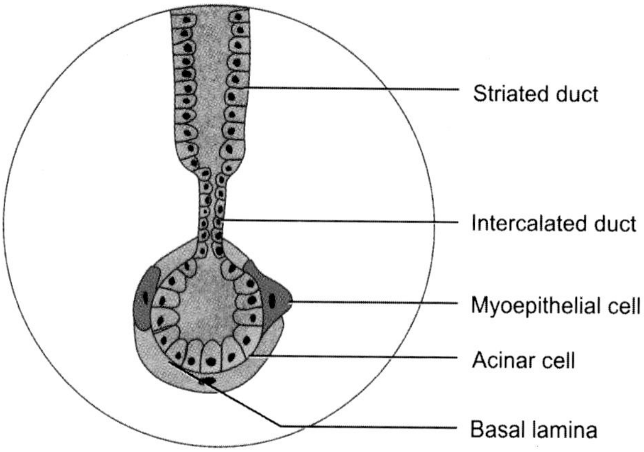
Striated duct
Intercalated duct
Myoepithelial cell
Acinar cell
Basal lamina

Fig. 30.6: Structure of ducts and acini

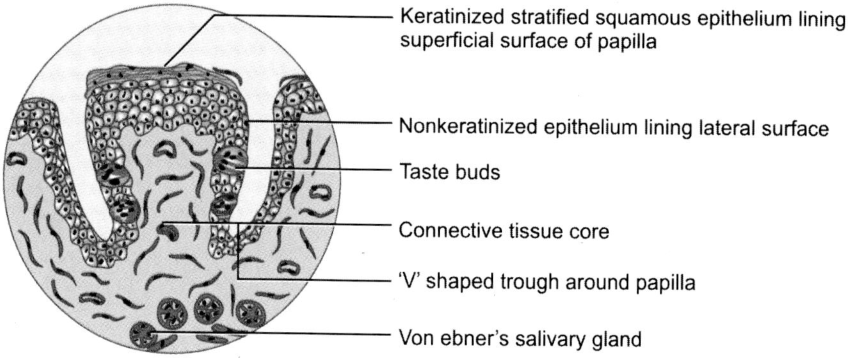
Keratinized stratified squamous epithelium lining superficial surface of papilla
Nonkeratinized epithelium lining lateral surface
Taste buds
Connective tissue core
'V' shaped trough around papilla
Von ebner's salivary gland

Fig. 30.7: Circumvallate papilla

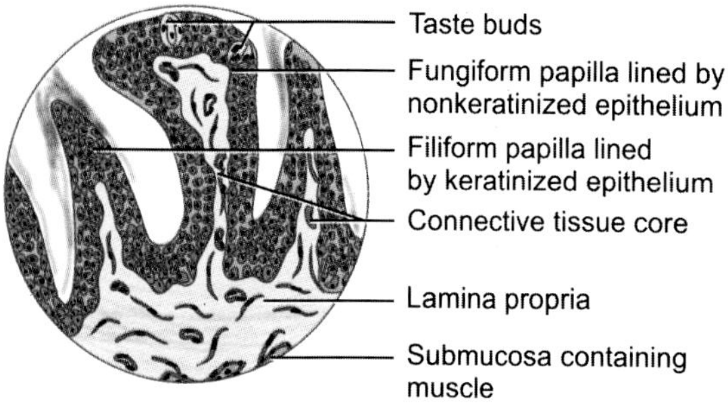
Taste buds
Fungiform papilla lined by nonkeratinized epithelium
Filiform papilla lined by keratinized epithelium
Connective tissue core
Lamina propria
Submucosa containing muscle

Fig. 30.8: Fungiform and filiform papilla

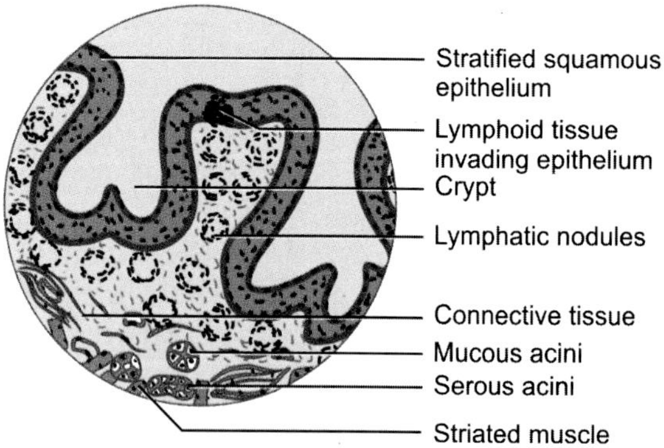
Stratified squamous epithelium
Lymphoid tissue invading epithelium
Crypt
Lymphatic nodules
Connective tissue
Mucous acini
Serous acini
Striated muscle

Fig. 30.9: Palatine tonsil

Plate 3

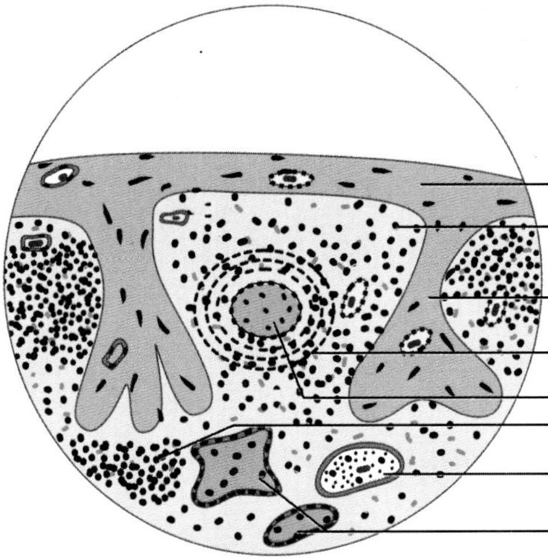

Capsule
Subcapsular sinus
Trabeculum with capillaries
Cortical nodule
Germinal center
Medullary cords
Trabecular sinus
Medullary lymph sinus

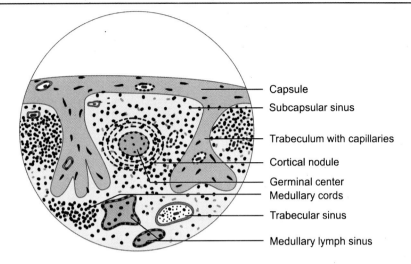

Fig. 30.10: Lymph node

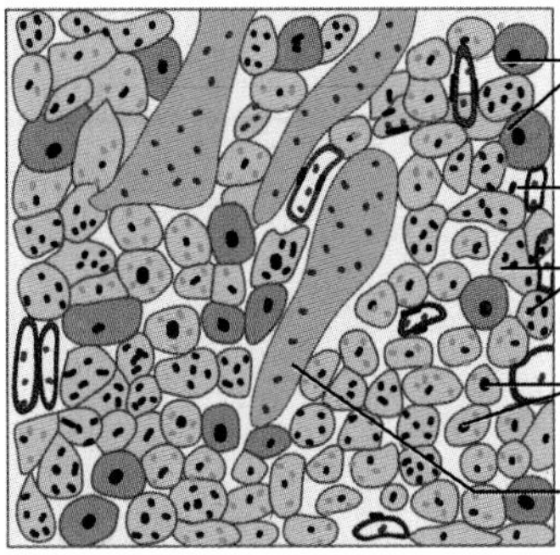

Chromophobes
Blood capillaries
Basophils
Acidophils
Sinusoid

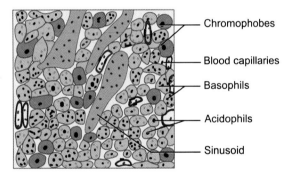

Fig. 30.11: Pituitary gland

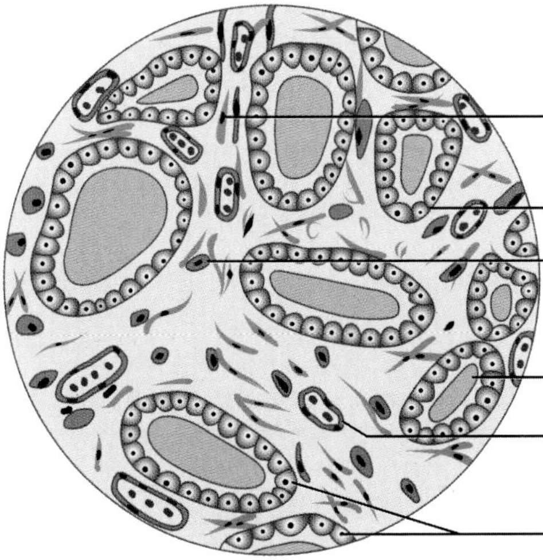

Interlobular connective tissue
Cuboidal epithelium lining follicles
Parafollicular cells
Colloid
Sinusoidal capillary
Follicles

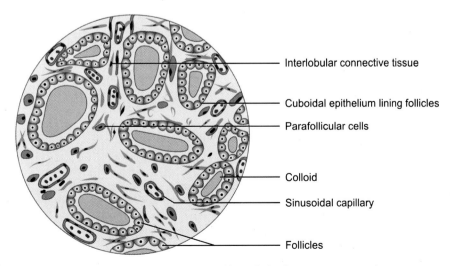

Fig. 30.12: Thyroid gland

Plate 4

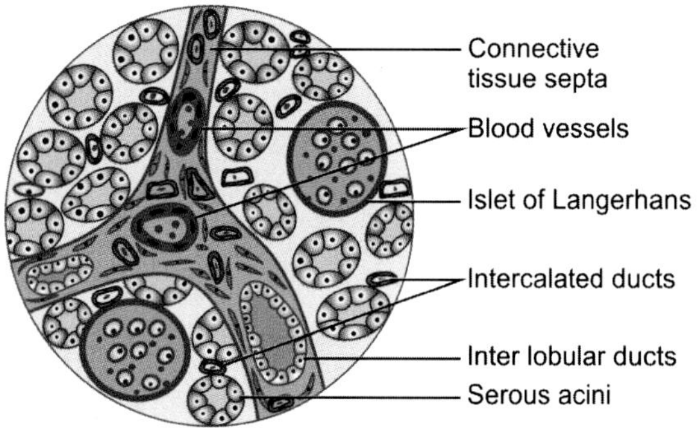

Connective tissue septa
Blood vessels
Islet of Langerhans
Intercalated ducts
Inter lobular ducts
Serous acini

Fig. 30.13: Pancreas

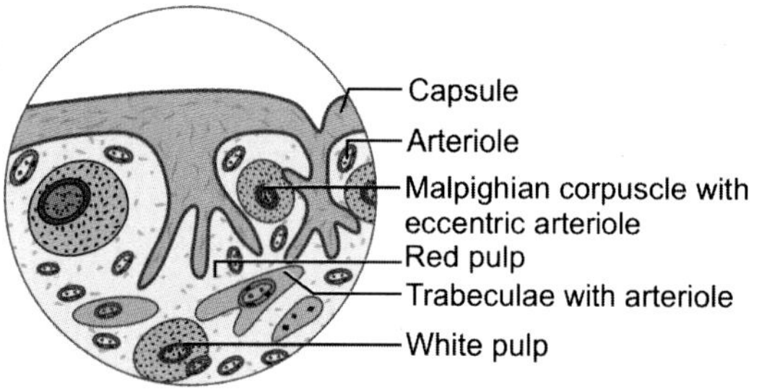

Capsule
Arteriole
Malpighian corpuscle with eccentric arteriole
Red pulp
Trabeculae with arteriole
White pulp

Fig. 30.16: Spleen

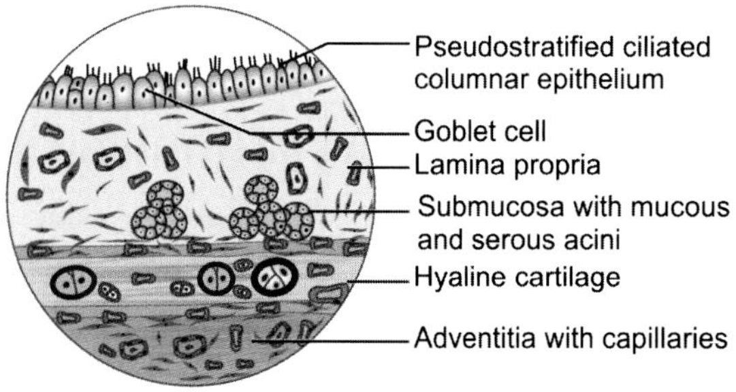

Pseudostratified ciliated columnar epithelium
Goblet cell
Lamina propria
Submucosa with mucous and serous acini
Hyaline cartilage
Adventitia with capillaries

Fig. 30.14: Trachea

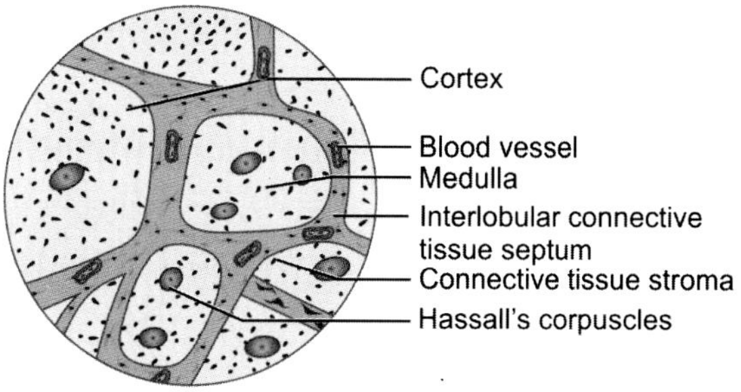

Cortex
Blood vessel
Medulla
Interlobular connective tissue septum
Connective tissue stroma
Hassall's corpuscles

Fig. 30.17: Thymus

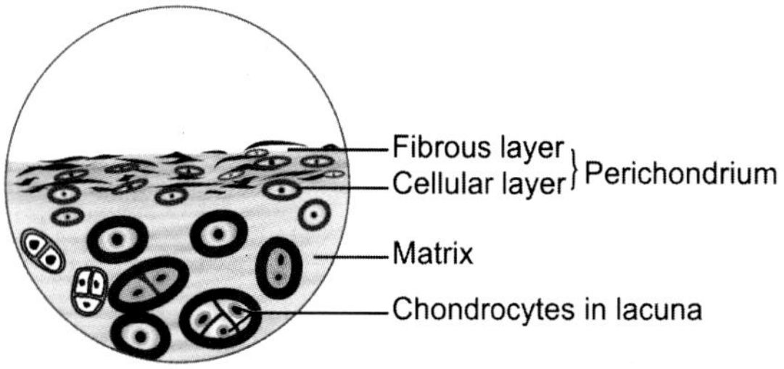

Fibrous layer
Cellular layer
Perichondrium
Matrix
Chondrocytes in lacuna

Fig. 30.15: Hyaline cartilage

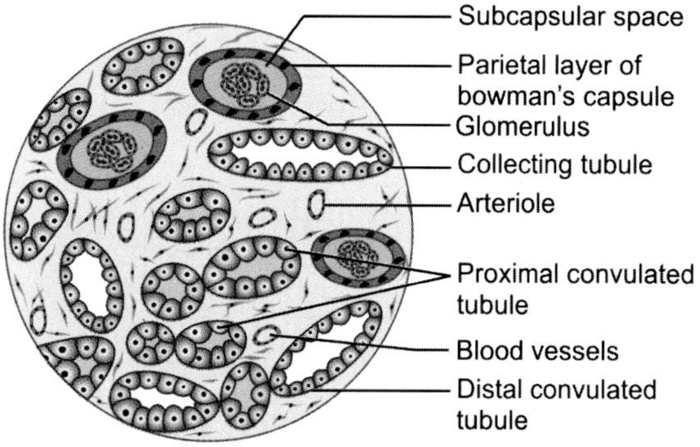

Subcapsular space
Parietal layer of bowman's capsule
Glomerulus
Collecting tubule
Arteriole
Proximal convulated tubule
Blood vessels
Distal convulated tubule

Fig. 30.18: Kidney

1 Scalp

SCALP

The soft tissue covering the vault of skull is known as scalp.

Extent

Anterior : Superaciliary arches
Posterior : External occipital protuberance and superior nuchal lines.
Lateral : Superior temporal line on each side

Layers

Consists of five layers:
S : Skin
C : Connective tissue
A : Aponeurosis
L : Loose areolar tissue
P : Periosteum

Skin

Richly supplied with hair, sweat glands and sebaceous glands.

Connective Tissue (Superficial Fascia)

- Blood vessels of scalp lie in this layer.
- Any injury here results in profuse bleeding as it is richly supplied by blood vessels.
- It consists of fat bounded with fibrous septa which binds skin to the subjacent aponeurosis.

Aponeurosis

- Formed by the aponeurosis (a fibrous connective tissue that attaches muscle to bone or other tissue) of occipitofrontalis muscle over the bone of skull.
- Occipitofrontalis originates from two parts/bellies:
  i. Occipital belly
  ii. Frontal belly
- The fibers of both bellies are inserted into a central fibrous layer known as Galea Aponeurotica/ Epicranial apponeurosis.

Extent

Anterior : Root of nose
Posterior : External occipital protuberance and highest nuchal lines on either side
Lateral : Zygomatic arch

Loose Areaolar Tissue

- It lies below the aponeurotic layer.
- Responsible for the mobility of scalp.
- Surgeons mobilize flaps in this plane for reconstructive surgery.

Periosteum (Pericranium)

- Innermost layer which is loosely attached to the surface of bone.
- Firmly adherent to the suture lines.

DANGEROUS LAYER OF THE SCALP

1. This layer is called the dangerous layer of scalp as it lodges the emissary veins which do not have valves (Fig. 1.1).
2. Emissary veins connect the extracranial veins with the intracranial venous sinuses to equalize the pressure.
3. Hence, if there is any infection of scalp, it can travel along the emissary vein into the intracranial dural venous sinuses leading to thrombosis.

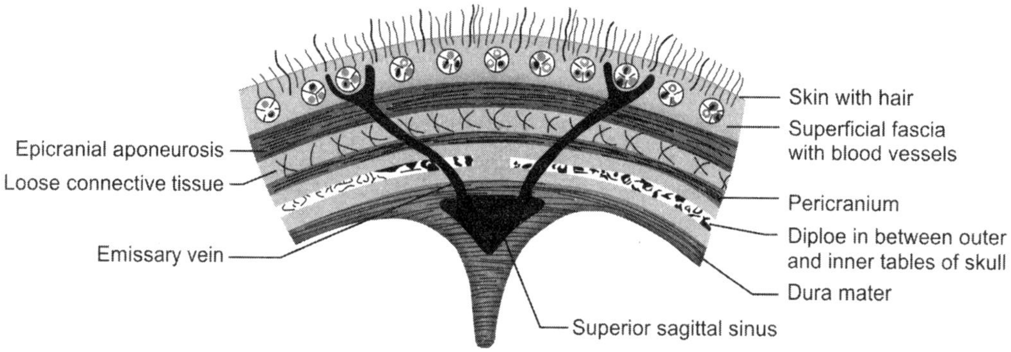
Skin with hair
Superficial fascia with blood vessels
Epicranial aponeurosis
Loose connective tissue
Pericranium
Diploe in between outer and inner tables of skull
Emissary vein
Dura mater
Superior sagittal sinus

Fig. 1.1: Layers of scalp

BLOOD SUPPLY

Arterial Supply – By Five Arteries

Front of Ear

1. Supratrochlear
2. Supraorbital
3. Superficial temporal

} Branch of ophthalmic artery

Behind the Ear

4. Posterior auricular
5. Occipital

} Branch of external carotid artery

Venous Supply—Veins Accompany the Arteries

- Supratrochlear
- Supraorbital
- Superficial temporal
- Posterior auricular
- Occipital

Nerve Supply

Sensory

Supplied by eight sensory nerves

Front of the Ear

1. Supratrochlear
2. Supraorbital
3. Zygomaticotemporal
4. Auriculotemporal

} Branch of trigeminal nerve

Behind the Ear

1. Great auricular
2. Lesser occipital
3. Greater occipital
4. Third occipital

} Arise from cervical plexus

Motor—By two nerves

1. Temporal
2. Posterior auricular

} Branch of facial nerve

Lymphatic Drainage

1. Preauricular lymph node—Drain anterior part of scalp.
2. Post-auricular lymph nodes—Drain posterior part of scalp.
3. Occipital lymph nodes.

Applied / Clinical Anatomy

1. Sebaceous cysts are common as sebaceous glands are abundant in the scalp.
2. Because of rich blood supply, the avulsed portion need not to be cut away, so it can be repositioned, sutured hence heals well.
3. The loose areolar tissue layer is the dangerous layer of scalp because emissary veins are lodged in this layer.
4. Wounds of the scalp bleed profusely because the vessels are prevented from retracting by the fibrous fascia.
5. Because of dense fascia, hemorrhages are never extensive hence, inflammation cause little swelling but much pain.
6. Black eye—Head injury results in collection of blood in connective tissue layer which causes generalized swelling. The blood may extend anteriorly into the root of nose and into the eyelids causing black eye.

   Figure 1.2 shows nerve and blood supply of scalp.

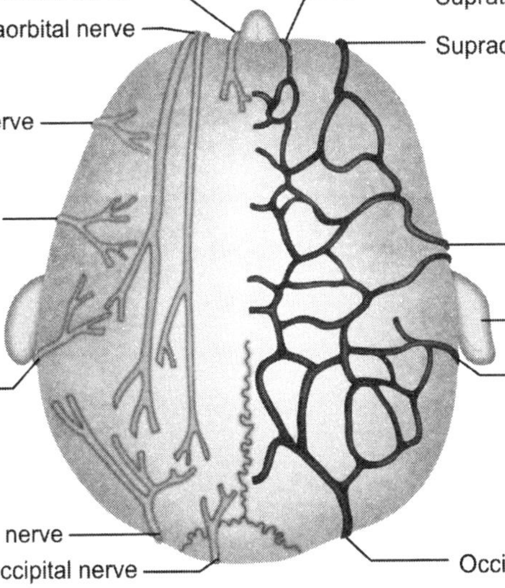
Supratrochlear nerve
Supraorbital nerve
Zygomatico-temporal nerve
Auriculotemporal nerve
Lesser occipital nerve
Greater occipital nerve
Third occipital nerve
Supratrochlear artery
Supraorbital artery
Superficial temporal artery
Pinna
Posterior auricular artery
Occipital artery

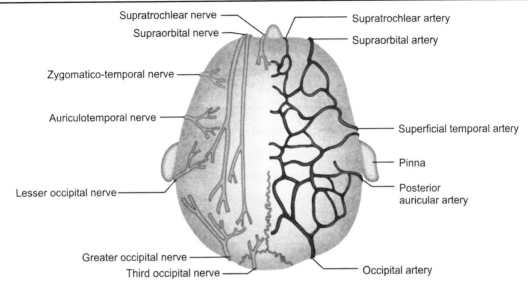

Fig. 1.2: Nerve and blood supply of scalp

PREVIOUS YEAR QUESTIONS

1. Describe scalp under following headings with diagrams:
   a. Layers
   b. Blood supply
   c. Nerve supply
   d. Lymphatic drainage
2. Write a short note on dangerous area of scalp.
3. Describe applied anatomy of scalp.

MULTIPLE CHOICE QUESTIONS

1. Following are the layers of scalp except:
   a. Superficial fascia
   b. Aponeurosis
   c. Pericranium
   d. Endocranium
2. Which layer is known as the "Dangerous area of scalp":
   a. Skin
   b. Pericranium
   c. Loose areolar tissue
   d. Deep fascia
3. Most of the movements of scalp occur between:
   a. Aponeurosis and pericranium
   b. Superficial fascia and deep fascia
   c. Skin and superficial fascia
   d. Loose areolar tissue and pericranium
4. All are true about emissary veins of scalp except:
   a. Valveless
   b. Connect extracranial veins with intracranial venous sinuses
   c. Principal vein of scalp
   d. Present in loose areolar tissue
5. Which of the following arteries does not supply scalp:
   a. Supratrochlear
   b. Supraorbital
   c. Facial
   d. Occipital
6. Lymph from scalp drains into:
   a. Parotid nodes
   b. Submandibular nodes
   c. Submental nodes
   d. Jugular nodes

Answers

1. (d) 2. (c) 3. (a) 4. (c) 5. (c) 6. (a)

2 Face

FACE

Extent

Superior : Hair line of scalp
Inferior : Chin and base of mandible
Lateral : Tragus of ear on either side
Face consist of two layers of soft tissue:

Skin

a. Rich vascular supply, thus wounds bleed profusely but heals rapidly
b. Numerous sweat and sebaceous glands present
c. Facial skin is thick and elastic, provides attachment to facial muscle

Superficial Fascia or Subcutaneous Tissue

It consists of:
i. Facial muscles
ii. Vessels
iii. Nerves
iv. Fat—abundant over cheeks and forms the buccal pad of fat especially in infants. It is absent over the eyelids.

There is no deep fascia in the face except over the parotid gland and buccinator muscle.

Facial Muscles / Muscles of Facial Expression (Fig. 2.1)

- Developed from 2nd branchial arch.

Group	*Muscles*	*Action*
Muscles of scalp	Occipitofrontalis (Front part)	Raises eyebrows upwards
Muscle of eyelid	• Orbicularis oculi—three Parts i. Palpebral ii. Orbital iii. Lacrimal	• Acts in closure of eyelids both voluntary or while blinking • Aids in transport of lacrimal fluid by dilating lacrimal sac
	• Corrugator supercilii	Pulls eyebrows medially and downwards
	• Levator palpebrae superioris	Elevates the eyelids
Muscle of nose	• Procerus	Act during frowning
	• Depressor septi	Dilatation of anterior nasal aperture
	• Orbicularis oris	• Closure of lips. • Protrusion of lips • Help in mastication as it compresses lip against gums and teeth
Muscles around the mouth	• Levator labii superioris aleque nasi	• Elevates and everts the upper lip
		• Dialates nostril
	• Levator labii superioris	• Elevates and everts the upper lip

Contd...

Contd...

Group	*Muscles*	*Action*
	• Levator anguli oris	• Raises angle of mouth
	• Depressor labii inferioris	• Pulls lower lip downwards and laterally
	• Depressor anguli oris	• Pulls angle of mouth downwards and laterally
	• Zygomaticus Major	• Pulls angle of mouth upwards and laterally
	• Zygomaticus Minor	• Elevates and evert upper lip
	• Mentalis	• Puckers the chin
	• Risorius	• Pulls angle of mouth downwards and laterally
	• Buccinator Main muscle of cheek Covered by buccopharyngeal membrane Not involved in facial expression	• Flattens cheek against the gums and teeth which helps during mastication • Helps in blowing out air through mouth • Whistling muscle
Muscles of neck	Platysma	• Depresses mandible • Pulls angle of mouth downwards as in horror or surprise

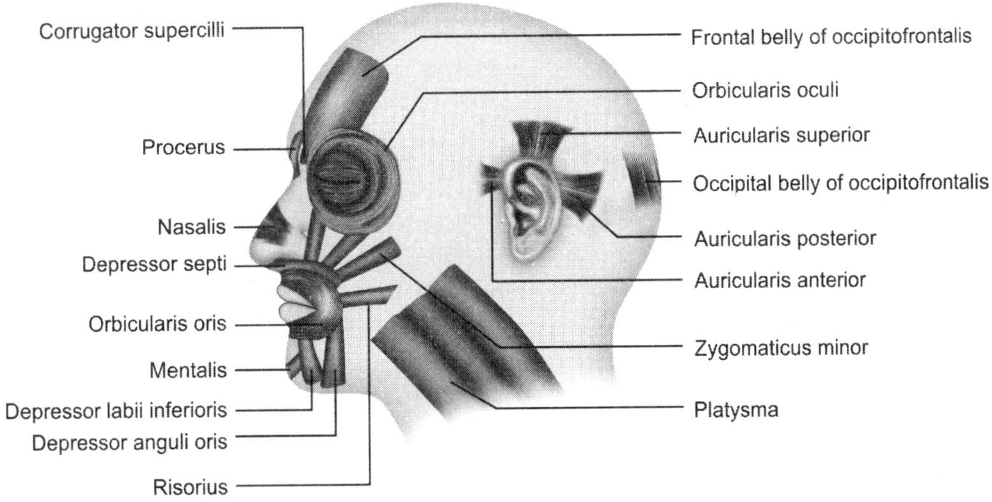
Corrugator supercilli
Procerus
Nasalis
Depressor septi
Orbicularis oris
Mentalis
Depressor labii inferioris
Depressor anguli oris
Risorius
Frontal belly of occipitofrontalis
Orbicularis oculi
Auricularis superior
Occipital belly of occipitofrontalis
Auricularis posterior
Auricularis anterior
Zygomaticus minor
Platysma

Fig. 2.1: Muscles of facial expression

- All are supplied by facial nerve except levator palpebrae superioris which is supplied by oculomotor nerve.

BLOOD SUPPLY OF FACE

Arterial Supply (Fig. 2.2)

1. Facial artery—Chief artery of face which arises from external carotid artery.
   a. It is divided into → Superior labial
   → Inferior labial
   → Lateral nasal
2. Transverse facial artery—branch of superficial temporal artery.
3. Arteries that accompany the cutaneous nerves.

Venous Supply

Facial Vein (Fig. 2.3)

- Main vein of the face
- Begins as the angular vein at the angle of eye formed by supratrochlear and supraorbital vein

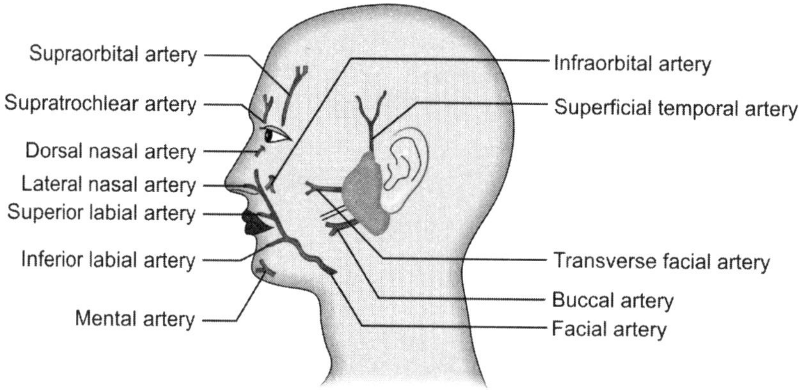
Supraorbital artery
Supratrochlear artery
Dorsal nasal artery
Lateral nasal artery
Superior labial artery
Inferior labial artery
Mental artery
Infraorbital artery
Superficial temporal artery
Transverse facial artery
Buccal artery
Facial artery

Fig. 2.2: Arterial supply of face

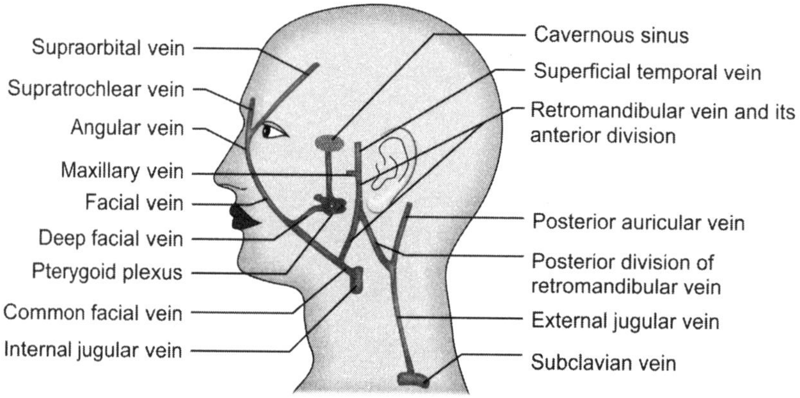
Supraorbital vein
Supratrochlear vein
Angular vein
Maxillary vein
Facial vein
Deep facial vein
Pterygoid plexus
Common facial vein
Internal jugular vein
Cavernous sinus
Superficial temporal vein
Retromandibular vein and its anterior division
Posterior auricular vein
Posterior division of retromandibular vein
External jugular vein
Subclavian vein

Fig. 2.3: Vein supply of face

Retromandibular Vein

- Anterior division joins with angular vein and forms the common facial vein which drains into the internal jugular vein.
- Posterior division joins with post auricular vein and form external jugular vein and drains into subclavian vein.

Supratrochlear vein ↘ ↙ **Supraorbital vein**

Angular vein

Takes straight course and pierces deep fascia ↓ ← Anterior division of retromandibular vein

Common facial vein

↓

Drains into the internal jugular vein

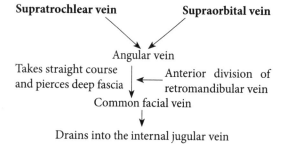

Clinical and Applied Anatomy

The area of face drained by the facial vein is the dangerous area of the face (Fig. 2.4):

- It comprises of lower part of nose, upper lip and the adjoining cheek.
- The facial vein communicates with the cavernous sinus via two routes:
  i. Angular or ophthalmic veins
  ii. Deep facial vein → pterygoid plexus of veins cavernous → emissary veins cavernous sinus.

NERVE SUPPLY OF THE FACE

- Facial vein does not contain valves.
- Facial nerve rests directly on the muscles of facial expression.

Lymphatic Drainage		
S. no.	*Part*	*Drains into*
1.	**Upper group** – Lateral half of forehead – Eyelids – Upper part of cheek – Lateral part of mandible	Parotid lymph node
2.	**Middle group** – Middle of forehead – Middle part of eyelid – Medial part of cheek – Medial part of mandible – Upper lip – Lateral part of lower lip	Submandibular lymph nodes
3.	**Lower group** – Central part of lower lip – Central part of chin	Submental lymph nodes

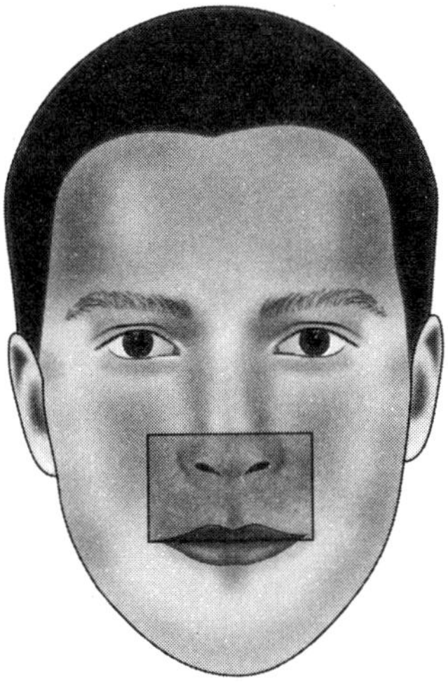

Fig. 2.4: Dangerous area of face

- Contraction of these muscle aids the retrograde spread of infective emboli from an infected part.
- Thus, emboli reach the cavernous sinus and cause thrombosis, which can be fatal.

Sensory Supply (Fig. 2.5)

1. Trigeminal nerve
   a. Ophthalmic division
      i. Lacrimal nerve
      ii. Supraorbital
      iii. Supratrochlear
      iv. Infratrochlear
      v. External nasal
   b. Maxillary division
      i. Infraorbital
      ii. Zygomatico facial
      iii. Zygomatico temporal
   c. Mandibular division
      i. Mental
      ii. Buccal
      iii. Auriculotemporal
2. Greater Auricular Nerve (C_2)
   Supplies the area of skin over the angle of mandible.

Motor Supply (Fig. 2.6)

- Derived from facial nerve
- It has five branches:
  i. Temporal
  ii. Zygomatic
  iii. Buccal
  iv. Marginal mandibular
  v. Cervical

FACIAL NERVE

- It is the 7th cranial nerve
- Mixed nerve containing both sensory and motor fibers.

Nuclear Origin

1. Motor nucleus of facial nerve
2. Superior salivatory nucleus

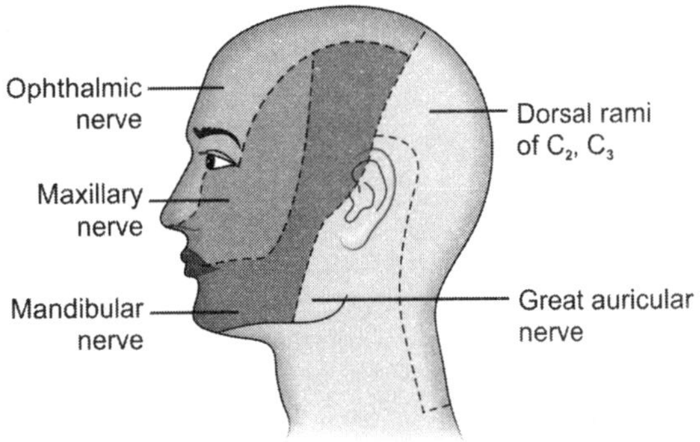

Ophthalmic nerve
Maxillary nerve
Mandibular nerve
Dorsal rami of C_2, C_3
Great auricular nerve

Fig. 2.5: Sensory supply of face

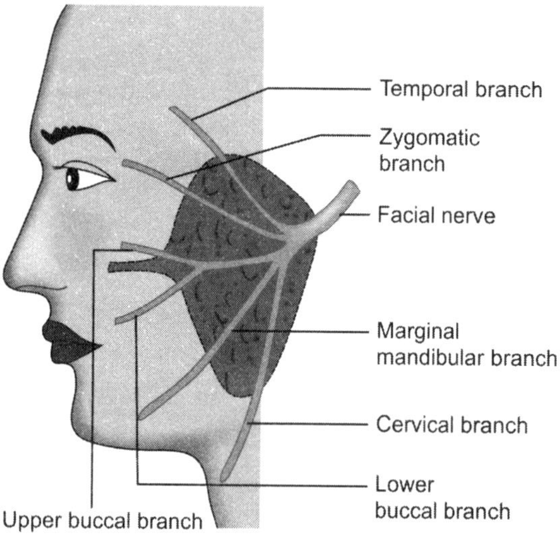
Temporal branch
Zygomatic branch
Facial nerve
Marginal mandibular branch
Cervical branch
Lower buccal branch
Upper buccal branch

Fig. 2.6: Motor supply of face

3. Nucleus of tractus solitarius
4. Spinal nucleus of trigeminal nerve.

Functional Components

1. Special visceral efferent is motor to muscles of facial expression.
2. Special visceral afferent—Carries taste sensation from anterior 2/3rd of tongue and palate.
3. General visceral efferent—Provides secretomotor fibers to:
   a. Submandibular and sublingual salivary gland
   b. Lacrimal gland
   c. Mucous glands of nose, palate and pharynx.
4. General somatic afferent—for sensory impulses from muscles of facial expression and external auditory meatus.

Intracranial Course

Facial nerve arises from brain stem by two roots (Fig. 2.7)

1. Motor Root : Larger and arises from the lower pons
2. Sensory Root : Arises from the lateral groove between pons and medulla. It is also known as nervous intermedius

Course

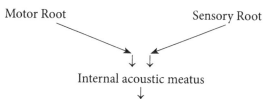

Motor Root → ↓ ← Sensory Root

Internal acoustic meatus
↓
Facial canal in the petrous temporal bone
↓
Epitympanic part of the middle ear
↓
Turns sharply backwards making an acute bend called Genu or Knee of facial nerve (Geniculate ganglion present on this Genu)
↓
Runs horizontally backwards in a bony canal
↓
Reaches junction of medial and posterior walls of middle ear
↓
Turns downwards and continues vertically in facial canal
↓
Emerges out of the skull through stylomastoid foramen

Extracranial Course

Stylomastoid foramen
↓
Curves forwards around the styloid process
↓
Parotid gland
↓
Divides into its terminal branches

Branches of Facial Nerve

1. Greater petrosal nerve
2. Lesser petrosal nerve
3. Nerve to stapedius
4. Chorda tympani nerve
   a. *Carries*: Taste fibers from anterior 2/3rd of tongue except from vallate papillae.
   b. Secretomotor fibers to the submandibular and sublingual salivary glands.

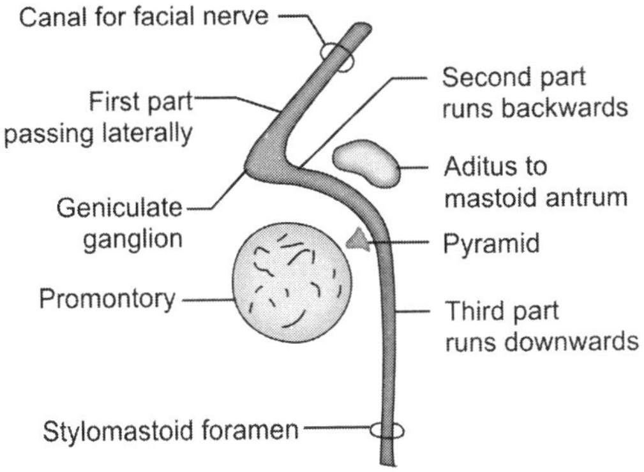
Canal for facial nerve
First part passing laterally
Second part runs backwards
Aditus to mastoid antrum
Geniculate ganglion
Pyramid
Promontory
Third part runs downwards
Stylomastoid foramen

Fig. 2.7: Intracranial course of facial nerve

5. Posterior auricular nerve
6. Nerve to posterior belly of digastric
7. Terminal branches – Five branches arise within the parotid gland
   a. Temporal—Supplies muscles of ear, frontal belly of occipitofrontalis and corrugator supercilli.
   b. Zygomatic—supplies orbicularis oculi.
   c. Buccal—Two in number:
      i. Upper supplies zygomaticus major and minor and levators of upper lip
      ii. Lower supplies buccinator and orbicularis oris.
   d. Marginal mandibular—supplies muscles of lower lip and chin
   e. Cervical—Supplies platysma
8. Communicating branches

Clinical and Applied Anatomy

Facial Palsy

- It is the paralysis of facial nerve
- It is of two types—Upper motor neuron type/Supranuclear palsy and lower motor neuron type/Infranculear palsy

Bell's Palsy

- It is unilateral, peripheral facial paralysis that has an abrupt onset.
- Cause may be cold exposure, trauma, tumor, familial occurrence as vascular damage, etc.

	Supranuclear palsy	*Infranculear palsy*
i.	It is caused by upper motor neuron lesion	It is caused by lower motor neuron lesion
ii.	Patient can make furrows on looking upwards	Furrows are lost on the side of face affected.
iii.	Lower part of face on the opposite side of lesion involved	Whole face and forehead of same side are involved
iv.	Lesion is situated above pons	Situated in pons or in the pathway from pons to its exit
v.	Isolated involvement is rare	Isolated lesion (idiopathic) are common e.g. Bell's Palsy

- It has following clinical features:
  i. Facial asymmetry
  ii. Loss of wrinkles on forehead
  iii. Inability to close the eye
  iv. Angle of mouth drops on affected side
  v. Loss of naso labial furrow
  vi. Accumulation of food into vestibule of mouth
  vii. Drooling of saliva from the angle of mouth
  viii. Loss of resistance while blowing out air in mouth
  ix. Skin folds are blunted on the affected side
- It is self-limiting disease and usually the patient recovers within 4 to 12 weeks.
- Treatment is symptomatic.

PREVIOUS YEAR QUESTIONS

1. Describe face under following headings:
   i. Development   ii. Nerve supply
   iii. Arterial supply   iv. Venous drainage
2. Describe in details the extracranial course of facial nerve.
3. Enumerate branches of facial nerve.
4. Describe facial nerve under following heads:
   i. Nuclei and course
   ii. Branches
   iii. Applied anatomy – Bell's palsy
5. Describe sensory nerve supply of face.
6. Write a short note on dangerous area of face.
7. Classify and name the muscles of facial expression.

MULTIPLE CHOICE QUESTIONS

1. There is no deep fascia in the face except over the
   a. Parotid gland
   b. Submandibular gland
   c. Sublingual gland
   d. All
2. The facial nerve
   a. Arises from medulla oblongata
   b. Transverses through parotid gland
   c. Supplies muscle of mastication
   d. Carries no taste fibers
3. Facial artery is a branch of
   a. Internal carotid artery
   b. External carotid artery
   c. Superficial temporal artery
   d. Maxillary artery
4. Danger area of face is called because of connection of facial veins to cavernous sinus through
   a. Transverse facial vein
   b. Maxillary vein
   c. Superior ophthalmic vein
   d. Ethmoidal vein
5. Largest vein of face is
   a. Facial vein
   b. Retromandibular vein
   c. Posterior auricular vein
   d. Supratrochlear vein
6. All muscles of facial expression are supplied by facial nerve except
   a. Orbicularis oris
   b. Levator palpebrae superioris
   c. Orbicularis oculi
   d. Levator anguli oris
7. Nerve supply of buccinator
   a. Mandibular nerve
   b. Facial nerve
   c. Maxillary nerve
   d. Auriculotemporal nerve
8. Facial nerve is
   a. Motor b. Sensory
   c. Parasympathetic d. Mixed
9. Following part of face drains into submandibular lymph node except
   a. Upper lip
   b. Lateral part of lower lip
   c. Medial part of mandible
   d. Central part of lower lip
10. Smiling and frowning are actions produced by following nerves:
    a. Mastication; trigeminal (V cranial) nerve
    b. Mastication; facial (VII cranial) nerve
    c. Facial expression; trigeminal (V cranial) nerve
    d. Facial expression; facial (VIII cranial) nerve
11. All the following muscle are innervated by facial nerve except
    a. Occipitofrontalis
    b. Rigorous
    c. Anterior belly of digastric
    d. Procerus
12. Facial muscles are derived from:
    a. 1st branchial arch
    b. 2nd branchial arch
    c. 3rd branchial arch
    d. 4th branchial arch
13. Which of the following is correctly matched:
    a. Doubt-mentalis
    b. Surprise-frontals
    c. Grief-depressor angulii oris
    d. All

Answers

1. (a) 2. (b) 3. (b) 4. (c) 5. (a) 6. (b) 7. (b) 8. (d) 9. (d) 10. (d)
11. (c) 12. (b) 13. (d)

3 Orbit

EYELIDS

- Eyelids are the movable curtains present in front of the eyeball.
- They protect the eye from injury, foreign bodies and bright light.
- Helps to keep the cornea moist and clean.
- Each eyelid – upper and lower are made up of five layers:
  i. Skin
  ii. Superficial fascia
  iii. Palpebral fascia (orbital septum)
  iv. Tarsal plate (meibomian/tarsal glands)
  v. Conjunctiva (palpebral part)

CONJUNCTIVA

Transparent mucous membrane consist of two parts

1. Palpebral conjunctiva
   - Lines inner aspect of eyelid
   - Highly vascular
2. Bulbar conjunctiva
   - Covers the sclera of the eyeball

LACRIMAL APPARATUS

The structures concerned with secretion and drainage of lacrimal or tear fluid constitute the lacrimal apparatus (Fig. 3.1).

Components of Lacrimal Apparatus

Lacrimal Gland and its Duct

- It is serous gland situated in lacrimal fossa.
- Dozen ducts from gland open into conjunctiva and pour lacrimal fluid into sac.
- Supplied by lacrimal branch of ophthalmic artery
- Innervated by lacrimal nerve which has both sensory and secretomotor fibers.

Conjunctival Sac

- Potential sac present between palpebral and bulbar conjunctiva.
- Most of the fluid evaporates and the remaining fluid is drained by lacrimal canaliculi.

Lacrimal Pancta and Canaliculis

- Each lacrimal canaliculus begins from a lacrimal punctum located at the medial end of the eyelid.
- Superior canaliculus

  \> Common canaliculus → Lacrimal sac

  Lower canaliculus
- Each is 10 mm long

Lacrimal Sac

- Membranous sac, 12 mm long and 8 mm wide.
- Located in lacrimal groove on the medial wall of the orbit
- It continues inferiorly with the nasolacrimal duct.

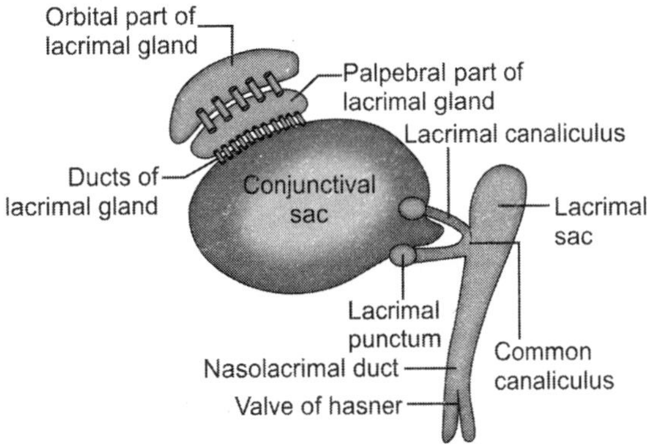

Orbital part of lacrimal gland
Palpebral part of lacrimal gland
Lacrimal canaliculus
Ducts of lacrimal gland
Conjunctival sac
Lacrimal sac
Lacrimal punctum
Common canaliculus
Nasolacrimal duct
Valve of hasner

Fig. 3.1: Lacrimal apparatus

Nasolacrimal Duct

- Membranous duct, 18 mm long which runs downwards, backwards and laterally from the lacrimal sac and opens in the inferior meatus of nose.
- Drains lacrimal fluid from lacrimal sac to the nose
- Its opening in the nose is guarded by lacrimal fold/ valve of Hasner.
- This prevent retrograde entry of air and nasal secretion into the eye.

Applied Anatomy

- Inflammation of lacrimal sac is known as Dacryocystitis.
- It hampers the drainage of lacrimal fluid into the nose which course from the conjunctival sac on to the face, a condition called Epiphora.
- Stye is the suppurative inflammation of zies gland.
- Chalazion (Internal stye) is the inflammation of meibomian gland.

BONY ORBIT

- Orbits are a pair of bony cavities, situated one on either side of root of the nose
- Each orbit is four sided pyramid with its apex directed behind at the optic canal and base in front, represented by orbital margins.

BOUNDARIES OF THE ORBIT

Medial Wall (Thinnest)

1. Frontal process of maxilla
2. Lacrimal bone
3. Orbital plate of ethmoid
4. body of sphenoid

Lateral Wall (Strongest)

1. Zygomatic bone
2. Greater wing of sphenoid.

Floor

1. Body of maxilla
2. Zygomatic bone
3. Palatine bone

Roof

1. Frontal bone
2. Lesser wing of sphenoid

Superior Orbital Fissure

It connects the orbit to middle cranial fossa.

Boundaries

Superior	:	Lesser wing of sphenoid
Inferior	:	Greater wing of sphenoid
Medial	:	Body of sphenoid

Structures passing through (Fig. 3.2)

- In superolateral compartment
  - Lacrimal, trochlear and frontal nerve.
  - Superior ophthalmic vein.
  - Recurrent meningeal branch of lacrimal artery.
- In intermediate compartment
  - Occulomotor nerve.
  - Nasociliary nerve.
  - Abducent nerve.
- In inferomedial compartment
  - Inferior ophthalmic vein

Inferior Orbital Fissure

It connects the orbit to the infratemporal and pterygopalatina fossa.

Boundaries

Anteromedial	:	Posterior border of maxilla
Posterolateral	:	Lower margin of greater wing of sphenoid
Lateral	:	Zygomatic bone
Medial	:	Medial end of the superior orbital fissure

Structures Passing through

- Infraorbital vessles
- Infraorbital nerve
- Zygomatic nerve
- Orbital branch of pterygopalatine ganglion
- Inferior ophthalmic veins and pterygoid venous plexus.

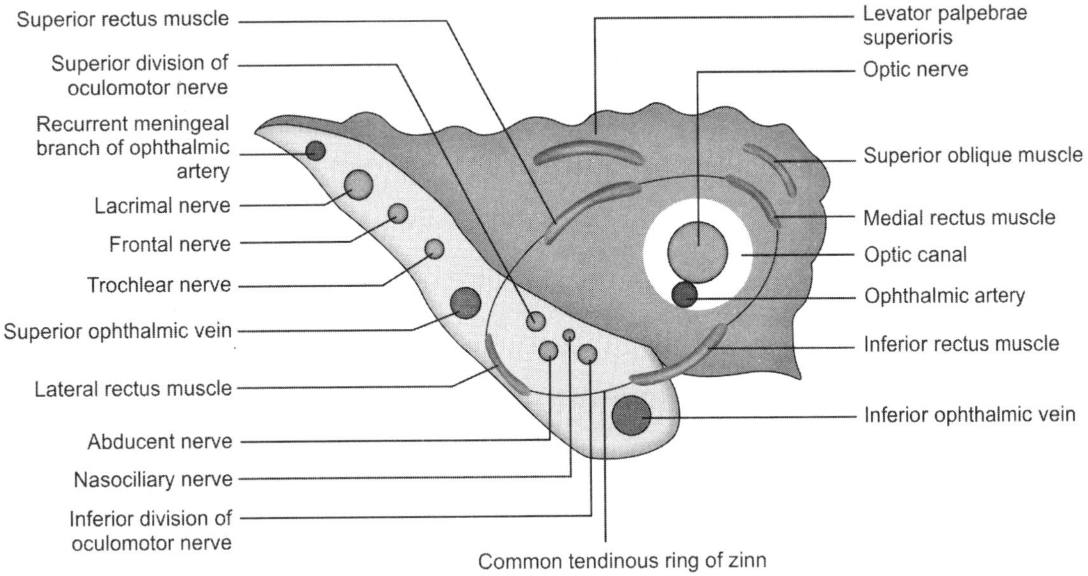
Superior rectus muscle
Superior division of oculomotor nerve
Recurrent meningeal branch of ophthalmic artery
Lacrimal nerve
Frontal nerve
Trochlear nerve
Superior ophthalmic vein
Lateral rectus muscle
Abducent nerve
Nasociliary nerve
Inferior division of oculomotor nerve
Common tendinous ring of zinn
Levator palpebrae superioris
Optic nerve
Superior oblique muscle
Medial rectus muscle
Optic canal
Ophthalmic artery
Inferior rectus muscle
Inferior ophthalmic vein

Fig. 3.2: Structures passing through superior orbital fissure

CONTENTS OF ORBIT

- Eyeball
- Muscles of orbit
- Fascia bulbi
- Nerves
  - Optic nerve
  - 3rd, 4th and 6th cranial nerve
  - Ophthalmic nerve
- Ophthalmic artery
- Superior and inferior ophthalmic veins
- Lacrimal gland
- Orbital fat

MUSCLES OF ORBIT

Seven voluntary and three involuntary muscles.

Extraocular Muscle of Eyeball (Fig. 3.3)

- Six muscles move the eyeball and one muscle move the upper eyelid.
- Consists of :
  1. Four recti muscles
     a. Superior rectus
     b. Inferior rectus
     c. Medial rectus
     d. Lateral rectus

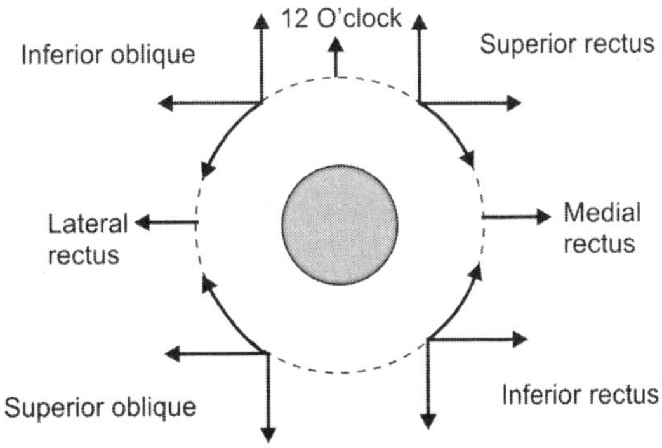
12 O'clock
Inferior oblique
Superior rectus
Lateral rectus
Medial rectus
Superior oblique
Inferior rectus

Fig. 3.3: Actions of extraocular muscles of eyeball

  2. Two oblique muscles (Fig. 3.4)
     a. Superior oblique
     b. Inferior oblique

Involuntary Extraocular Muscles

- Superior tarsal muscle
- Inferior tarsal muscle
- Orbitalis muscles

All are supplied by superior cervical Ganglia.

Clinical and Applied Anatomy

- Unilateral paralysis of an individual muscle due to involvement of corresponding nerve, produces

Muscle	*Origin*	*Insertion*	*Nerve Supply*	*Action*
• **Four recti:**				
i. Superior recti ii. Inferior recti iii. Medial recti iv. Lateral recti	Common tendinous ring	Sclera a little posterior to limbus	Occulomotor nerve except lateral rectus which is supplied by abducent (VI) nerve (LR6)	• Superior – Upward, medial rotation (adduction) and intortion • Inferior – Depression, adduction and extortion • Medial – Adduction (medial rotation) Abduction (Lateral rotation) • Lateral
• **Two oblique**				
i. Superior oblique ii. Inferior oblique iii. Levator palpebral superioris	• Body of sphenoid • Anteromedial angle of floor of the orbit lateral to lacrimal groove • Lesser wing of sphenoid above the common tendinous ring	• Sclera between the superior and lateral rectus • Into sclera a little below and posterior to insertion of superior oblique – Upper lamellae – skin of upper eyelids – Intermediate lamella – upper margin of superior tarsus – Lower lamellae superior fornix of conjunctiva	Trochlear nerve (IV) (SO 4) • Oculomotor nerve • Oculomotor nerve	Depression, abduction, intortion Elevation, abduction, extortion Elevation of upper eyelids

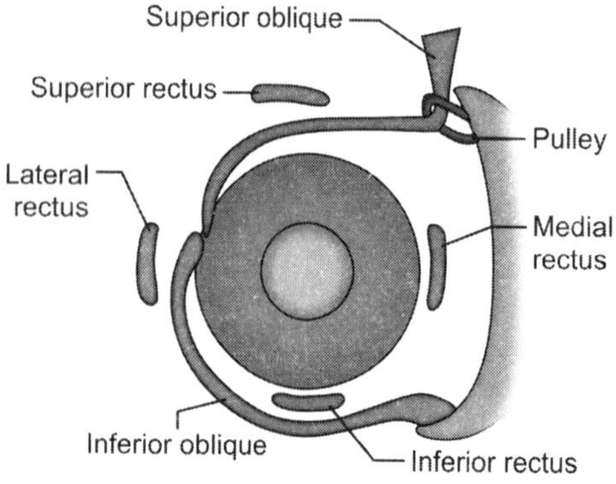
Superior oblique
Superior rectus
Lateral rectus
Pulley
Medial rectus
Inferior oblique
Inferior rectus

Fig. 3.4: Oblique of eyeball muscles

Strabismus/Squint and may result in Diplopia (double vision).

- Paralysis of levator palpebrae superior leads to ptosis i.e. drooping of upper eyelid. This can be due to either, involvement of occulomotor nerve or cervical sympathetic chain (as in Horner's syndrome).

FACIAL SHEATH OF EYEBALL (BULBAR FASCIA)

- Tenon's capsule form a thin, loose membranous sheath around the eyeball.
- The eyeball can freely move within this sheath.
- Sheath is pierced by:
  - i. Tendons of extraocular muscles
  - ii. Ciliary vessles and nerve
- Sheath gives off three expansion
  - i. Tubular sheath
  - ii. Medial check ligament
  - iii. Lateral check ligament
- Lower part of Tenon's capsule is thickened, and named as Suspensory ligament of eye or suspensry ligament of Lockwood.
- It is expanded in the center and narrow at its extremities.
- It is slung like a hammock below the eyeball.
- It is formed by union of margins of sheaths of inferior rectus and inferior oblique muscle with medial and lateral check ligaments (Fig. 3.5)
- It supports the eyeball.

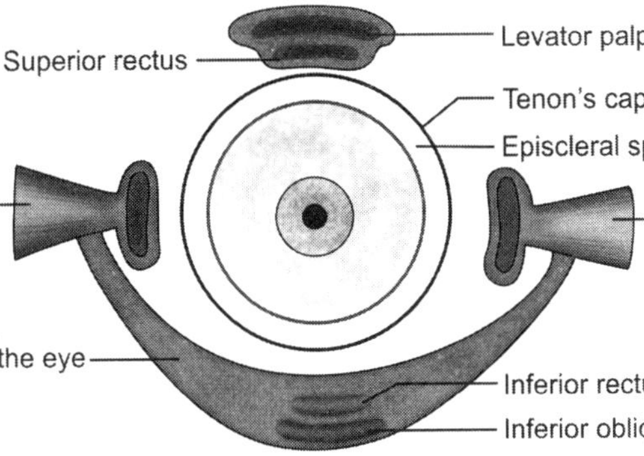
Superior rectus
Levator palpebrae superioris
Tenon's capsule
Episcleral space
Lateral check ligament
Medial check ligament
Suspensory ligament of the eye
Inferior rectus muscle
Inferior oblique muscle

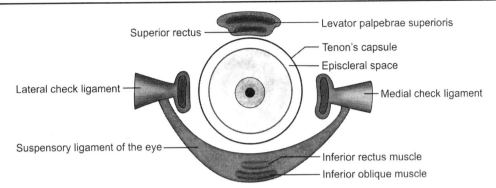

Fig. 3.5: Ligaments of eye

OCULOMOTOR NERVE

It is 3rd cranial nerve.

Functional Components

- General visceral efferent—Constriction of pupil and accommodation.
- General somatic efferent—Motor to extraocular muscles.
- General somatic afferent—Receives sensory impulse from muscles of eyeball.

Nuclear Origin

This nuclear complex consists of two components:

- Somatic efferent—Supplies all extraocular muscles except superior Oblique and lateral rectus.
- Visceral efferent (Nucleus of Edinger – westphal)
  - These fiber relay in the ciliary ganglion.
  - They supply sphincter pulillae and muscles

Course

Oculomotor sulcus of crus cerebri

↓

Nerve passes between superior and posterior cerebellar arteries

↓

Cavernous sinus

↓

Descends to lateral wall of the sinus

↓

In the anterior part of sinus, nerve divides into upper and lower division

↓

Both division enter orbit though middle part of superior orbital fissure

Distribution

1. Smaller upper division ascends on the lateral side of optic nerve and supplies superior rectus and levator palpebrae superioris.
2. Larger lower division divideds into three branches.
   a. Supply medial rectus
   b. Supply inferior rectus
   c. Supply inferior oblique (longest of these and it gives motor root to .... ciliary ganglion).

Clinical Anatomy

1. Total paralysis of IIIrd nerve results in
   a. Ptosis
   b. Lateral squint
   c. Dilation of pupil
   d. Loss of accommodation
   e. Proptosis
   f. Diplopia
2. A mildbrain lesion causing contralateral hemiplegia and ipsilateral paralysis of the third nerve is known as Weber's syndrome.
3. Supranuclear paralysis of third nerve causes loss of conjugate movement of the eyes.

CILIARY GANGLION

Definition

It is peripheral parasympathetic ganglion. Placed in the course of oculomotor nerve (Figs 3.6 and 3.7).

Location

Near the apex of orbit between the optic nerve and tendon of lateral rectus muscles.

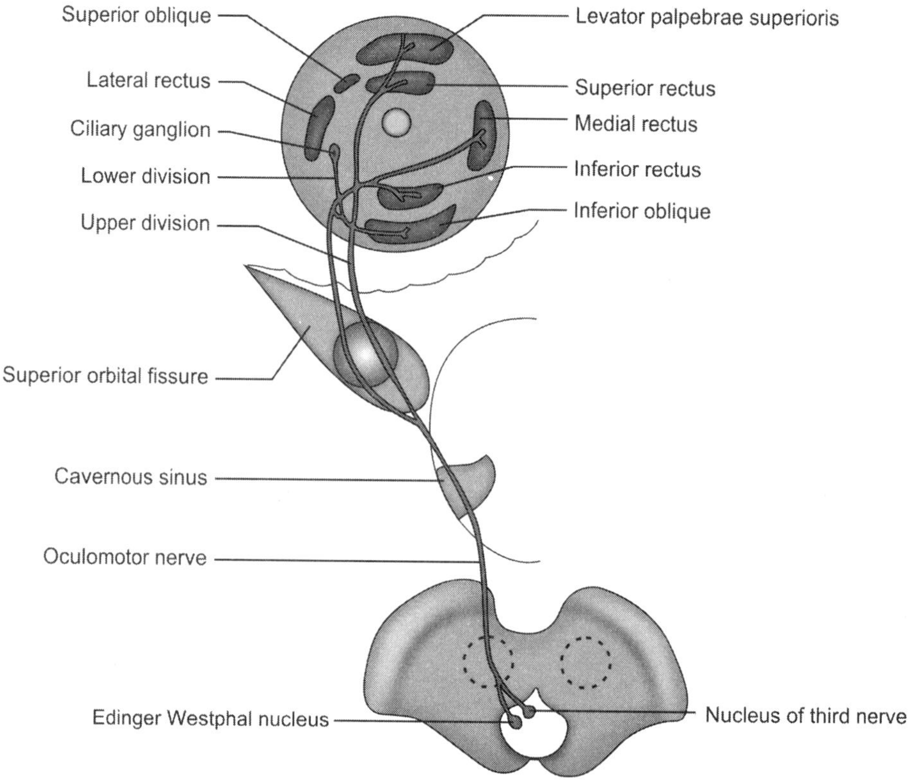
Superior oblique
Levator palpebrae superioris
Lateral rectus
Superior rectus
Ciliary ganglion
Medial rectus
Lower division
Inferior rectus
Upper division
Inferior oblique
Superior orbital fissure
Cavernous sinus
Oculomotor nerve
Edinger Westphal nucleus
Nucleus of third nerve

Fig. 3.6: Oculomotor nerve

Roots

Motor Root: Arises from nerve to inferior oblique

- Contains preganglionic fiber that begin in the Edinger Westphal nucleus and relay in the ganglion.
- Postgraunglionic fiber arise in the ganglion and supply the sphincter pulillae and ciliaris muscle.

Sensory Root: Comes from nasociliary nerve

These sensory fibers do not relay in the ganglion

- *Sympathetic Root:* Branch from the internal carotid
  a. Contains postganglionic fibers arising in superior plexus cervical ganglion which do not relay in this ganglion.
  b. These supply blood vessels of the eyeball and dilator pupillae.

Branches

- It gives 8 to 10 ciliary nerves which divide into 15 to 20 branches.
- Then they pierce the sclera.

VESSELS OF THE ORBIT

Ophthalmic Artery

Origin

Branch of cerebral part of the internal carotid artery given off medial to the anterior clinoid process.

Branches

1. Central artery of retina
2. Lacrimal artery
3. Posterior ciliary arteries
4. Supraorbital artery

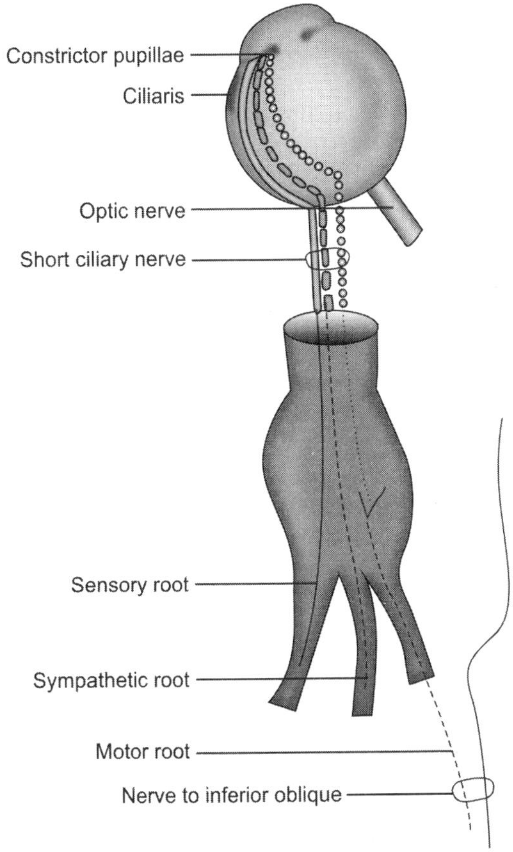

Constrictor pupillae
Ciliaris
Optic nerve
Short ciliary nerve
Sensory root
Sympathetic root
Motor root
Nerve to inferior oblique

Fig. 3.7: Ciliary ganglion

5. Posterior ethmoidal artery
6. Anterior ethmoidal artery
7. Dorsal nasal artery
8. Supratrochlear artery
9. Medial palpebral branches

Clinical Anatomy

The central artery of retina is an end artery. Obstruction of this artery by an embolism or pressure results in sudden total blindness.

Ophthalmic Veins

Superior Ophthalmic Vein

- Accompanying the ophthalmic artery and runs above the optic nerve.
- Passes through superior orbital fissure and drains into the cavernous sinus.
- Communicates anteriorly with supraorbital and angular vein.

Inferior Ophthalmic Vein

- It runs below the optic nerve
- It drains either by joining the superior ophthalmic vein or directly into cavernous sinus.
- It communicates with pterygoid venous plexus.

PREVIOUS YEAR QUESTIONS

1. Write short notes on supports of eyeball.
2. Write a note on oblique muscles of eyeball.
3. Describe the origin, insertion, nerve supply and action of extraocular muscles.
4. Describe occulomotor nerve and mention its applied anatomy.
5. Write a short note an ciliary ganglion.

MULTIPLE CHOICE QUESTIONS

1. Which of the following is the weakest part of orbit
   a. Medial wall
   b. Lateral wall
   c. Floor of orbit
   d. Roof of orbit
2. Which structure pass through inferior orbital fissure
   a. Superior ophthalmic vein
   b. Ophthalmic artery
   c. Trochlear nerve
   d. Zygomatic nerve
3. Nasolacrimal duct is directed
   a. Downward, medially, backwards
   b. Downward, laterally, backwards (DLB)
   c. Downward, laterally, forwards
   d. Downward, medially, forwards
4. Lacrimal gland is supplied by which of the following ganglion
   a. Otic
   b. Ciliary
   c. Sphenopalatine
   d. Submandibular
5. Nasolacrimal duct opens into
   a. Superior meatus
   b. Middle meatus
   c. Inferior meatus
   d. None of the above

6. Dacrycystitis is caused by the inflammation of
   a. Submandibular gland
   b. Parotid gland
   c. Sublingual gland
   d. Lacrimal gland
7. Ptosis may occur due to
   a. Trochlear nerve
   b. Occulomotor nerve
   c. Trigeminal nerve
   d. Superior oblique muscle
8. Occulomotor supplies all the muscles of eye except
   a. Lateral rectus
   b. Superior oblique
   c. Superior rectus
   d. A and B both
9. All of the following are true about upper eyelid except
   a. Muscles which close the eyelid are supplied by facial nerve
   b. Muscles which open the eyelid are supplied by trigeminal nerve
   c. Sensory supply is by the Vth cranial nerve
   d. Blood supply is by the lacrimal and ophthalmic arteries.
10. Which of the following is not a branch of ophthalmic nerve
    a. Frontal
    b. Lacrimal
    c. Nasociliary
    d. Medial ethmoid
11. Cliliary ganglion is located
    a. Between optic nerve and lateral rectus
    b. Apex of orbit
    c. Between apex of orbit and superior rectus
    d. Apex of orbit between optic nerve and lateral rectus
12. Abduction of eyeball is by the action of
    a. Lateral rectus, superior oblique and inferior oblique
    b. Medial rectus, superior rectus and inferior rectus
    c. Superior oblique and superior rectus
    d. Inferior oblique and inferior rectus

Answers

1. (a) 2. (d) 3. (b) 4. (c) 5. (c) 6. (d) 7. (b) 8. (d) 9. (b). 10. (d)
11. (d) 12. (a)

4 Temporal and Infratemporal Region

TRIGEMINAL NERVE

- It is the Vth cranial nerve
- It is called trigeminal because it consists of three division:
  1. Ophthalmic nerve
  2. Maxillary nerve
  3. Mandibular nerve

Functional Component

- *General somatic afferent:* Receives sensations from the skin of face, mucosal surfaces and muscle of mastication.
- *Special visceral afferent:* Motor to muscles of 1st branchal arch.

Nuclear Origin

1. Sensory nuclei:
   a. Chief sensory nucleus
   b. Spinal nucleus
   c. Mesencephalic nucleus
2. Motor nucleus

Course

Large sensory root ↓ / Small motor root ↓

Pass forward in posterior cranial fossa

↓ ↓

Invaginate the dura of posterior cranial fossa forming the trigeminal cave

↓ ↓

Sensory root joins trigeminal ganglion / Motor root lies deep but does not join ganglion

↓

Passes out to join the mandibular nerve

TRIGEMINAL GANGLION

- Semilunar in shape
- Lies in relation to apex of petrous temporal bone in middle cranial fossa
- Covered by double fold of dura mater known as trigeminal cave
- Contains pseudounipolar neurons

Distribution

1. Ophthalmic
2. Maxillary
3. Mandibular

OPHTHALMIC NERVE

Smallest and purely sensory.

Course and Origin

Medial part of trigeminal ganglion

↓

Pierces the Dura Mater of trigeminal cave

↓

Enters the lateral wall of cavernous sinus

↓

Finally enters orbit through superior **orbital fissure**

↓

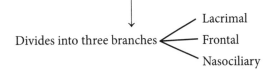

Divides into three branches → Lacrimal, Frontal, Nasociliary

Branches

1. Lacrimal nerve
2. Frontal nerve
   a. Supraorbital
   b. Supratrochlear

3. Nasociliary nerve
   a. Sensory communicating branch to ciliary ganglion.
   b. Long ciliary nerve
   c. Posterior ethmoidal nerve
   d. Anterior ethmoidal nerve
   e. Infratrochlear nerve

MAXILLARY NERVE

- Second division of trigeminal nerve
- Purely sensory

Course

Arises from trigeminal ganglion
↓
Pierces the dura mater of trigeminal cave
↓
Leaves middle cranial fossa through **foramen rotundum**
↓
Reaches pterygopalatine fossa
↓
Enters orbit through **inferior orbital fissure** where it is called as **infraorbital nerve**
↓
Runs in infraorbital groove and canal
↓
Appears on face through **infraorbital faramen**

Branches

a. In middle cranial fossa	i. Meningeal branch
b. In pterygopalatine fossa	ii. Ganglionic branches iii. Zygomatic nerve • Zygomaticotemporal • Zygomaticofacial iv. Posterior superior alveolar N
c. In orbit (Infraorbital canal)	i. Middle superior alveolar nerve ii. Anterior superior alveolar nerve
d. On the face	i. Palpebral ii. Nasal iii. Superior labial

Pterygopalatine Ganglion (Sphenopalatine Ganglion) (Fig. 4.1)

- Largest peripheral ganglion of parasympathetic system
- Serves as **relay station** for the secretomotor fibers of the lacrimal glands and mucous glands of the nose, palate, pharynx and paranasal sinuses.
- Topographically, it is related to maxillary nerve.
- Functionally, related to facial nerve.
- Lies in the pterygopalatine fossa.

Relation

Posterior	:	Pterygoid canal
Medial	:	Pharyngeal artery
Lateral	:	Artery of pterygoid canal
Superior	:	Maxillary nerve

Root

1. Motor or parasympathetic root
2. Sympathetic root
3. Sensory root

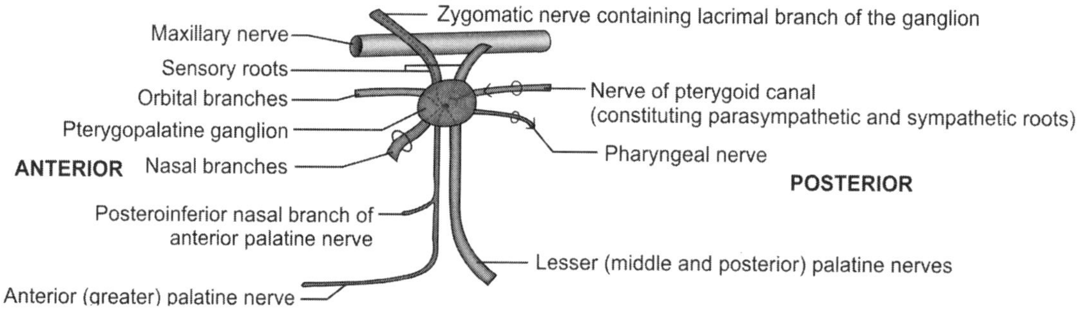
Zygomatic nerve containing lacrimal branch of the ganglion
Maxillary nerve
Sensory roots
Orbital branches
Pterygopalatine ganglion
ANTERIOR
Nasal branches
Posteroinferior nasal branch of anterior palatine nerve
Anterior (greater) palatine nerve
Nerve of pterygoid canal (constituting parasympathetic and sympathetic roots)
Pharyngeal nerve
POSTERIOR
Lesser (middle and posterior) palatine nerves

Fig. 4.1: Pterygopalatine ganglion

Branches

- Orbital
- Palatine
  - Greater palatine nerve
  - Lesser palatine nerve
- Nasal
  - Lateral nasal
  - Medial nasal
- Pharyngeal

MANDIBULAR NERVE (FIG. 4.2)

- Largest
- Nerve of the 1st branchial arch
- Consists of both sensory and motor fibers

Functional Component

1. General somatic afferent
2. Special visceral afferent

Origin

Formed by two roots
1. Larger sensory root—from trigeminal ganglion
2. Small motor root—from pons

Course

Both roots pass through foramen ovale
↓
Join to form main trunk
↓
Lies in infratemporal fossa, main trunk divides into
↙ ↘
Small anterior | Large posterior

Relations of trunk of mandibular nerve

Medial	:	Tensor veli palatini
Lateral	:	Lateral pterygoid
Anterior	:	Otic ganglion, tensor palati
Posterior	:	Middle meningeal artery

APPLIED ANATOMY

Trigeminal Neuralgia

- The neuralgic pain or facial pain occurring in territory of a trigeminal nerve is termed as trigeminal neuralgia.
- It is a pain syndrome recognized by patient history.
- It is characterized by pain often accompanied by a brief facial spasm.
- Triggered by touching, washing of face, shaving teeth, brushing, cold breeze, eating and talking, etc.
- Trigger zone:
  - Vermilion border of lip
  - Ala of nose
  - Cheeks
  - Around eyes

SUBMANDIBULAR GANGLION

- Parasympathetic ganglion
- Relay station for secretomotor fibers that supply the submandibular and sublingual salivary glands
- Topographically, it is connected to lingual nerve
- Functionally, connected to facial nerve
- Pin head size
- Fusiform shape
- Lies on outer surface of hyoglossus muscle in submandibular region
- Suspended from lingual nerve by two roots

Relations

Above	:	Lingual nerve
Below	:	Submandibular duct
Medial	:	Submandibular gland
Lateral	:	Hyoglossus muscle

Roots

- Parasympathetic root
- Sympathetic root

Branches

- Postganglionic parasympathetic fibers
  - Supplies submandibular gland
- Postganglionic sympathetic fibers
  - Are vasomotor to submandibular and sublingual glands

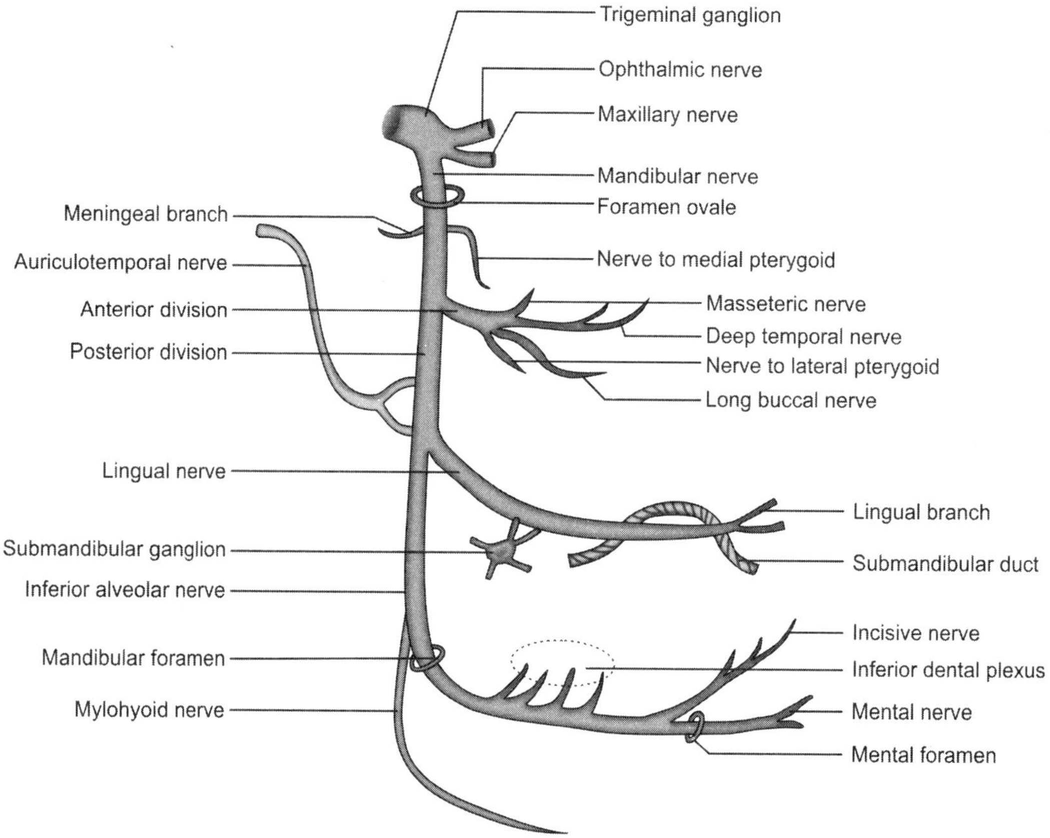
Trigeminal ganglion
Ophthalmic nerve
Maxillary nerve
Mandibular nerve
Foramen ovale
Meningeal branch
Auriculotemporal nerve
Nerve to medial pterygoid
Anterior division
Masseteric nerve
Deep temporal nerve
Posterior division
Nerve to lateral pterygoid
Long buccal nerve
Lingual nerve
Lingual branch
Submandibular ganglion
Submandibular duct
Inferior alveolar nerve
Incisive nerve
Mandibular foramen
Inferior dental plexus
Mylohyoid nerve
Mental nerve
Mental foramen

Fig. 4.2: Mandibular nerve

OTIC GANGLION (FIG. 4.3)

- Parasympathetic ganglion
- Connects mandibular division of trigeminal nerve which provide relay station to secretomotor fibers of the parotid gland.
- Topographically connected to mandibular nerve
- Functionally, connected to glossopharyngeal nerve
- Pin head size
- Oval in shape
- Lies in infratemporal fossa, just below foramen ovale

Relations

Anterior	:	Medial pterygoid muscle
Posterior	:	Middle meningeal artery
Lateral	:	Trunk of mandibular nerve
Medial	:	Tensor veli palatine

Roots or connection

1. Parasympathetic root:
   a. Obtained from lesser petrosal nerve
   b. Preganglionic fibers arise in inferior salivatery nucleus, pass via glossopharyngeal nerve, lesser petrosal nerve to relay in otic ganglion.
2. Sympathetic root:
   a. Conveys postganglionic fibers from the superior cervical ganglion
   b. Fibers do not relay in ganglion
3. Somatic motor root:
   a. Pass through ganglion without relay

Branches and Distribution

1. Communicating branches to auriculo temporal nerve – Convey fibers to the parotid gland.
2. Communicating branches to chorda tympani

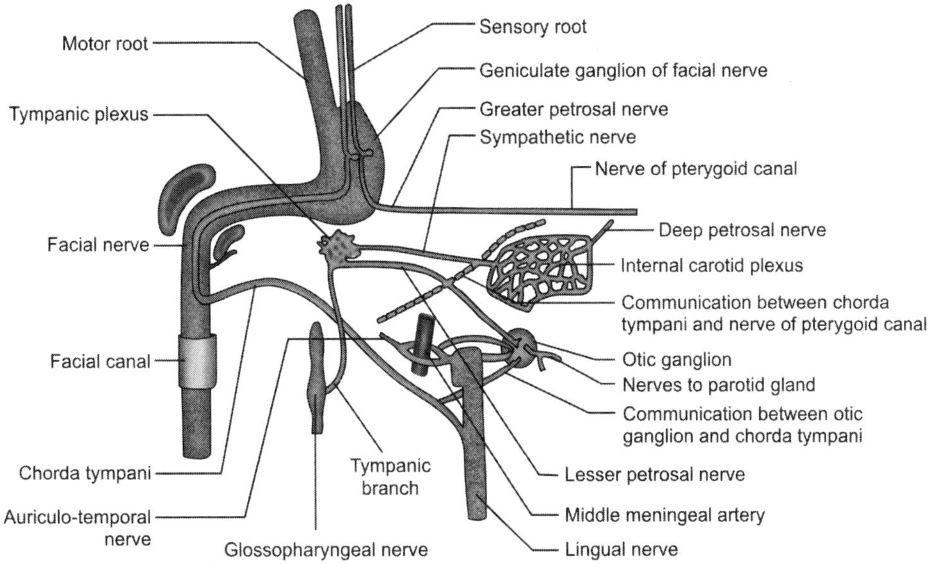
Motor root
Sensory root
Geniculate ganglion of facial nerve
Tympanic plexus
Greater petrosal nerve
Sympathetic nerve
Nerve of pterygoid canal
Deep petrosal nerve
Facial nerve
Internal carotid plexus
Communication between chorda tympani and nerve of pterygoid canal
Facial canal
Otic ganglion
Nerves to parotid gland
Communication between otic ganglion and chorda tympani
Chorda tympani
Tympanic branch
Lesser petrosal nerve
Auriculo-temporal nerve
Middle meningeal artery
Glossopharyngeal nerve
Lingual nerve

Fig. 4.3: Connections of otic ganglion

Division	*Branches*	*Supply*
Main trunk	• Nervous spinosus (Meningeal branch) • Nerve to medial pterygoid	• Dura mater of middle cranial fossa • Medial pterygoid, tensor palati, tensor tympani, muscles
Anterior division (3 motor and 1 sensory)	**Motor branches:** • Deep temporal nerve (two) • Nerve to lateral pterygoid • Masseteric nerve **Sensory branch** • Buccal nerve	 • Temporalis muscle (Deep surface) • Lateral pterygoid muscle • Masseter muscle • Supplies skin and mucous membrane of cheek
Posterior division (3 sensory) (ALI)	• Auriculo-temporal nerve – Auricular – Articular – Superficial temporal – Communicating • Inferior alveolar nerve – Larger terminal branch – Mixed nerve – Enters mandibular amen and traverses the mandibular canal	 • Pinna, external acoustic meatus • Temporomandibular joint (TMJ) • Area of skin over temple • Parotid gland
Posterior	• Inferior dental plexus • Incisive • Mental • Nerve to mylohyoid	• Molar and premolar teeth and adjoining gums • Canine and incisor teeth and adjoining gum • Skin of chin and lower lip • Mylohyoid and anterior belly of digastrics
	• Lingual nerve–Small terminal branches a. Sensory branches b. Communicating branches i. With chorda tympani ii. With hypoglossal nerve	 • Mucous membrane of anterior 2/3rd of tongue, floor of mouth and adjoining gums • Taste sensation from anterior 2/3rd of tongue • Proprioceptive sensations from lingual muscle

MAXILLARY ARTERY / INTERNAL MAXILLARY ARTERY

Larger terminal branch of external carotid artery (Fig. 4.4).

Course

Begins behind the neck of mandible
↓
Crosses the lower head of lateral pterygoid
↓
Emerges between the two heads of lateral pterygoid
↓
Enter the pterygopalatine fossa through pterygo maxillary fissure
↓
Gives off terminal branches

Parts (Table 4.1)

Divided into three parts by the lower head of lateral pterygoid muscle

a. First part
b. Second part
c. Third part

Characteristics of Branches

- Branches from 1st and IInd part accompany mandibular nerve
- Branches from IIIrd part accompany maxillary nerve
- Branches fro 2nd part are muscular only

Clinical and Applied Anatomy

- Middle meningeal artery sometimes form in fracture of side of skull. This results in extradural

Table 4.1: Parts of internal maxillary artery

First Part 5 Branches	*Second Part 4 Branches*	*Third Part 6 Branches*
1. Deep auricular	1. Deep temporal	1. Posterior superior alveolar
2. Anterior tympanic	2. Pterygoid branches	2. Infra orbital
3. Middle meningeal (Frontal, Parietal)	3. Masseteric	3. Greater palatine
	4. Buccal	4. Pharyngeal
4. Accessory meningeal		5. Artery of Pterygoid canal
5. Inferior alveolar		6. Sphenopalatine artery

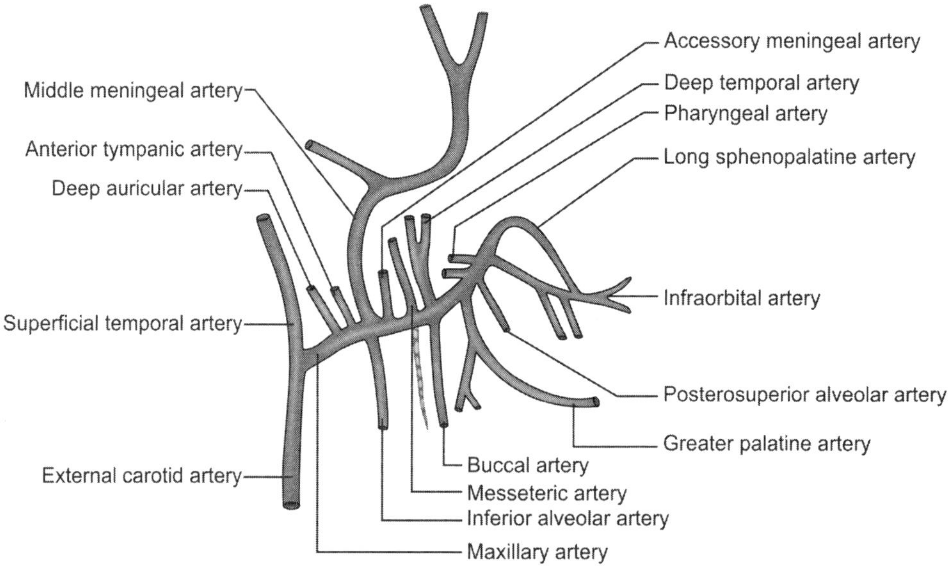
Accessory meningeal artery
Deep temporal artery
Pharyngeal artery
Long sphenopalatine artery
Middle meningeal artery
Anterior tympanic artery
Deep auricular artery
Infraorbital artery
Superficial temporal artery
Posterosuperior alveolar artery
Greater palatine artery
Buccal artery
External carotid artery
Messeteric artery
Inferior alveolar artery
Maxillary artery

Fig. 4.4: Internal maxillary artery and its branches

hematoma → compression of brain → paralysis of opposite half of the body.

PREVIOUS YEAR QUESTIONS

1. Write a note on maxillary artery and enumerate its branches.
2. Mention distribution of mandibular nerve and its applied anatomy in reference to neuralgia.
3. Write a short note on otic ganglion.
4. Write extracranial course of mandibular nerve.
5. Describe mandibular nerve with its branches and applied anatomy.
6. Write a short note on pterygopalatine ganglion.
7. Enumerate branches of 3rd part of maxillary artery.
8. Comment on trigeminal ganglion.
9. Write a note on submandibular ganglion.

MULTIPLE CHOICE QUESTIONS

1. Secretomotor supply of parotid gland is through:
   a. Otic ganglion
   b. Gasserian ganglion
   c. Geniculate ganglion
   d. Submandibular ganglion
2. Inferior dental artery is a branch of:
   a. Mandibular artery
   b. Maxillary artery
   c. Pterygomandibular plexus
   d. None
3. All of the following are supplied by mandibular nerve except:
   a. Masseter
   b. Buccinator
   c. Medial pterygoid
   d. Anterior belly of digastric
4. Sphenopalatine ganglion does not supply:
   a. Nasal mucosa
   b. Sublingual gland
   c. Ciliary ganglion
   d. Both B and C
5. How many nuclei does the Trigeminal nerve have in the CNS:
   a. Three
   b. Four
   c. Five
   d. Six
6. Masseteric nerve is a branch of:
   a. Long buccal nerve
   b. Mandibular division of trigeminal nerve
   c. Maxillary division of trigeminal nerve
   d. Motor branch of facial nerve
7. Maxillary nerve innervates all of the following except:
   a. Ala of nose and lower eyelids
   b. Upper cheek
   c. Gingiva of maxilla
   d. Temporomandibular joint
8. All are true about mandibular nerve except:
   a. Sensory branch arises from anterior trunk
   b. Supplies muscles of mastication by main trunk
   c. Buccal nerve innervates buccinator muscle
   d. Nerve to medial pterygoid arises from main trunk

Answers

1. (a) 2. (b) 3. (b) 4. (d) 5. (b) 6. (b) 7. (d) 8. (b)

5 Temporomandibular Joint and Muscles of Mastication

TEMPOROMANDIBULAR JOINT (TMJ)

- It is the joint formed between the head of mandible and the articular fossa of temporal bone
- Synovial joint of the condylar variety.

Articular Surfaces (Fig. 5.1)

- Covered by a fibrocartilage and not hyaline cartilage which is present in most synovial joint
- It has two articular surface:
  i. Upper—mandibular fossa or articular eminence of temporal bone.
  ii. Lower—condylar process of mandible.

Articular Disc

- It is an oval fibrocartilaginous plate that divides the joint space into two compartments.
  i. Upper compartment—permits gliding movement
  ii. Lower compartment—permits gliding and rotary movement
- Disc is attached with fibrous capsule at its periphery

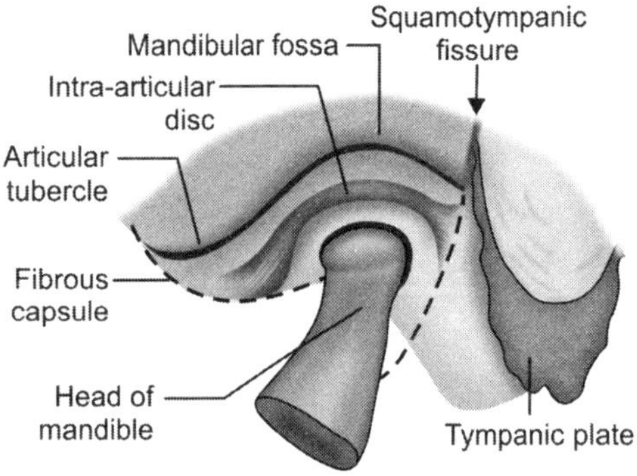
Mandibular fossa
Squamotympanic fissure
Intra-articular disc
Articular tubercle
Fibrous capsule
Head of mandible
Tympanic plate

Fig. 5.1: Articular surface of TMJ

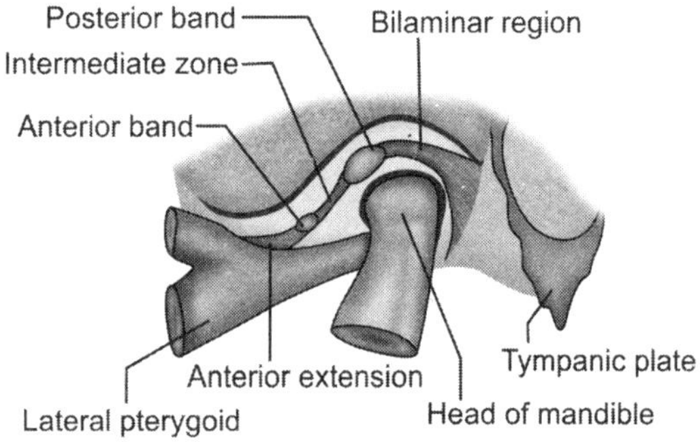
Posterior band
Bilaminar region
Intermediate zone
Anterior band
Anterior extension
Tympanic plate
Lateral pterygoid
Head of mandible

Fig. 5.2: Components of articular disc

- Composition (Fig. 5.2)
  i. Anterior extension
  ii. Anterior thick band
  iii. Intermediate zone
  iv. Posterior thick band
  v. Bilamellar region
- Disc represents degenerated primitive insertion of lateral pterygoid.

LIGAMENT (FIG. 5.3)

Fibrous Capsule

- Capsule attaches above to the articular tubercle and below to the neck of the mandible
- Synovial membrane lines the fibrous capsule and neck of the mandible.

Lateral or Temporomandibular Ligament

- Formed by thickening of lateral part of the capsular ligament
- It is attached to the articular tubercle and to the posterolateral aspect of the neck of the mandible.

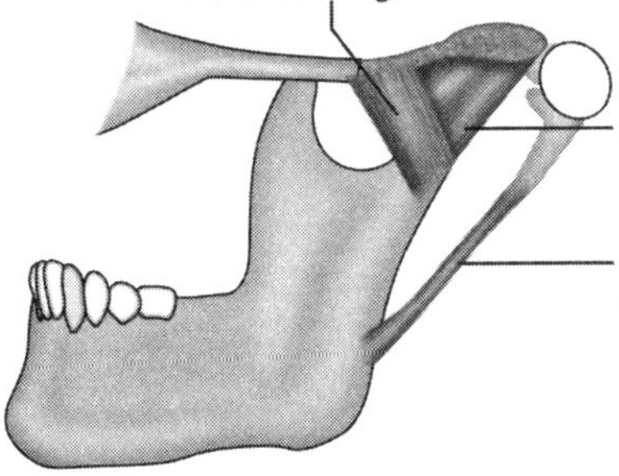
Lateral temporo-
mandibular ligament
Joint capsule
Stylomandibular
ligament

Fig. 5.3: Ligaments of TMJ

Sphenomandibular Ligament

- Originates from spine of sphenoid and inserted into the lingula of the mandible below.
- It represents the remnant of 1st arch or Meckel's cartilage.
- It is an accessory ligament.

Stylomandibular Ligament

- It is an another accessory ligament
- Originates from tip of styloid process and is inserted to the angle of mandible.

Relations (Table 5.1)

Anterior : Lateral pterygoid muscle, masseteric nerve and vessels

Posterior : Parotid gland, external auditory meatus, superficial temporal vessels, auriculotemporal nerve

Medial : Spine of sphenoid, sphenomandibular ligament, auriculotemporal nerve, chorda tympani nerve, middle meningeal artery

Lateral : Skin
Fasciae
Parotid gland
Facial nerve

Superior : Middle cranial fossa

Inferior : Maxillary artery and vein

Nerve Supply

- Auriculotemporal nerve
- Masseteric nerve

Blood Supply

- Superficial temporal artery
- Maxillary artery veins follow the arteries

Stability of the joint: By following factors

- Articular tubercles
- Lateral temporol—mandibular ligament
- Muscles
- Position of mandible is most stable when mouth is closed or slightly open.

CLINICAL AND APPLIED ANATOMY

- **Dislocation of Mandible:** During excessive opening of the mouth or during convulsion, head of the mandible of one or both sides may slip into the infratemporal fossa. As a result, there is inability to close mouth.

Table 5.1: Movement of TMJ

Movements	*Mechanism of Movement*	*Muscle Involved*
Depression	Gliding movement in upper compartment and rotatory movement in lower compartment	Lateral pterygoid Geniohyoids Mylohyoid
Elevation	Reversal of depression	Masseter Medial pterygoid Temporalis
Protrusion	Gliding movement in upper compartment	Medial pterygoid Lateral pterygoid
Retraction	Reversal of protrusion	Posterior fibres of temporalis
Chewing	Gliding movement in upper compartment of one joint and rotatory movement in lower compartment of other joint simultaneously	Alternative action of medial and lateral pterygoid of each side

- **Derangement of the articular disc:** May result from an injury, like over closure or malocclusion. This gives rise to clicking and pain.

Muscles of Mastication

- Four pairs of muscle move the mandible during mastication
- Located in infratemporal region
- Inserted in the ramus of mandible
- Innervated by branches of anterior division and trunk of mandibular nerve
- All acts on temporomandibular joint.

ACCESSORY MUSCLE OF MASTICATION—BUCCINATOR

Buccinator muscle helps during mastication by preventing accumulation of food in the vestibule of mouth.

Origin

- Upper fibers : Alveolar process of maxilla opposite the molar teeth
- Middle fibers : Pterygomandibular raphe
- Lower fibers : Alveolar process of mandible opposite the molar teeth

Insertion

- Upper fibers : Upper lip
- Middle fibers : Both the upper and lower lips
- Lower fibers : Lower lip

Nerve Supply

Buccal branch of the facial nerve

Actions

- Flattens the cheek against the gum and teeth
- Prevent accumulation of food in the mouth
- Helps in whistling.

Clinical and Applied Anatomy (Table 5.2)

Buccal branch of mandibular nerve is sensory. It pierces the buccinator muscle but does not supply it.

PREVIOUS YEAR QUESTIONS

- Describe TMJ under following headings.
  - Type and articular surfaces

Table 5.2: Subsections of TMJ

Muscle	*Origin*	*Insertion*	*Nerve Supply*	*Action*
• **Temporalis** – Fan-shaped	• Floor of the temporal fossa • Undersurface of temporal fossa	• Tip and medial surface of coronoid process • Anterior border of ramus of mandible	Two deep temporal branches from anterior division of mandibular nerve	• Anterior and middle fibers–elevate mandible • Posterior fibers—retract the mandible • Helps in side-to-side movements
• **Medial Ptery goid** – Quadrilateral shape	• Superficial head—maxiliary tuberosity and adjoining palatine bone • Deep head—larger-arise from medial surface of lateral pterygoid plate	• Medial surface of ramus of mandible • Inner aspect of angle of mandible	Nerve to medial pterygoid, branch of main trunk of mandibular nerve	• Elevation of mandible • Protrussion of mandible • Helps in side-to-side movements of jaw
• **Lateral Ptergoid** – Key muscle of the fossa	• Upper head—infratemporal surface and greater wing of sphenoid bone • Lower head—larger-lateral surface of lateral pterygoid plate	• Pterygoid fovea in the neck of mandible • Articular disc and capsule of TMJ	A branch from anterior division of mandibular nerve	• Depression of mandible • Protrussion of mandible • Side-to-side movements
• **Masseter** – Quadrilateral in shape	Lower border of zygomatic arch	Outer surface of ramus	Massetric nerve from the anterior division of mandibular nerve	• Elevation of mandible • Retraction of mandible • Clenching of teeth • Protussion

  - Ligaments
  - Muscle producing movements
  - Applied anatomy
- Write a short note on muscles of mastication.
- Write a note on masseter muscle.
- Write a short note on buccinator muscle.
- Write about movements of TMJ and muscles involved in it.
- Describe muscles of mastication with their attachments, action, nerve supply and blood supply.

MULTIPLE CHOICE QUESTIONS

1. Anterior limit of infratemporal fossa:
   a. Lateral pterygoid plate
   b. Maxillary posterior wall
   c. Pterygomaxillary fissure
   d. Mastoid process
2. Muscle which pulls the disc of TMJ downwards:
   a. Lateral pterygoid
   b. Medial pterygoid
   c. Digastric
   d. Mylohyoid
3. TMJ is supplied by following arteries:
   a. Superficial temporal
   b. Maxillary
   c. Internal carotid
   d. a and b
4. Which of the following muscle is depressor of mandible?
   a. Temporalis
   b. Lateral pterygoid
   c. Masseter
   d. Medial pterygoid
5. Articular disc of TMJ is:
   a. Fibrocartilagenous
   b. Bony
   c. Hyaline
   d. Elastic
6. Following are muscles of mastication except:
   a. Buccinator
   b. Masseter
   c. Temporalis
   d. Pterygoids
7. Temporalis muscle originates from:
   a. Side of skull
   b. Zygomatic process
   c. Ramus of mandible
   d. Pterygopalatine fossa
8. Muscles of mastication are supplied by:
   a. 2nd part of maxillary artery
   b. 3rd part of maxillary artery
   c. 1st part of maxillary artery
   d. Facial artery
9. Retraction of mandible is achieved by:
   a. Lateral pterygoid
   b. Temporalis
   c. Medial pterygoid
   d. Masseter
10. Medial pterygoid muscle is attached to:
    a. Medial surface of lateral pterygoid plate
    b. Lateral surface of medial pterygoid plate
    c. Medial surface of medical pterygoid plate
    d. Lateral surface of lateral pterygoid plate

Answers

1. (b) 2. (a) 3. (d) 4. (b) 5. (a) 6. (a) 7. (a) 8. (a) 9. (b) 10. (a)

6 Parotid Region

SALIVARY GLANDS

- Number of salivery glands are scattered throughout the oral cavity
- There are three pairs of large salivary glands
  a. Parotid—beside the ear
  b. Submandibular—below the mandible
  c. Sublingual—below the tongue
- Secretions/saliva from all these glands helps keep the oral cavity moist and begin the process of digestion.

PAROTID GLAND

- Para = near and otic = ear
- Largest salivary gland located in parotid bed
- Pyramidal in shape
- It weighs 25 gm
- Facial nerve divides the gland into the superficial and deep lobe connected by isthmus.

Boundaries (Fig. 6.1)

1. Anterior : Posterior border of ramus of mandible
2. Posterior : Mastoid process, sternocleidomastoid muscle
3. Superior : External acoustic meatus, TMJ
4. Inferior : Posterior belly of digastric, stylohyoid

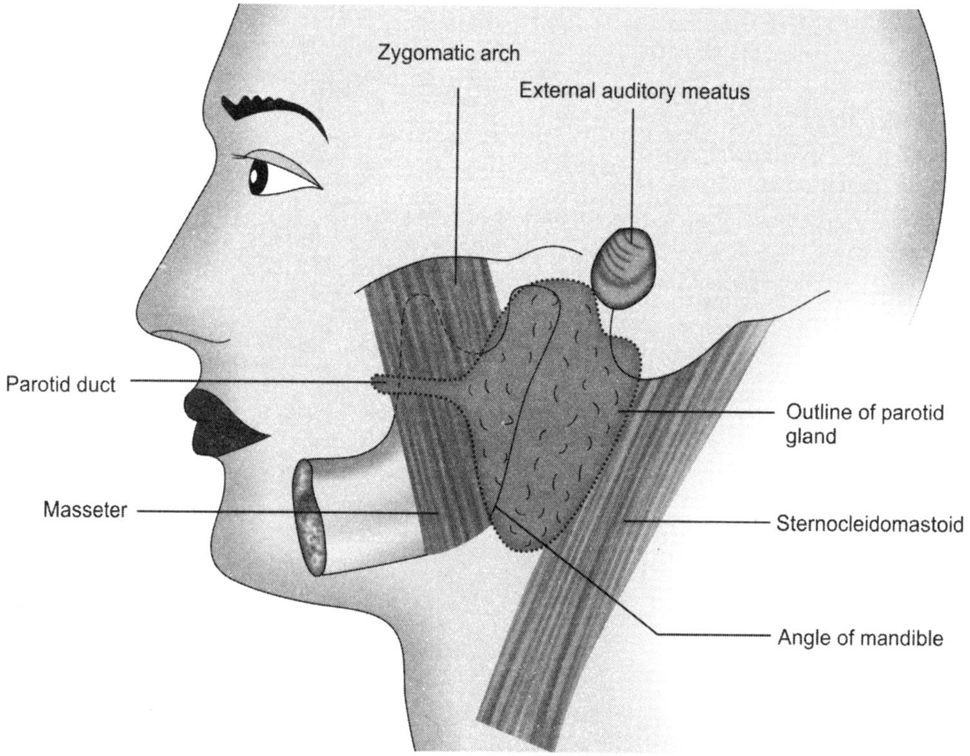

Zygomatic arch
External auditory meatus
Parotid duct
Outline of parotid gland
Masseter
Sternocleidomastoid
Angle of mandible

Fig. 6.1: Boundaries of parotid gland

5. Medial : Styloid process, styloglossus, stylohyoid

ANATOMICAL FEATURES (TABLE 6.1)

Capsules of Parotid Gland

1. False capsule
   - Formed by tough investing layer of deep cervical fascia
2. Truc capsule
   - Formed by the condensation of fibrous tissue of parotid gland

Structures Present within the Parotid Gland

Facial Nerve and its Branches (Fig. 6.2)

- Emerges from the stylomastoid foramen and enters gland by piercing its posteromedial surface and divides into two trunks

a. Temporofacial trunk
   - → Temporal nerve
   - → Zygomatic nerve

Table 6.1: Anatomical Features of Parotid Gland

	Features	*Relation*
Apex	Overlaps the posterior belly of digastric and adjoining carotid triangle	• Structure passing through it – Cervical branch of facial nerve – Two divisions of retromandibular vein
Superior surface/ base	• Concave • Related to external acoustic meatus and TMJ	• Structure passing through it – Temporal branch of facial nerve – Superficial temporal vessels – Auriculotemporal nerve.
Lateral surface	Largest	• Related to – Skin – Superficial fascia – Platysma
Anteromedial surface	• Deeply groved by ramus of mandible • Structure emerging – Branches of facial nerve – Transverse facial artery	• It is related to – Masseter – Medial pterygoid – Posterior border of ramus – Lateral surface of TMJ
Posteromedial surface	• Structures entering the gland through this are: – External carotid artery—in lower part – Facial nerve trunk—in upper part	• Related to – Mastoid process with sternocleidomastoid and posterior belly of digastric – Styloid process and styloid group of muscle
Anterior border	Thin border Present between superficial and anteromedial surfaces	• Structure emerging are: – Zygomatic branch of facial nerve – Transverse facial vessels – Upper buccal branch of facial nerve – Parotid duct – Lower buccal branch of facial nerve – Marginal mandibular branch of facial nerve
Posterior border	Separate the superficial surface from the posteromedial surface	• Structure emerging are: – Posterior auricular vessel – Posterior auricular branch of facial nerve
Medial border	Separate the anteromedial surface from posteromedial surface	It is related to the lateral wall of the pharynx

b. Cervico facial trunk → Buccal nerve; → Marginal mandibular nerve; → Cervical nerve

- They leave through anterior border of gland, resembles the foot of goose. Hence, known as Pes Anserinus.

2. Retromandibular Vein

3. External Carotid Artery

4. Deep Parotid Lymps Nodes

Histology of Parotid Gland

- Compound tubuloalveolar gland
- Acini are lined by seromucinous cells which open into collecting duct.

Parotid Duct

- 5 mm long
- Emerges from middle of the anterior border of gland
- Runs over masseter
- Pierces four layers of cheek:
  a. Buccal pad of fat
  b. Buccopharyngeal fascia
  c. Buccinator muscle
  d. Buccal mucosa
- Opens into the vestibule of mouth opposite the 2nd upper molar tooth.

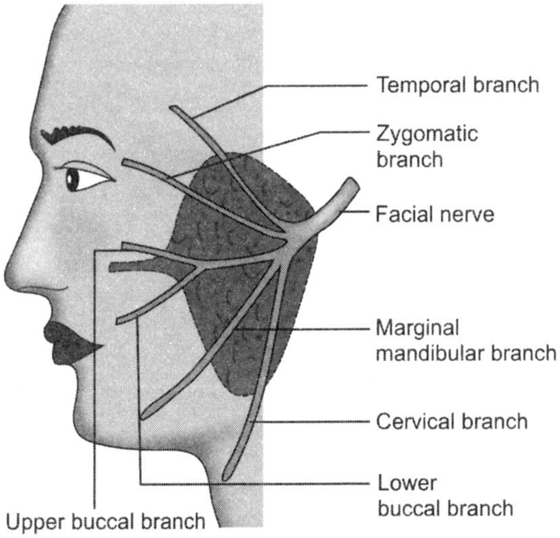
Temporal branch
Zygomatic branch
Facial nerve
Marginal mandibular branch
Cervical branch
Lower buccal branch
Upper buccal branch

Fig. 6.2: Facial nerve and its branches

Blood Supply

Artery : Branches of external carotid artery
Vein : External jugular vein

Lymphatic Drainage

1. Superficial parotid group
2. Deep parotid group

→ Drains into deep cervical lymph nodes

Nerve Supply

Parasympathetic

Preganglionic fibers arise from inferior salivatory nucleus
↓
Pass through glassopharyngeal nerve, lesser petrosal nerve
↓
Relay in otic ganglion

- Postgonglionic fiber pass through auriculotemparal nerve to supply parotid gland
- It is secretomotor and results in watery secretion.

Sympathetic

- Derived from the sympathetic plexus around the external carotid artery
- Formed by postganglionic fibers from superior cervical sympathetic ganglion
- It is secretomotor and results in mucinous secretion.

Sensory

a. Auriculotemporal nerve
b. Greater auricular nerve
c. C_2

Clinical and Applied Anatomy

1. **Mumps** is a viral infection which has special affinity for the parotid glands and result in swollen and painful glands
2. **Infection** of parotid gland is consequence of retrograde bacterial infection from mouth through the parotid duct
3. During surgical removal of gland, facial nerve is preserved by removing gland into two parts.

PREVIOUS YEAR QUESTIONS

1. Write a short note on parotid duct.
2. Describe parotid gland under the following:
   a. Surfaces with relations
   b. Nerve supply
   c. Applied anatomy
3. Briefly describe anatomy of parotid gland and add a note on blood supply and nerve supply.
4. Write a note on secretomotor fibers of parotid gland.

MULTIPLE CHOICE QUESTIONS

1. Following structures are within parotid gland except:
   a. External carotid artery
   b. Facial nerve
   c. Retromandibular vein
   d. Facial artery
2. Parotid duct pierces muscle:
   a. Risorius
   b. Massetor
   c. Buccinator
   d. Zygomaticus major
3. The secretomotor supply of parotid gland comes from:
   a. Greater petrosal nerve
   b. Auriculotemporal nerve
   c. Maxillary nerve
   d. Chorda tympani
4. The orifice of parotid duct is located:
   a. At the hamular notch
   b. In proximity to the incisive papilla
   c. On the buccal mucosa near the maxillary second molars
   d. Slightly posterior to mandibular incisors
5. Surgical excision of parotid gland endanger which of the following structure?
   a. Hypoglossal nerve
   b. Motor nerve of muscles of matriculation
   c. External carotid artery, auriculotemporal nerve and facial nerve
   d. Lesser occipital and spinal accessory nerve
6. Duct of parotid gland is:
   a. Stenson's duct
   b. Wharton's duct
   c. Nasolacrimal duct
   d. Bartholin's duct.

Answers

1. (d) 2. (c) 3. (b) 4. (c) 5. (c) 6. (a)

7 Submandibular Region

SUBMANDIBULAR SALIVARY GLAND (FIG. 7.1)

- It is below the mandible in the anterior part of the digastric triangle
- It is about the size of walnut
- Roughly J-shaped.

Anatomical Features

Indented by the posterior border of mylohyoid which divides it into:

i. Large superficial part
ii. Smaller deep part

Superficial Part

- Fills the anterior part of the digastric triangle
- It has two ends and three surfaces

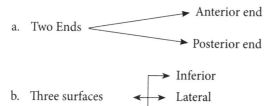

a. Two Ends → Anterior end; Posterior end

b. Three surfaces → Inferior; Lateral; Medial

Relations (Fig. 7.2)

Surfaces	*Parts*	*Related to*
Inferior Surface	-	• Skin • Superficial fascia containing platysma and cervical branch of facial nerve • Deep fascia • Facial vein • Submandibular lymph nodes
Lateral Surface	-	• Submandibular fossa • Medial pterygoid muscle • Facial artery
Medical Surface	Divided into 3 parts • Anterior part • Intermediate part • Posterior part	• Mylohyoid muscle, nerve and vessels • Hyoglossus muscle • Lingual and hypoglossal nerve • Submandibular ganglion • Styloglossus muscle • Stylohyoid ligament • Glossopharyngeal nerve

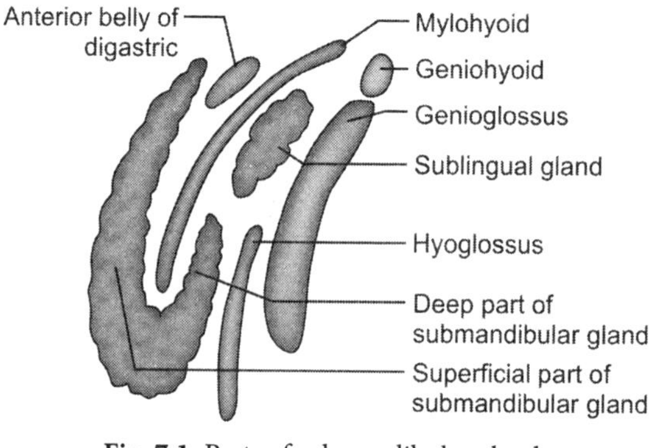
Anterior belly of digastric
Mylohyoid
Geniohyoid
Genioglossus
Sublingual gland
Hyoglossus
Deep part of submandibular gland
Superficial part of submandibular gland

Fig. 7.1: Parts of submandibular gland

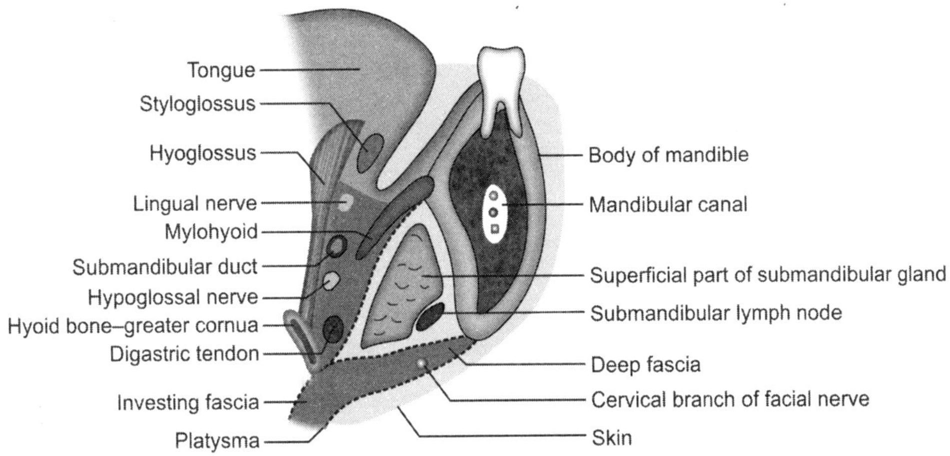
Tongue
Styloglossus
Hyoglossus
Lingual nerve
Mylohyoid
Submandibular duct
Hypoglossal nerve
Hyoid bone–greater cornua
Digastric tendon
Investing fascia
Platysma
Body of mandible
Mandibular canal
Superficial part of submandibular gland
Submandibular lymph node
Deep fascia
Cervical branch of facial nerve
Skin

Fig. 7.2: Relations of submandibular gland

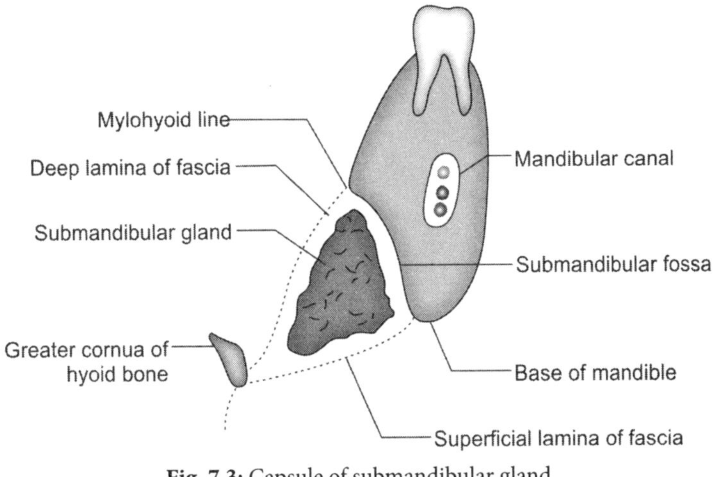
Mylohyoid line
Deep lamina of fascia
Submandibular gland
Greater cornua of hyoid bone
Mandibular canal
Submandibular fossa
Base of mandible
Superficial lamina of fascia

Fig. 7.3: Capsule of submandibular gland

Deep Part

- Smaller in size
- Lies on the hyoglossus muscle, deep to mylohyoid

Relations

Medial	:	Hyoglossus muscle
Lateral	:	Mylohyoid muscle
Superior	:	Lingual nerve and submandibular ganglion
Inferior	:	Hypoglossal nerve

Capsule of Submandibular Gland (Fig. 7.3)

- Investing layer of deep fascia splits to cover the superficial part of gland
- Superficial layer gets attached to base of mandible and deep layer to mylohyoid line on mandible.

Submandibular Duct / Wharton's Duct

- 5 cm long
- Emerges at the anterior end of the deep part and runs forward on the hyoglossus muscle, between lingual and hypoglossal nerve

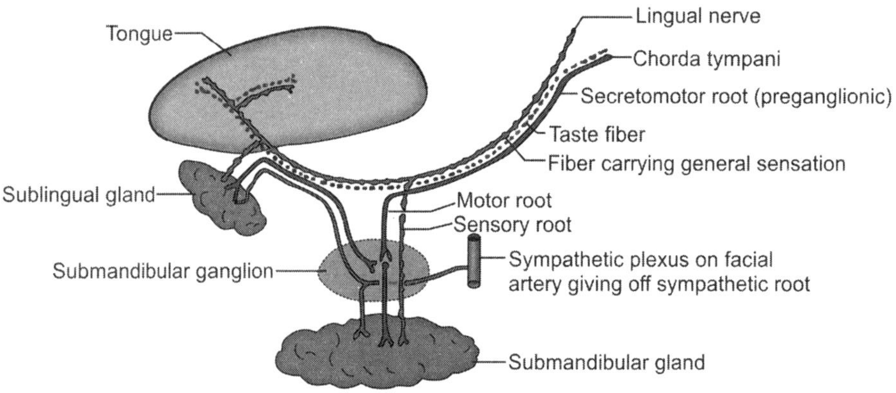
Tongue
Lingual nerve
Chorda tympani
Secretomotor root (preganglionic)
Taste fiber
Fiber carrying general sensation
Sublingual gland
Motor root
Sensory root
Submandibular ganglion
Sympathetic plexus on facial artery giving off sympathetic root
Submandibular gland

Fig. 7.4: Nerve supply of submandibular gland

- It opens on the floor of mouth, on the summit of the sublingual papilla, at the side of the tongue.

Blood Supply

- Arterial – Branches of facial and lingual artery
- Venous – Internal jugular vein.

Lymphatic Drainage

Submandibular lymph node

Nerve Supply (Fig. 7.4)

a. Parasympathetic/Secretomotor

Preganglionic fibers arise from superior salivatory nucleus

↓

Pass through facial nerve, chroda tympani nerve, lingual nerve

↓

Relay into the submandibular ganglion

↓

Postganglionic fibers arises from the ganglion

↓

Supplies directly the gland

↓

It is secretomotor causes watery secretion

b. Sympathetic
   - Derived from the sympathetic plexus around facial artery.
   - Formed by postganglionic fibers from superior cervical sympathetic ganglion.

c. Sensory
   - Lingual nerve

SUBLINGUAL SALIVARY GLAND

- Smallest of three pairs
- Lies immediately below the mucosa of the floor of the mouth
- Almond-shaped
- Rest in sublingual fossa
- Separated from the base of tongue by the submandibular duct
- Glands pour—its secretion by a series of duct 10-15 in number on the sublingual fold into the oral cavity.

Applied Anatomy of Salivary Gland

1. Sialoliths are commonly seen with submandibular salivary gland because of its location
2. Viral and bacterial infections cause the inflammation of salivary gland known as sialoadenitis.

SUPRAHYOID MUSCLES

Suprahyoid muscles are:

i. Digastric
ii. Stylohyoid
iii. Mylohyoid
iv. Geniohyoid

HYOGLOSSUS MUSCLE (FIG. 7.5)

- It is muscle of tongue
- Thin quadrilateral muscle

Muscle	Origin	Insertion	Nerve Supply	Actions
• **Digastric**	• Anterior belly—from digastric fossa of mandible • Posterior belly—From mastoid notch of temporal bone	Both heads meet, perforate stylohyoid and held by a fibrous pulley to the hyoid bone	• Nerve to mylohyoid • Facial	• Depresses mandible when mouth is open • Elevate hypoid bone
• **Stylohyoid**	Styloid process	Junction of body and greater cornua of hyoid bone	Facial nerve	• Pulls hyoid bone backwards and upwards • With other muscles fixes the hyoid bone
• **Mylohyoid** – Triangular muscle – Two mylohyoids form the floor of mouth	Mylohyoid line of mandible	Posterior fibers—Body of hyoid bone Middle and anterior fibers median raphe between mandible and hyoid bone	Nerve to mylohyoid	• Elevates floor of mouth in first stage of deglutition • Helps in depression of mandible • Elevation of hyoid bone
• **Geniohyoid**	Genial tubercle	Body of hyoid bone	C1 through hypoglossal nerve	Elevates hyoid bone

Relations

	Superficial	*Deep*
Posterior belly of digastric	• Mastoid process with sternocleidomastoid • Stylohyoid • Parotid gland • Submandibular gland and lymph node • Angle of mandible	• Transverse process of the atlas • Internal and external carotid artery • Internal jugular vein • Vagus, accessory and hypoglossal nerve (10th, 11th and 12th) • Hyoglossus muscle
Mylohyoid	• Anterior belly of digastric • Submandibular gland • Mylohyoid nerves and vessels • Submental branch of facial artery	• Hyoglossus with its superficial relations • Genioglossus with its superficial relations

Origin

Greater cornu and lateral part of body of hyoid bone.

Insertion

Side of tongue between styloglossus and inferior longitudinal muscle of tongue.

Nerve Supply

Hypoglossal (XII) nerve

Action

1. Depresses the tongue
2. Helps in retracting protruded tongue.

Relations

Superficial Relation	*Deep Relation*
Styloglossus Lingual nerve Submandibular gland Submandibular ganglion Submandibular duct Hypoglossal nerve	Inferior longitudinal muscle of tongue Genioglossus Middle constricter of pharynx Glossopharyngeal nerve Stylohyoid ligament lingual artery

Structure passing through

1. Glossophryngeal nerve
2. Stylohyoid ligament
3. Lingual artery

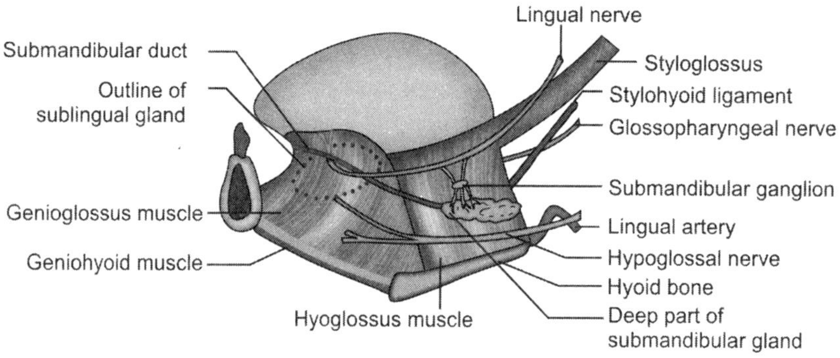
Lingual nerve
Submandibular duct
Outline of sublingual gland
Styloglossus
Stylohyoid ligament
Glossopharyngeal nerve
Submandibular ganglion
Genioglossus muscle
Lingual artery
Geniohyoid muscle
Hypoglossal nerve
Hyoid bone
Hyoglossus muscle
Deep part of submandibular gland

Fig. 7.5: Relations of hyoglossus muscle

PREVIOUS YEAR QUESTIONS

1. Write short note on digastric muscle.
2. Write briefly on posterior belly of digastric.
3. Describe submandibular gland and write a note on secretomotor fibers of it.
4. Describe submandibular gland under headings
   a. Deep relations.
   b. Innervation/nerve supply.
5. Draw the labeled diagram to show relations of hyoglossus muscle.
6. Write about hyoglossus muscle and add a note on relations of it.
7. Write a short note on mylohyoid muscle.

MULTIPLE CHOICE QUESTIONS

1. Submandibular gland is situated in:
   a. Digastric triangle
   b. Carotid triangle
   c. Muscular triangle
   d. Deep to hyoglossus
2. Sublingual gland lies:
   a. Superior to mylohyoid
   b. Inferior to mylohyoid
   c. Deep to genioglossus
   d. Deep to geniohyoid
3. Submandibular gland is divided into superficial and deep part by:
   a. Stylohyoid b. Geniohyoid
   c. Digastric d. Mylohyoid
4. The nerve supplying submandibular gland are:
   a. V b. IX
   c. VII d. XII
5. Deep surface of hyoglossus is related to:
   a. Lingual nerve
   b. Hypoglossal nerve
   c. Submandibular ganglion
   d. Glossopharyngeal nerve
6. Mylohyoid muscle:
   a. Arises from hyoid bone
   b. Developed from 2nd pharyngeal arch
   c. Depresses the hyoid
   d. Elevates the hyoid
7. Oral diaphragm/floor of mouth is formed by:
   a. Genioglossus b. Mylohyoid
   c. Orbicularis oris d. Buccinator
8. Which of the following muscle has dual nerve supply?
   a. Digastric b. Lateral pterygoid
   c. Massetor d. Temporalis
9. The action of digastric muscle is:
   a. Depression of mandible
   b. Protrusion of mandible
   c. Side-to-side movement
   d. Depressing the floor of mouth
10. All of the following muscles are elevator of hyoid bone except:
    a. Digastric b. Hyoglossus
    c. Mylohyoid d. Geniohyoid

Answers

1. (a) 2. (a) 3. (d) 4. (c) 5. (d) 6. (d) 7. (b) 8. (a) 9. (a) 10. (b)

8 Side of the Neck

- Neck is that part of the body which connects the head to the upper part of trunk
- It is cylindrical in shape.

ANATOMICAL FEATURES OF NECK

It consists of three layers - Skin
- Superficial fascia
- Deep fascia of neck

Skin

Supplied by IInd, IIIrd and IVth cervical nerves.

Superficial Fascia

A thin sheet of muscle fiber known as the platysma is present in this facial.

Platysma

- Quadrilateral shaped
- Striated muscle.

Origin

Fascia over the deltoid and pectoralis major up to 2nd rib.

Insertion

Lower border of body of mandible.

Fibers

- Lies over the superficial vein and nerve.
- Cover the sternocleidomastoid.

Nerve Supply

Cervical branch of facial nerve.

Actions

1. Contractions aid in venous return
2. Depresses the mandible
3. Pulls the angle of mouth downwards and laterally.

DEEP CERVICAL FASCIA (FASCIA COLLI) (FIG. 8.1)

Consists of six layers:

1. Investing
2. Pretracheal
3. Prevertebral
4. Carotid sheath
5. Buccopharyngeal fascia
6. Pharyngobasilar fascia.

Investing Layer

- Lies deep to platysma
- Surround the neck like a collar
- Forms the roof of the posterior triangle.

Attachment

Features of the Investing Layer

a. Between the angle of mandible and mastoid process fascia splits to enclose the parotid gland.

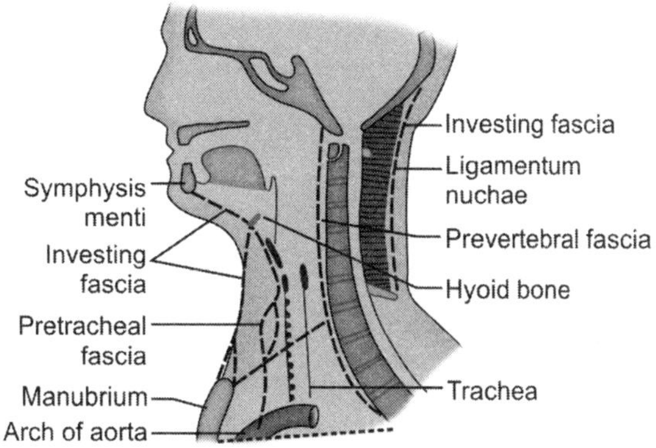
Investing fascia
Ligamentum nuchae
Symphysis menti
Prevertebral fascia
Investing fascia
Hyoid bone
Pretracheal fascia
Manubrium
Trachea
Arch of aorta

Fig. 8.1: Deep cervical fascia (fascia colli)

Boundaries	Attachments
Superiorly	• External occipital protuberance • Superior nuchal line • Mastoid process • Lower border of zygomatic arch and body of mandible.
Inferiorly	• Upper border of spine of scapular • Acromian process of scapula • Upper surface of clavicle • Suprasternal notch of manubrium sterni.
Posteriorly	• Ligamentum nuchae • Spine of C7 vertebra.
Anteriorly	• Symphysis menti • Hyoid bone • Manubrium sterni.

- The superficial lamina named as parotid fascia is thick and dense and attached to the zygomatic arch
- Deep lamina is thin and attached to the styloid process and mandible.

b. This fascia splits to enclose two muscles

i. Trapezius ii. Sternocleidomastoid

2 Glands → Parotid, Submandibular

2 Spaces → Suprasternal, Supraclavicular

c. It also forms pulleys to bind the tendons of the digastric and omohyoid muscles.

Pretracheal Fascia

- Lies over the trachea
- Encloses and suspends the thyroid gland and forms its false capsule.

Attachment

Boundaries	Attachments
Superiorly	• Hyoid bone • Thyroid cartilage • Cricoid cartilage.
Inferiorly	• Encloses the inferior thyroid veins • Blends with the arch of aorta.
Either side	• Fuses with front of the carotid sheath.

Other Features of Pretracheal Fascia

1. Posterior layer of thyroid capsule is thick on either side to form a suspensory ligament for the thyroid gland known as Ligament of Berry.
   a. Ligaments are attached chiefly to the cricoid cartilage and may extend to thyroid cartilage.
   b. They support the thyroid gland, and do not let it sink into the mediastinum.
2. Fascia provides a slippery surface for the free movements of the trachea during swallowing.

Prevertebral Fascia

- Lies in front of the prevertebral muscle
- Forms the floor of the posterior triangle.

Attachment

Boundaries	Attachments
Superiorly	Base of the skull
Inferiorly	• Anterior longitudinal ligament • Body of fourth thoracic vertebra.
Anteriorly	Separated from the pharynx and buccopharyngeal fascia by the retropharyngeal space.
Laterally	Lost deep to the trapezius.

Features of Prevertebral Fascia

1. Cervical and brachial plexuses lie behind this fascia and pierced by four coetaneous branches of cervical plexus.
2. The trunks of branchial plexus and the subclavian artery carry with them a covering of this fascia which is known as auxiliary sheath which extends into the axilla.
3. Fascia provides a fixed base for the movements of the pharynx, the esophagus and the control sheaths during swallowing.

Carotid Sheath

The deep cervical fascia forms a tubular sheath around the major vessels of the neck known as carotid sheath.

Extend

From the base of skull above to the arch of aorta below.

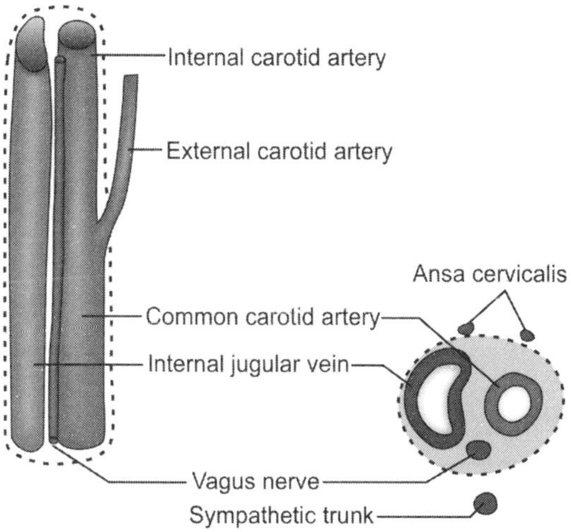
Internal carotid artery
External carotid artery
Ansa cervicalis
Common carotid artery
Internal jugular vein
Vagus nerve
Sympathetic trunk

Fig. 8.2: Carotid sheath and its contents

Contents (Fig. 8.2)

1. Common carotid artery in lower part
2. Internal carotid artery in upper part
3. Internal jugular vein
4. Vagus nerve.

Features

1. Formed by condensation of fibroaereolar tissue
2. Attached to the pretracheal and prevertebral fascia
3. Ansa carvicalis is embedded in its anterior layer
4. Cervical sympathetic chain lies close to the posterior layer in front of the prevertebral fascia.

Buccopharyngeal Fascia

- Fascia covers the superior constrictor muscle externally
- Extends on to the buccinater muscle.

Pharyngobasilar Fascia

- It lies deep to the pharyngeal muscle
- Especially thickened between the upper border of superior constrictor muscle and base of skull.

Clinical and Applied Anatomy

1. Parotid swellings are very painful due to unyielding nature of the parotid fascia.
2. Thyroid gland and all thyroid swellings move with deglutition because the thyroid is attached to the larynx by the suspensory ligament of Berry.
3. While excising the submandibular gland, the external carotid artery should be secured before dividing it.
4. Neck infections behind the prevertebral fascia arise usually from tuberculosis of the cervical vertebrae.

POSTERIOR TRIANGLE

Posterior triangle is a space on the side of the neck situated behind the sternocleidomastoid muscle.

Boundaries (Fig. 8.3)

Anterior	:	Posterior border of sternocleidomastoid
Posterior	:	Anterior border of trapezius
Base	:	Middle third of the clavicle
Apex	:	Meeting joint of sternocleidomastoid and trapezius
Roof	:	Investing layer of deep cervical fascia
Floor	:	Muscular, formed by six muscles: a. Semispinalis capitis b. Splenius capitus c. Levator scapulae d. Scalenus posterior e. Scalenus medius f. Outer border of 1st rib.

- Prevertebral layer of deep cervical fascia covers all the muscles of the floor.

Division of the Posterior Triangle

It is subdivided by the inferior belly of the omohyoid into.

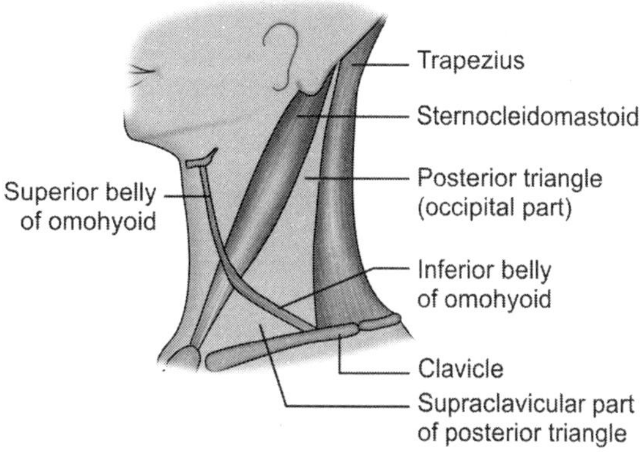
Trapezius
Sternocleidomastoid
Superior belly of omohyoid
Posterior triangle (occipital part)
Inferior belly of omohyoid
Clavicle
Supraclavicular part of posterior triangle

Fig. 8.3: Boundaries of posterior triangle

Contents	*Occipital triangle*	*Subclavian triangle*
• **Nerves**	• Spinal accessary nerve • Four cutaneous branches of cervical plexus – Lesser occipital – Great curricular – Anterior cutaneous nerve – Supraclavicular nerve. • Muscular branches: – Two branches to levator scapulae – Two branches to trapezius – Nerve to rhomboideus. • Upper part of the brachial plexus	• Three trun of brachial plexus • Nerve to serratus anterior • Nerve to subclavius • Suprascapular nerve.
• **Vessels**	• Transverse cervical artery and vein • Occipital artery.	• Third part of subclavian artery and subclavian vein • Suprascapular artery and vein • Commencement of transverse cervical artery • Lower part of external jugular vien.
• **Lymph nodes**	Along the posterior border of the sternocleido-mastoid, supraclavicular nodes occipital nodes.	Few number of supraclavicular chain

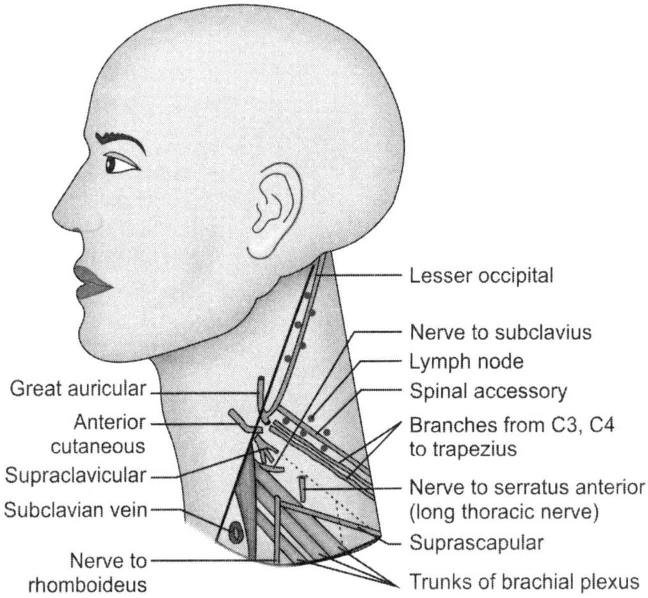
Lesser occipital
Nerve to subclavius
Lymph node
Spinal accessory
Branches from C3, C4 to trapezius
Nerve to serratus anterior (long thoracic nerve)
Suprascapular
Trunks of brachial plexus
Great auricular
Anterior cutaneous
Supraclavicular
Subclavian vein
Nerve to rhomboideus

Fig. 8.4: Contents of posterior triangle

1. ***Occipital triangle***—Larger upper part
2. ***Supraclavicular/Subclavian triangle***—Smaller lower part.

Contents of the Posterior Triangle (Fig. 8.4)

Features of Posterior Triangle

1. **Spinal accessory nerve** emerges a little above the middle of the sternocleidomastoid muscle.
2. **Four cutaneous branches of the cervical plexus** pierce the fascia covering the floor of triangle.
3. **Muscular branches** to levator scapulae and to the trapezius appear at middle of sternocleidomastoid.
4. **Nerve to subclavius** descends in front of the brachial plexus and subclavian vessels.
5. **Suprascapular nerve** arises from the upper trunk of brachial plexus.

6. **Three trunks of brachial plexus** emerge between the scalenus anterior and medius, carrying the axially sheath around them.
7. **Subclavian artery** passes behind the tendons of scalenous anterior and subclavian vein passes in front of the tendon.
8. **Transverse cervical artery** is a branch of the thyrocervical trunk.

STERNOCLEIDOMASTOID MUSCLE (STERNOMASTOID)

Largest superficial muscle of neck.

Origin

1. Sternal head – Superolateral part of manubrium, sterni (Tendinous)
2. Clavicular head – Medial 1/3rd of clavicle (Muscylotendinous).

Insertion

1. Thick tendon into lateral surface of mastoid process
2. Think aponeurosis into lateral half of superior nuchal line of occipital bone.

Nerve Supply

1. Spinal accessory nerve
2. Branches from ventral rami of C_2
3. Proprioceptive.

Blood Supply

- Anterior : 1. Superior thyroid artery
  2. Suprascapular arery
  3. Occipital artery.
- Veins follow the arteries.

Action

1. When one muscle contract –
   a. Turns chin to opposite side
   b. Tilt head towards the shoulder.
2. When both muscles contract together –
   a. Draw the head forwards
   b. With longus coli, they flex the neck against resistance
   c. Reverse action helps in forced inspiration.

Relations

- It is enclosed in investing layer of deep cervical fascia and pierced by accessory nerve and four sternocleidomastoid arteries.

Superficial Relations

1. Skin
2. Superficial fascia and superficial lamina of deep fascia
3. Platysma
4. External jugular vein
5. Superficial cervical lymph node ↔
   - → Great curricular
   - → Transverse cutaneous
   - → Medial supraclavicular
6. Parotid gland overlaps the muscle.

Deep Relations

1. Bones and joint
   - → Mastoid process
   - → Sternoclavicular joint
2. Carotid sheath
3. Muscles
   - → Sternohyoid
   - → Sternothyroid
   - → Omohyoid
   - → 3 scaleni
   - → Levator scapulae
   - → Splenius capitis
   - → Posterior belly of digastric
4. Arteries
   - → Common carotid, internal and
   - → External carotid
   - → Sternomastoid
   - → Occipital
   - → Subclavian
   - → Suprascapular
   - → Transverse cervical
5. Veins
   - → Internal jugular
   - → Anterior jugular
   - → Facial
   - → Lingual
6. Nerves
   - → Vagus
   - → Accessory
   - → Cervical plexus
   - → Bronchial plexus
   - → Phrenic
   - → Ansa cervicalis
7. Lymph nodes, deep cervical

Clinical and Applied Anatomy

1. Most common swelling in the posterior triangle is due to enlargement of the supraclavicular lymph nodes.
2. Torticollis or wry neck is a deformity in which head is bent to one side and the chin points to other side.
   a. This is a result of spasm of muscles supplied by the spinal accessory nerve, these being the sternocleidomastoid and trapezius.
   b. Type- 1. Rheumatic – Due to cold
      2. Reflex – Due to inflamed cervical lymph node
      3. Congenital – Due to birth injury
      4. Spasmodic – Due to central irritation
3. **Block dissection** of the neck for malignant disease is the removal of cervical lymph nodes along with involved structures.

Muscles of the Side

1. Sternocleidomastoid
2. Digastric – Anterior and posterior belly
3. Stylohyoid
4. Mylohyoid
5. Geniohyoid
6. Sternohyoid
7. Omohyoid
   → Superior belly
   → Inferior belly
8. Sternothyroid
9. Thyrohyoid.

PREVIOUS YEAR QUSTIONS

1. Describe briefly the investing layer of deep cervical fascia.
2. Write a short note on sternomastoid muscle.
3. Write a short note on boundaries and contents of subclavian triangle.
4. Write a short note on carotid sheath.
5. Mention boundaries and contents of posterior triangle of the neck.

MULTIPLE CHOICE QUESTIONS

1. Carotid sheath contains all except:
   a. Vagus nerve
   b. Internal carotid artery
   c. Internal jugular vein
   d. External carotid artery
2. Contents of posterior triangle are these except:
   a. Brachial plexus
   b. Thyrocervical trunk
   c. Subclavian artery
   d. Omohyoid
3. Wry neck deformity is due to damage of:
   a. Platysma
   b. Sternohyoid
   c. Sternocleidomastoid
   d. Omohyoid
4. Vein related to superficial surface of sternocleidomastoid is:
   a. External jugular vein
   b. Internal jugular vein
   c. Anterior jugular vein
   d. Facial vein.
5. Surgical excision of submandibular gland, endanger which of the following structures:
   a. Internal carotid artery
   b. External carotid artery
   c. Common carotid artery
   d. Facial artery
6. The occipital bone provides attachment to all except:
   a. Trapezius
   b. Ligamentum nuchae
   c. Sternocleidomastoid
   d. Rectus capitus

Answers

1. (d) 2. (d) 3. (c) 4. (a) 5. (b) 6. (c)

9 Back of the Neck

Posterior aspect of neck is primarily muscular.

LIGAMENTUM NUCHAE (FIG. 9.1)

- Triangular fibrous sheet that separates muscles of the two sides of the neck.
- In the median plane beneath the deep fascia, a fibrous sheath attached to the spines of the cervical vertebrae.
- It is attached above to the external occipital protuberance and crest.
- Divides neck into two parts.
- Each half is covered by muscles which lie between the deep cervical fascia and posterior aspect of cervical vertebrae.

MUSCLES OF BACK

Arranged in two groups on each side of the midline.

Superficial Group

Primarily involved in the movements of upper limb:

a. Trapezius
b. Levator scapulae
c. Rhomboideus major and minor

Deep Intrinsic Group

- These muscle maintain the upright posture of head
- Intrinsic muscles are arranged in three groups from superficial for deep.

a. **Splenius group:** Outermost
   i. Splenius capitis
   ii. Splenius cervicis.
b. **Erector spinae group:** Larger muscles, chief extensor
   i. Spinalis, medially
   ii. Longissimus, intermediate
   iii. Iliocostocervicalis, laterally.
c. **Transverse:** Spinalis group
   i. Semispinalis (cause extension of head)
   ii. Multifidus
   iii. Rotators.

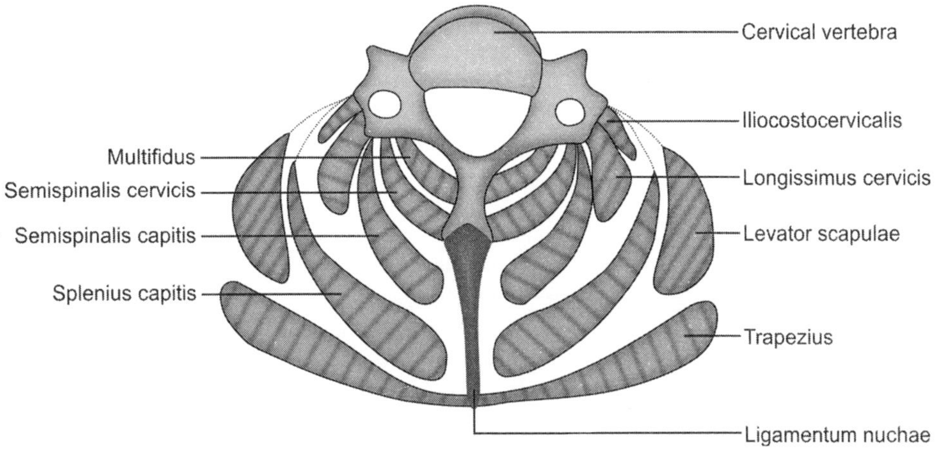

Cervical vertebra
Iliocostocervicalis
Multifidus
Longissimus cervicis
Semispinalis cervicis
Semispinalis capitis
Levator scapulae
Splenius capitis
Trapezius
Ligamentum nuchae

Fig. 9.1: Ligamentum nuchae

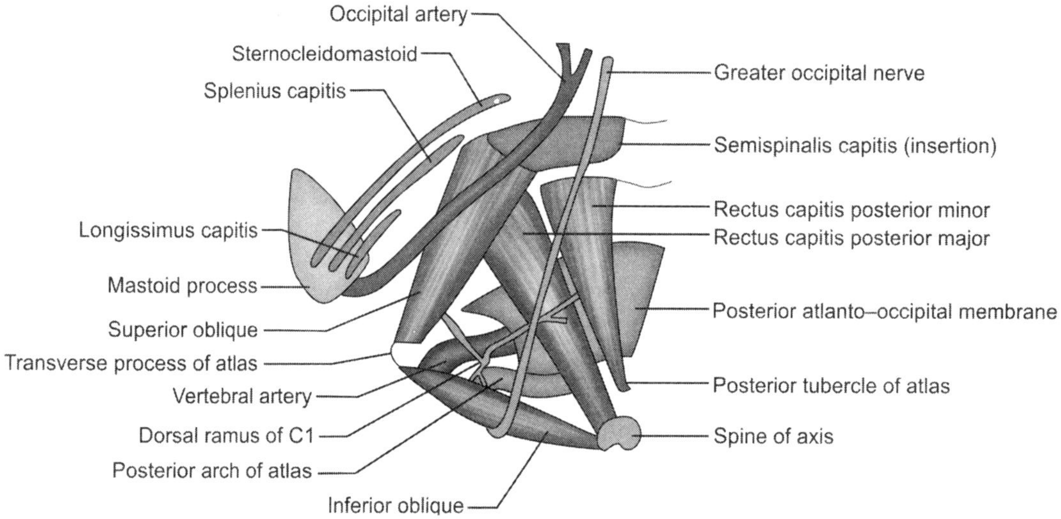
Occipital artery
Sternocleidomastoid
Splenius capitis
Longissimus capitis
Mastoid process
Superior oblique
Transverse process of atlas
Vertebral artery
Dorsal ramus of C1
Posterior arch of atlas
Inferior oblique
Greater occipital nerve
Semispinalis capitis (insertion)
Rectus capitis posterior minor
Rectus capitis posterior major
Posterior atlanto–occipital membrane
Posterior tubercle of atlas
Spine of axis

Fig. 9.2: Boundaries and content of suboccipital triangle

d. **Other deep muscles**
   i. Interspinalis
   ii. Inter transversii
   iii. Suboccipital.

Nerve Supply

Deep muscles of neck are supplied by the respective dorsal rami of cervical nerves.

SUBOCCIPITAL TRIANGLE (FIG. 9.2)

- A pair of muscular triangles situated deep in the suboccipital region one on either side of midline.
- Bounded by four suboccipital muscles.

Boundaries

Superomedial - Rectus capitis posterior major
Rectus capitis posterior minor

Superolateral - Superior oblique

Inferior - Inferior oblique

Roof

Medially - Dense fibrous tissue covered by the semispinalis capitis

laterally - Longissimus capitis

Muscle	*Origin*	*Insertion*	*Actions*
• **Rectus capitis posterior major**	Spine of axis	Lateral part of area below the inferior nuchal line	• Mainly postural • Acting alone – turns chin to same side • Acting together two muscles extend the head
• **Rectus capitis posterior minor**	Posterior tubercle of atlas	Medial part of area below the inferior nuchal line	• Postural • Extend the head
• **Oblique capitis superior (Superior oblique)**	Transverse process of atlas	Lateral area between the nuchal lines	• Postural • Extend the head • Flex head laterally
• **Oblique capitis inferior (Inferior oblique)**	Spine of axis	Transverse process of atlas	• Postural • Turn chin for same side

Floor

i. Posterior arch of atlas
ii. Posterior atlanto-occipital membrane.

Content

i. Third part of vertebral artery
ii. Dorsal ramus of C1 (suboccipital nerve)
iii. Suboccipital plexus of veins.

SUBOCCIPITAL MUSCLES

- Groups of small muscles
- Situated in upper most part of back of the neck below semispinalis capitis
- Form the boundaries of suboccipital triangle
- Supplied by suboccipital nerve [dorsal ramus C_1].

Clinical and Applied Anatomy

1. **Neck rigidity** seen in cases with meningitis is due to spasm of the extensor muscles.
2. **Cisternal puncture** is done when lumbar puncture fails.
3. **Neurosurgeons approach** the posterior cranial fossa through this region.

PREVIOUS YEAR QUESTIONS

1. Write a note on contents of suboccipital triangle.
2. Describe boundaries and contents of suboccipital triangle.

MULTIPLE CHOICE QUESTIONS

1. Sternocleidomastoid and trapezius are supplied by:
   a. Cranial accessory
   b. Vagus
   c. Spinal accessory
   d. Glossopharyngeal
2. All are true for ligamentum nuchae except:
   a. Fibrous sheet that separate neck into two parts
   b. Attached above to external occipital protuberance
   c. Lies in median plane beneath deep fascia
   d. Lies between deep fascia and superficial fascia.
3. All the following muscles extend the head except:
   a. Rectus capitis posterior major
   b. Rectus capitis posterior minor
   c. Oblique capitis superior
   d. Oblique capitis inferior

Answers

1. (c) 2. (d) 3. (d)

10 Front of the Neck

- Side of the neck has anterior and lateral surfaces
- It is rectangular in shape
- Divided into two triangles by sternocleidomastoid muscle as:
  i. Anterior triangle
  ii. Posterior triangle

ANTERIOR TRIANGLE

- It lies between the midline of the neck and sternocleidomastoid muscle
- It is subdivided into smaller triangles.

Boundaries (Fig. 10.1)

Anterior	:	Anterior midline of neck extending from symphysis menti to middle of suprasternal notch.
Posterior	:	Anterior border of sternocleidomastoid.
Base	:	Lower border of body of mandible and line joining angle of mandible with mastoid process.
Apex	:	Suprasternal notch—Meeting point between sternocleidomastoid and anterior midline.

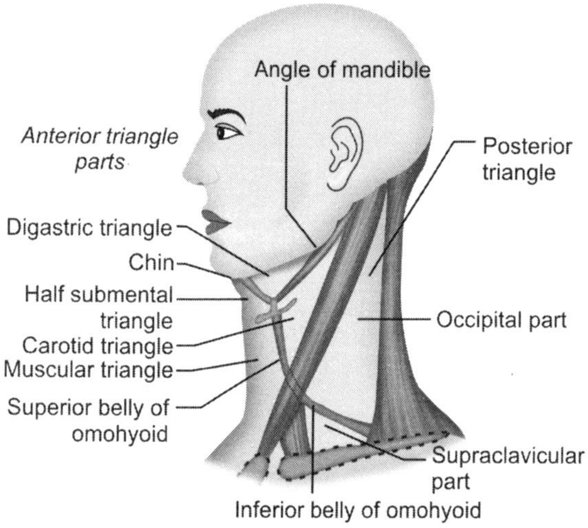

Angle of mandible
Anterior triangle parts
Posterior triangle
Digastric triangle
Chin
Half submental triangle
Carotid triangle
Muscular triangle
Superior belly of omohyoid
Occipital part
Supraclavicular part
Inferior belly of omohyoid

Fig. 10.1: Boundaries and subdivisions of anterior triangle

Subdivisions of Anterior Triangle

It is subdivided by the diagastric muscle and superior belly of omohyoid into four triangles:

i. Submental triangle
ii. Digastric triangle
iii. Carotid triangle
iv. Muscular triangle

Submental Triangle

It is complete only when the neck is seen from front.

Boundaries (Fig. 10.2)

On each side	:	Anterior belly of digastric
Base	:	Body of hyoid bone
Apex	:	Symphysis manti (Chin)
Floor	:	Oral diaphragm formed by mylohyoid muscle.

Contents

1. Submental lymph nodes
2. Submental veins
3. Anterior jugular veins.

Digastric Triangle

- Area between the body of mandible and hyoid bone is known as the submandibular region.
- Superficial structures lies in:
  - Submental triangle
  - Digastric triangle

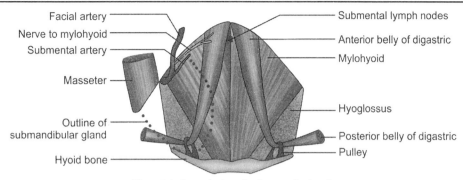

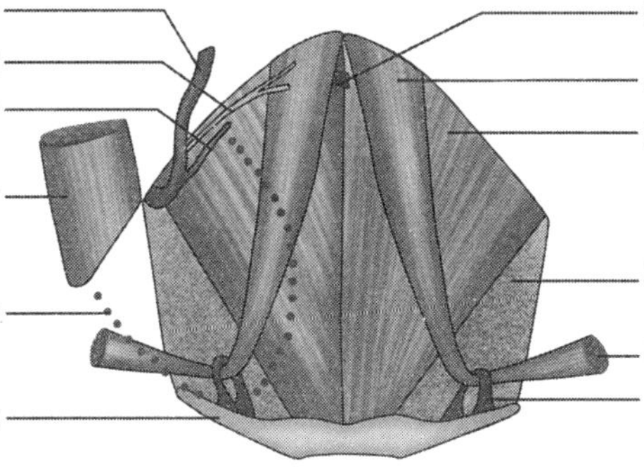
Facial artery
Nerve to mylohyoid
Submental artery
Masseter
Outline of submandibular gland
Hyoid bone
Submental lymph nodes
Anterior belly of digastric
Mylohyoid
Hyoglossus
Posterior belly of digastric
Pulley

Fig. 10.2: Boundaries of submental triangle

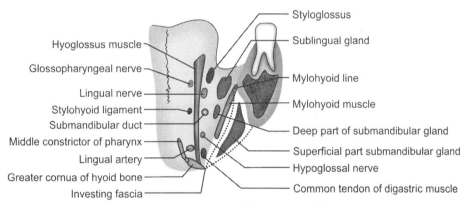

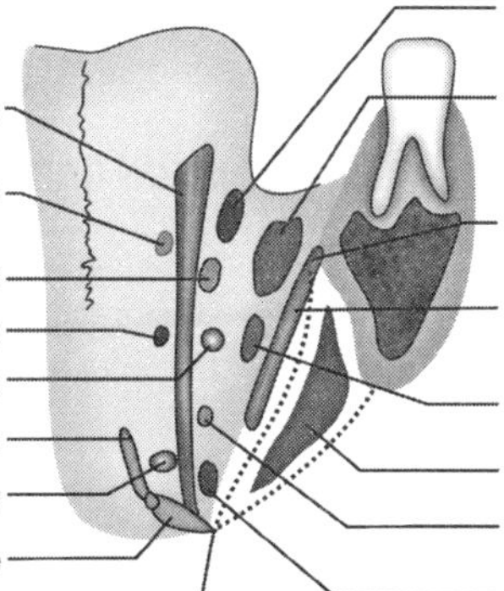
Hyoglossus muscle
Glossopharyngeal nerve
Lingual nerve
Stylohyoid ligament
Submandibular duct
Middle constrictor of pharynx
Lingual artery
Greater cornua of hyoid bone
Investing fascia
Styloglossus
Sublingual gland
Mylohyoid line
Mylohyoid muscle
Deep part of submandibular gland
Superficial part submandibular gland
Hypoglossal nerve
Common tendon of digastric muscle

Fig. 10.3: Contents of digastric triangle

Boundaries

Antero-inferior	:	Anterior belly of digastric
Postero-inferior	:	Posterior belly of digastric
Base	:	Body of mandible Line joining angle of mandible and mastoid process
Apex	:	Intermediate tenden of digastric muscle
Floor	:	Mylohyoid muscles Hyoglossus Middle constrictor
Roof	:	Investing layer of deep cervical fascia skin, superficial fascia

Contents (Fig. 10.3)

1. Submandibular gland – superficial part
2. Submandibular lymph nodes
3. Hypoglossal nerve
4. Submental artery and vein
5. Mylohyoid nerves and vessels
6. External carotid artery
7. Carotid sheath with its contents
8. Structures passing between the external and internal carotid arteries are:
   a. Styloid process
   b. Styloglossus muscle
   c. Stylopharyngeus muscle
   d. Glossopharyngeal nerve
   e. Lower end of parotid gland
   f. Pharyngeal branch of vagus nerve.

Carotid Triangle

Boundaries

Superior	:	Posterior belly of digastric and stylohyoid.
Antero-inferior	:	Superior belly of omohyoid.

Posterior : Anterior border of sternocleidomastoid.

Roof : Investing layer of deep cervical fascia.

Floor : Formed by five muscles:
- a. Thyrohyoid
- b. Hyoglossus
- c. Middle constrictor of pharynx
- d. Inferior constrictor of pharynx.

Contents (Fig. 10.4)

1. Common carotid artery with its terminal branches:
   - a. Internal carotid artery
   - b. External carotid artery.
2. Internal jugular vein
3. Occipital vessels
4. Facial vessels
5. Lingual vessels
6. Superior thyroid vessels
7. Pharyngeal vessels
8. Cranial nerves:
   - a. Vagus
   - b. Spinal accessory
   - c. hypoglossal.
9. Sympathetic chain
10. Cervical part of deep cervical lymph nodes.

Muscular Triangle

Boundaries

Anterior : Anterior midline of the neck

Anterosuperior : Superior belly of omohyoid

Posteroinferior : Anterior border of sternocleidomastoid

Contents

1. Infrahyoid muscles – Form the floor
   - a. Superior group
     - → Sternohyoid
     - → Omohyoid
   - b. Deep group
     - → Sternohyoid
     - → Thyrohyoid

COMMON CAROTID ARTERY

- Chief artery supplying head and neck
- It is present in a pair, one on the right and one on the left side.

Origin

1. Right common carotid - From brachiocephalic trunk
2. Left common carotid - From arch of aorta directly

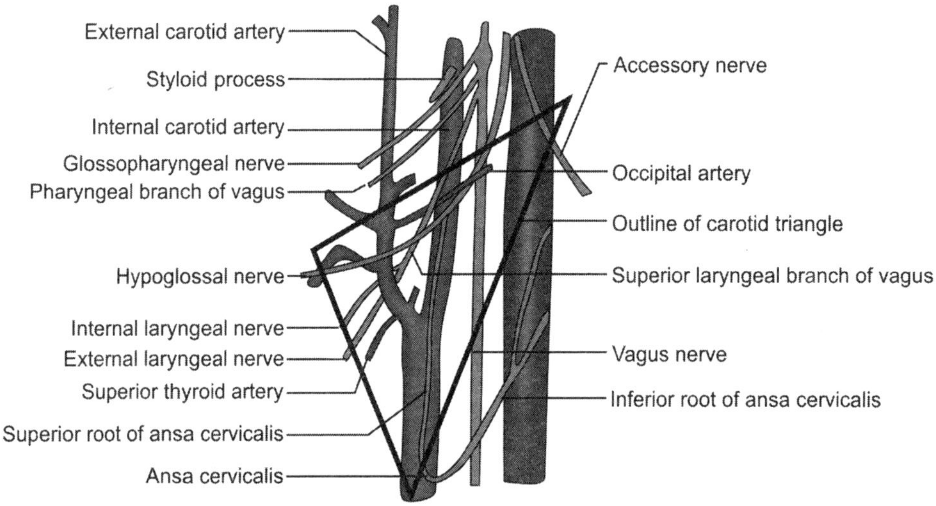

External carotid artery
Styloid process
Internal carotid artery
Glossopharyngeal nerve
Pharyngeal branch of vagus
Hypoglossal nerve
Internal laryngeal nerve
External laryngeal nerve
Superior thyroid artery
Superior root of ansa cervicalis
Ansa cervicalis
Accessory nerve
Occipital artery
Outline of carotid triangle
Superior laryngeal branch of vagus
Vagus nerve
Inferior root of ansa cervicalis

Fig. 10.4: Contents of carotid triangle

Termination

Each terminator at the level of the intervertebral disk between C_3 and C_4 vertebrae by dividing into its terminal branches.

Course

Left common carotid artery
↓
Ascends upwards
↓
Enter neck behind left sternoclavicular joint

Right common carotid artery ⟶ ↓

Runs upwards
↓
Reaches upper border of thyroid cartilage enclosed in carotid sheath

Relations

- ***Anterior*** (From within outwards)
  - Lateral part of thyroid gland
  - Infrahyoid strap muscles
  - Sternocleidomastoid
  - Anterior jugular vein
  - Deep fascia with platysma
  - Superficial fascia
  - Skin.
- ***Posterior*** (From within outwards)
  - Carotid body
  - Thoracic duct
  - Inferior thyroid artery
  - Sympathetic nerve trunk
  - Vertebral artery
  - Prevertebral muscles with fascia
  - Transverse processes of lower cervical vertebra.
- ***Lateral***
  - Vagus nerve
  - Internal jugular vein.
- ***Medial***
  - Thyroid gland
  - Recurrent laryngeal nerve
  - Trachea
  - Esophagus
  - Larynx and pharynx.

BRANCHES OF COMMON CAROTID ARTERY

- External carotid artery
- Internal carotid artery.

Carotid Sinus

- The termination of the common carotid artery, or the beginning of the internal carotid artery shows a slight dilatation, known as carotid sinus.
- In this region, tunica media is thin, but the adventitia is thick.

Infrahyoid muscles				
Muscle	*Origin*	*Insertion*	*Nerve Supply*	*Actions*
• **Sternohyoid**	• Manubrium sterni • Clavicle and posterior sternoclavicular ligament	Medial part hyoid bone	Ansa cervicalis	Depresses the hyoid bone
• **Sternothyroid**	• Manubrium sterni • First costal cartilage	Oblique line of thyroid cartilage	Ansa cervicalis	Depresses larynx
• **Thyrohyoid**	Oblique line of thyroid cartilage	Body and greater cornua of thyroid cartilage	C_1 through hypoglossal nerve	• Depresses hyoid bone • Elevate larynx
• **Omohyoid** – Inferior belly – Superior belly	• Upper border of scapular near suprascapular notch • Suprascapular ligament	Body of hyoid bone bound to clavicle by a facial pulley	Ansa cervicalis	Depresses the hyoid bnone

- Receives rich innervations from glossopharyngeal.
- It acts as "Baroreceptor" or "Pressure receptor".
- If regulates blood pressure.

Carotid Body

- It is small, oval reddish brown structure situated behind the bifurcation of common carotid artery.
- If receives a rich nerve supply mainly from glossopharyngeal nerve, vagus and sympathetic nerve.
- If acts as a "Chemoreceptor" and responds to changes in oxygen and carbon dioxide and pH content of the blood.
- Other allied chemoreceptors are found near:
  - i. Arch of aorta
  - ii. Ducts arteriosus
  - iii. Right subclavian artery.

  } Supplied by vagus nerve

EXTERNAL CAROTID ARTERY

Supplies structures present external to the skull and those in front of the neck.

Origin

Common carotid artery, at upper border of lamina of thyroid cartilage.

Termination

Ends by dividing into its terminal branches, at the level of the neck of mandible.

Course

External carotid artery
↓
Ascends upwards in curved manner
↓
Lies medial to internal carotid artery
↓
Crosses over it anteriorly
↓
Runs upwards in deep part of parotid gland
↓
Ends at the neck of mandible

Relations

Anterior

- Within the deep part of parotid gland:
  - a. Retromandibular vein
  - b. Facial nerve with its terminal branches
- Stylohyoid muscles
- Posterior belly of digastric muscle
- Hypoglossal nerve
- Lingual vein.

Posterior

- Constrictor muscles of pharynx
- Superior laryngeal nerve
- Internal carotid gland
- Styloid process
- Stylopharyngeus muscle
- Glossopharyngeal nerve
- Styloglossus muscle
- Part of parotid gland
- Pharyngeal branch of vagus nerve.

Branches of External Carotid Artery (Fig. 10.5)

It gives eight branches:

- i. Ascending pharyngeal artery
- ii. Superior thyroid artery
- iii. Lingual artery
- iv. Facial artery
- v. Occipital artery
- vi. Posterior auricular artery
- vii. Maxillary artery
- viii. Superficial temporal artery.

INTERNAL CAROTID ARTERY

- It is considered an upward continuation of the common carotid
- It supplies structures lying within the skull and in the orbit.

Origin

At the upper border of lamina of thyroid cartilage.

Termination

Internal carotid artery
↓

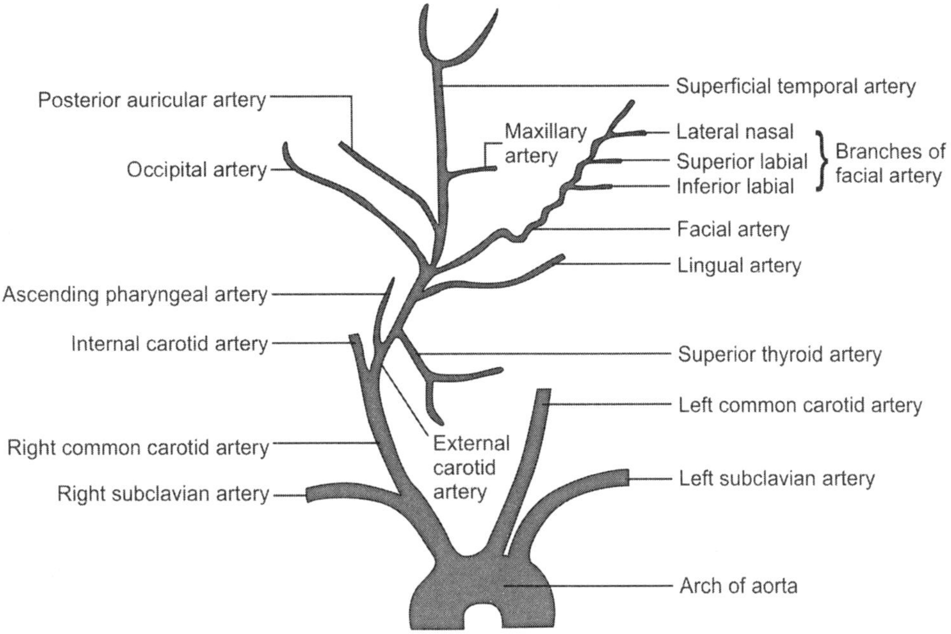
Posterior auricular artery
Occipital artery
Ascending pharyngeal artery
Internal carotid artery
Right common carotid artery
Right subclavian artery
Maxillary artery
External carotid artery
Superficial temporal artery
Lateral nasal
Superior labial
Inferior labial
Branches of facial artery
Facial artery
Lingual artery
Superior thyroid artery
Left common carotid artery
Left subclavian artery
Arch of aorta

Fig. 10.5: Branches of external carotid artery

Pass through foramen lacerum

↓

Enters cavernous sinus

↓

Ends below anterior perforated substance of brain

↙ ↘

Anterior cerebral artery   Middle cerebral artery

Structures Passing between External and Internal Carotid Arteries

1. Stylopharyngeus muscles
2. Glossopharyngeal nerve
3. Pharyngeal branch of vagus nerve
4. Styloid process
5. Deep part of parotid gland.

Course and Branches (Fig. 10.6)

Divided into four parts:

Cervical Part

- Ascends vertically upwards
- Lies in front of the transverse processes of upper cervical vertebrae
- In neck, enclosed in carotid sheath
- Lower part, is superficial and located in the carotid triangle
- Upper part, is deeply located and lies deep to the posterior belly of digastric, styloid process and parotid gland
- Structure passing between the internal jugular vein and internal carotid artery are four nerves as follows:
  - i. Glossopharyngeal
  - ii. Vagus
  - iii. Accessory
  - iv. hypoglossal
- Branch → No branch in neck.

Petrous Part

- Enter petrous part of temporal one in carotid canal
- Emerges in faramen lacerum
- Branches
  - i. Caroticotympanic branch to middle ear
  - ii. Pterygoid branch

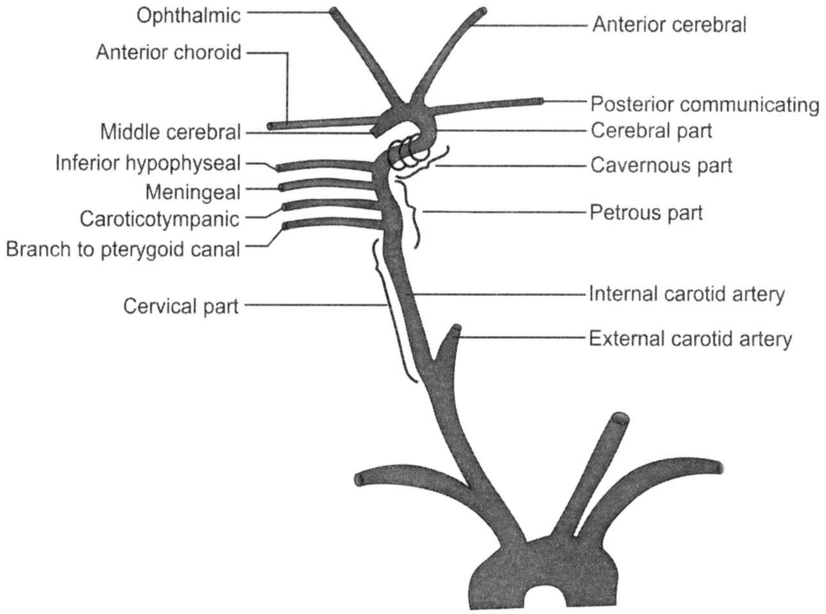
Ophthalmic
Anterior choroid
Middle cerebral
Inferior hypophyseal
Meningeal
Caroticotympanic
Branch to pterygoid canal
Cervical part
Anterior cerebral
Posterior communicating
Cerebral part
Cavernous part
Petrous part
Internal carotid artery
External carotid artery

Fig. 10.6: Branches of internal carotid artery

Cavernous Part

- Enters cavernous sinus
- Pierces the dural roof of sinus to reach the under-surface of cerebrum.
- Branches:
  - i. Cavernous branch to trigeminal ganglion
  - ii. Superior and inferior hypophyseal arteries.

Cerebral Part

- Runs the backwards in subarachnoid space and lies below optic nerve
- Reaches the anterior perforated substance of brain
- Ends by dividing into anterior and middle cerebral arteries.

Branches:

1. Ophthalmic
2. Anterior choroidal
3. Posterior communicating
4. Anterior cerebral
5. Middle cerebral

INTERNAL JUGULAR VEIN

Main venous channel of head and neck.

Extent

Base of skull in jugular foramen

↓

Ends behind the sternal end of clavicle by joining the subclavian vein

↓

Forms brachiocephalic vein

- Present with two dilatations:
  1. Superior bulb - In jugular fossa
  2. Inferior bulb - In lesser supraclavicular fossa

Course

Carotid sheath

↓

Passes vertically

↓

Lateral to internal carotid artery. Deep cervical lymph nodes are closely related to this vein

Tributaries of Internal Jugular Vein

1. Inferior petrosal sinus—connects cavernous sinus to superior bulb
2. Pharyngeal veins—from pharyngeal plexus

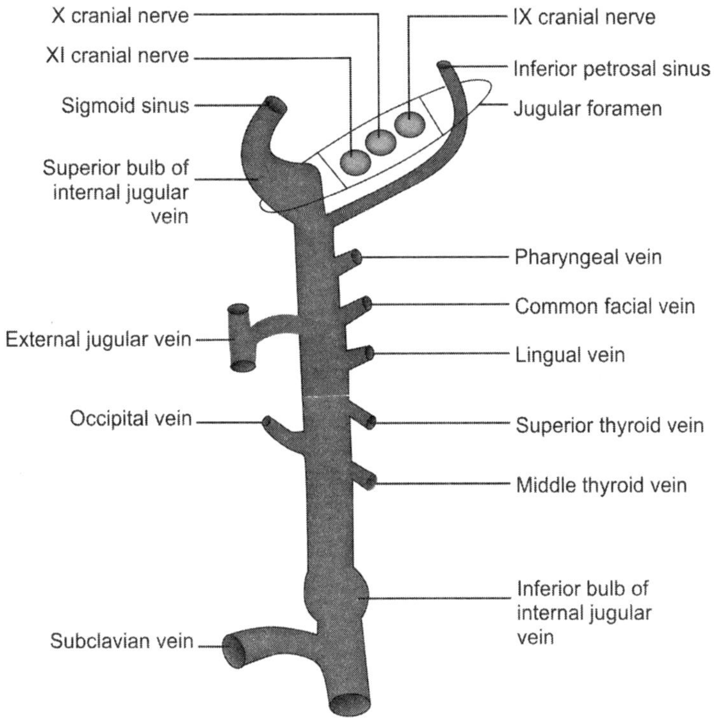
X cranial nerve
XI cranial nerve
Sigmoid sinus
Superior bulb of internal jugular vein
IX cranial nerve
Inferior petrosal sinus
Jugular foramen
Pharyngeal vein
Common facial vein
External jugular vein
Lingual vein
Occipital vein
Superior thyroid vein
Middle thyroid vein
Inferior bulb of internal jugular vein
Subclavian vein

Fig. 10.7: Internal jugular vein

3. Common facial vein
4. Superior thyroid vein—from upper part of thyroid gland
5. Middle thyroid vein—from middle of thyroid gland
6. Lingual vein
7. Occipital vein.

Clinical and Applied Anatomy

1. Internal jugular vein acts as a guide for surgeons during removal of deep cervical lymph nodes.
2. Vein can safely be connulated in cases of cardiovascular collapse.

EXTERNAL JUGULAR VEIN

It is a large vein present in the superficial fascia under cover of the platysma (Fig. 10.7).

Course

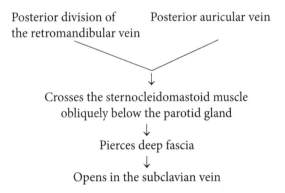

Posterior division of the retromandibular vein + Posterior auricular vein

↓

Crosses the sternocleidomastoid muscle obliquely below the parotid gland

↓

Pierces deep fascia

↓

Opens in the subclavian vein

Tributaries

1. Transverse cervical vein
2. Oblique jugular vein
3. Suprascapular vein

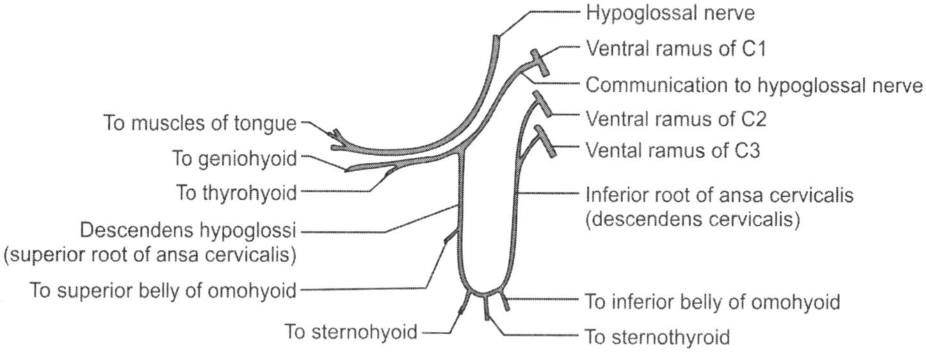
Hypoglossal nerve
Ventral ramus of C1
Communication to hypoglossal nerve
Ventral ramus of C2
Vental ramus of C3
Inferior root of ansa cervicalis (descendens cervicalis)
To inferior belly of omohyoid
To sternothyroid
To muscles of tongue
To geniohyoid
To thyrohyoid
Descendens hypoglossi (superior root of ansa cervicalis)
To superior belly of omohyoid
To sternohyoid

Fig. 10.8: Ansa cervicalis

4. Anterior jugular vein
5. Posterior external jugular vein

ANSA CERVICALIS (FIG 10.8)

- It is a thin nerve loop that lies embedded in the anterior wall of the carotid sheath over the larynx.
- It supplies the infrahyoid muscles.
- It has 2 roots.

Roots

Superior Root (Descendens Hypoglossi)

- Formed by the descending branch of the hypoglossal nerve.
- Carries the fibers of spinal nerve C1.
- Descends downwards over the internal and common carotid arteries.

Inferior Root (Descending Cervical Nerve)

- Derived from C2 and C3 spinal nerves.
- This root first descends and winds round the internal jugular vein.
- Then continues anteroinferiorly to join the superior root in front of common carotid artery.

PREVIOUS YEAR QUESTIONS

1. Write boundaries and contents of carotid triangle of neck.
2. Write a short note on ansa cervicalis.
3. Describe boundaries and contents of digastric triangle.
4. Enumerate the branches of external carotid artery.
5. Write short note on external jugular vein.

MULTIPLE CHOICE QUESTIONS

1. Which of the following subdivision of anterior triangle is unpaired:
   a. Muscular b. Digastric
   c. Submental d. Carotid
2. Common carotid artery divides at the level of:
   a. Hyoid bone
   b. Cricoid cartilage
   c. Superior border of thyroid cartilage
   d. Inferior border of thyroid cartilage
3. Right common carotid artery is branch of:
   a. Arch of aorta
   b. Subclavian artry
   c. Brachiocephalic artery
   d. Ascending aorta
4. Carotid body is richly supplied by:
   a. Facial nerve
   b. Glossopharyngeal nerve
   c. Abducent nerve
   d. Hypoglossal nerve
5. All of the following muscles form the boundaries of carotid triangle except:
   a. Anterior belly of digastric
   b. Posterior belly of digastric
   c. Sternomastoid
   d. Superior belly of omohyoid
6. Posterior boundary of carotid triangle is:
   a. Superior belly of omohyoid
   b. Posterior belly digastric
   c. Sternohyoid
   d. Sternocleidomastoid

7. Carotid artery may be palpated at:
   a. Hyoid bone
   b. Thyroid cartilage
   c. Transverse process of C_5
   d. Transverse process of C_3
8. Internal jugular vein is the continuation of:
   a. Cavernous sinus
   b. Sigmoidal sinus
   c. Superior sagittal sinus
   d. Transverse sinus
9. All the following are branches of external carotid artery except:
   a. Superior thyroid
   b. Anterior ehthmoidal
   c. Posterior auricular
   d. Occipital
10. Number of branches of internal carotid artery in the neck cervical region is:
    a. None b. One
    c. Two d. Four
11. External jugular vein:
    a. Lies deep to sternomastoid
    b. Drains into internal jugular vein
    c. Formed by union of posterior auricular and posterior division of retromandibular vein
    d. Pierces pretracheal layer of cervical fascia before termination
12. All of the following are supplied by ansa cervicalis except:
    a. Sternohyoid b. Omohyoid
    c. Sternothyroid d. Thyrohyoid
13. Motor supply of infrahyoid muscle is:
    a. Branches of cervical plexus
    b. Vagus nerve
    c. Glossopharyngeal nerve
    d. Mandibular nerve
14. Which is not an anterior triangle of neck:
    a. Digastric b. Subclavian
    c. Carotid d. Submental
15. Which of the following muscle separate carotid and digastric triangle:
    a. Anterior belly of digastric
    b. Posterior belly of digastric
    c. Superior belly of omohyoid
    d. Sternothyroid

Answers

1. (c)	2. (c)	3. (c)	4. (b)	5. (a)	6. (d)	7. (b)	8. (b)	9. (b)	10. (a)
11. (c)	12. (d)	13. (a)	14. (b)	15. (b)					

11 Deep Structures in the Neck

CONTENTS

- There are numerous deep structures in the neck
- They may be grouped as:
  1. Glands
     - Thyroid
     - Parathyroid
  2. Thymus
  3. Arteries
     - Subclavian
     - Carotid
  4. Veins
     - Subclavian
     - Internal jugular
     - Brachiocephalic
  5. Nerves
     - Glossopharyngeal
     - Vagus
     - Accessory
     - Hypoglossal
     - Sympathetic chain
     - Cervical plexus
  6. Lymph nodes and thoracic duct
  7. Viscera
     - Trachea
     - Esophagus
  8. Scalene muscles
  9. Cervical pleura and suprapleural membrane
  10. Styloid apparatus.

SUBCLAVIAN ARTERY (FIG. 11.1)

- Principal artery of the upper limb.
- It supplies the upper limb and a part of the neck and brain.

Origin

- Right subclavian artery (SCA): Brachrocephalic trunk behind the right stenoclavicular joint
- Left SCA: Arises from the arch of aorta.

Termination

At the outer border of 1st rib, it continues as the axillary artery.

Cause

Left subclacian artery runs upwards on left mediastinal pleura

↓

Makes groove on left lung

↓

Enters neck by passing behind left sternoclavicular joint

↓

Cervical part of each subclavian artery takes same course

↓

Extends to outer border of first rib

↓

Curved course over cervical pleura with convexity facing upwards.

Parts

- Each artery divides into three parts by scalenus anterior muscles
  - i. First part - Origin to medial border of muscle
  - ii. Second part - Lies behind the muscle
  - iii. Third part - Lateral border of muscle to outer border of first rib.

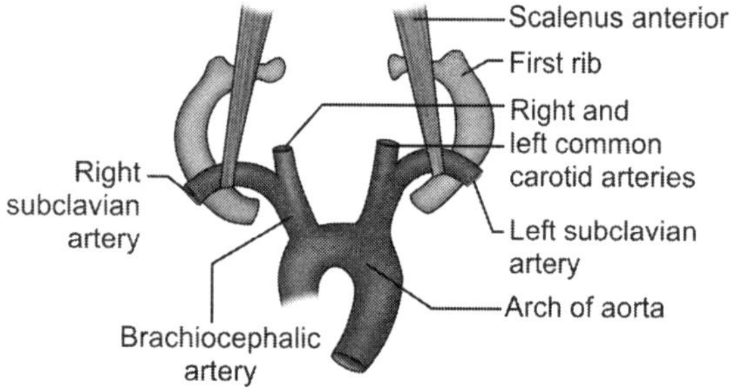
Scalenus anterior
First rib
Right and left common carotid arteries
Right subclavian artery
Left subclavian artery
Arch of aorta
Brachiocephalic artery

Fig. 11.1: Subclavian artery

Relations	First part	Second part	Third part
• **Anterior**	• Infrahyoid muscles • Anterior jugular vein	• Scalenus anterior muscle • Subclavian vein • Sternocleidomastoid muscle	• External jugular vein • Nerve to subclavius • Large thoracic nerve • Suprascapular artery • Clavicle • Deep and superficial facial • Platysma, skin
• **Posterior**	• Apex of lung with cervical pleura • Inferior cervical ganglion of sympathetic trunk	• Apex of lung with cervical pleura • Lower trunk of brachial plexus • Scalenus medius	• Lower trunk of brachial plexus • Scalenus medius
• **Above**	-	-	• Upper trunk of brachial plexus • Inferior belly of omohyoid
• **Below**	-	-	• Subclavian vein • Upper surface of 1st rib
• **Left side**	• Thoracic duct • Phrenic nerve	-	-
• **Right side**	• Right recurrent laryngeal nerve	• Phrenic nerve	-

Branches: Five branches (Fig. 11.2)

I. From first part
  a. Vertebral artery
  b. Internal thoracic artery
  c. Thyrocervical trunk
  d. Costocervical trunk (on left side only)

II. From second part: Costocervical trunk (on right side only)

III. From third part: Five Dorsal scapular artery

Vertebral Artery

Supplies brain, spinal cord meninges, surrounding bone and muscles

Origin: Upper aspect of 1st part of subclavian artery.

Course

Runs vertically upwards to enter the foramen transversarium of transverse process of C6 vertebra

↓

Passes through foramen

↓

After it emerges from the foramen transversarium of C1

↓

Winds backwards around atlas

↓

Enters foramen magnum to go into cranial cavity.

↓

It unites with vertebral artery of the other side at lower border of pons

↓

Forms the basilar artery

Parts: Subdivided into four parts (Fig. 11.3)

1. **First part**
   a. From origin to foramen transversarium of C6
   b. Lies in scalenovertebral triangle
2. **Second—Vertebral part:** Within foramen transversarium of upper 6 cervical vertebrae
3. **Third part**
   a. From foramen transversarium of C1 to foraman magnum
   b. Lies within the suboccipital triangle.
4. **Fourth part:** Intracranial part—from foramen magnum to lower part of pons.

Branches

I. In the neck (Cervical branches)
  a. Spinal
  b. Muscular.

II. In the cranial cavity (Cranial branches)
  a. Meningeal
  b. Posterior spinal artery

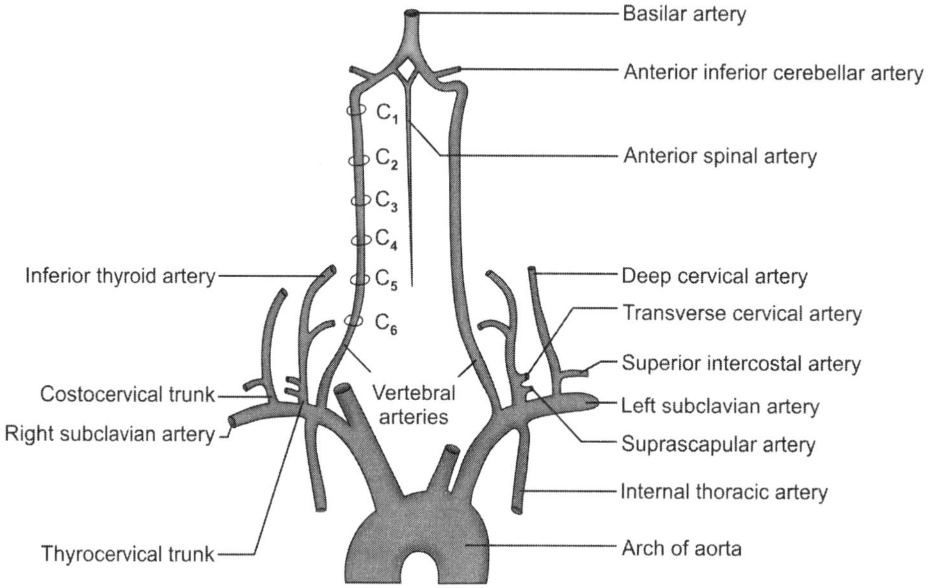
Basilar artery
Anterior inferior cerebellar artery
Anterior spinal artery
C1
C2
C3
C4
C5
C6
Inferior thyroid artery
Deep cervical artery
Transverse cervical artery
Superior intercostal artery
Costocervical trunk
Vertebral arteries
Left subclavian artery
Right subclavian artery
Suprascapular artery
Internal thoracic artery
Thyrocervical trunk
Arch of aorta

Fig. 11.2: Branches of subclavian artery

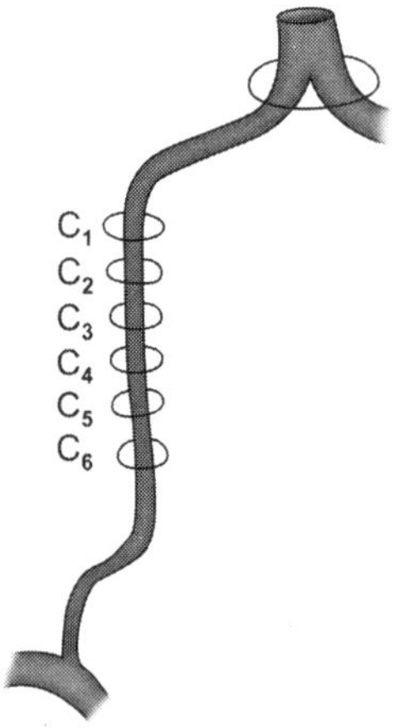
C1
C2
C3
C4
C5
C6

Fig. 11.3: Parts of vertebral artery

c. Posterior-inferior cerebellar artery
d. Anterior spinal artery
e. Medullar branches.

Relations

- Anterior - Lateral mass of atlas
- Posterior - Semi-spinalis capitis
- Lateral - Rectus capitis lateralis
- Medial - Ventral rami of 1st cervical nerve
- Inferior - Dorsal rami of 1st cervical nerve

Clinical and Applied Anatomy of Vertebral Artery

Subclavian Steal Syndrome

a. There is obstruction of subclavian artery proximal to origin of vertebral artery.
b. Thus, some blood from opposite vertebral artery can pass in a retrograde fashion to subclavian artery of affected side.
c. This provides collateral circulation.

Internal Thoracic Artery/Internal Mammary Artery

a. Arise from 1st part of subclavian artery opposite to thyrocervical trunk.
b. Enters the thorax behind the sternoclavicular joint.
c. At the level of 6th intercostal space it divides into 2 terminal branches:
   i. Musculophrenic
   ii. Superior epigastric.

Thyrocervical Trunk

a. Arises from the upper aspect of 1st part of subclavian artery.
b. Branches
   i. Inferior thyroid artery
      - Ascending cervical artery
      - Inferior laryngeal artery
      - Tracheal and esophageal artery
      - Glandular branches
   ii. Superficial cervical artery
   iii. Suprascapular artery

Costocervical Trunk

a. Arises from the posterior aspect of:
   i. 1st part of left side
   ii. 2nd part on right side.
b. It divides into:
   i. Deep cervical artery
   ii. Superior intercostal arteries.

Dorsal Scapular Artery

Arises from 3rd part of subclavian artery.

SUBCLAVIAN VEIN

Continuation of axillary vein.

Extent

- From 1st rib to medial border of scalenus anterior
- Then it joins internal jugular vein to form brachiocephalic vein.

Course

Subclavian vein
↓
Forms an arch across the pleura, below the arch of subclavian artery
↓
Two arches are separated from each other by scalenus anterior muscle
↓
Provides a pair of valves about 2 cm from its termination.

Relations (Fig. 11.4)

Anterior	• Clavicle • Subclavius muscle
Posterior	• Phrenic nerve • Scalenus anterior • Subclavian artery
Inferior	• 1st rib • Cupola of pleura

Tributaries

- External jugular vein
- Dorsal scapular vein
- Thoracic duct on left side.
  – Right lymphatic duct on right side
- Anterior jugular vein
- Cephalic vein.

Brachiocephalic Vein (Fig. 11.5)

- Internal jugular vein joins subclavian vein to form brachiocephalic vein.
- It is formed behind the sternoclavicular joint.

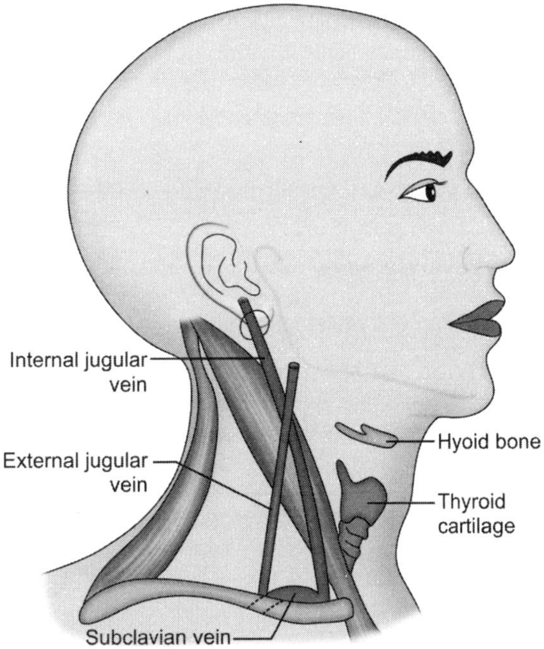
Internal jugular vein
External jugular vein
Hyoid bone
Thyroid cartilage
Subclavian vein

Fig. 11.4: Relation of internal and external jugular vein

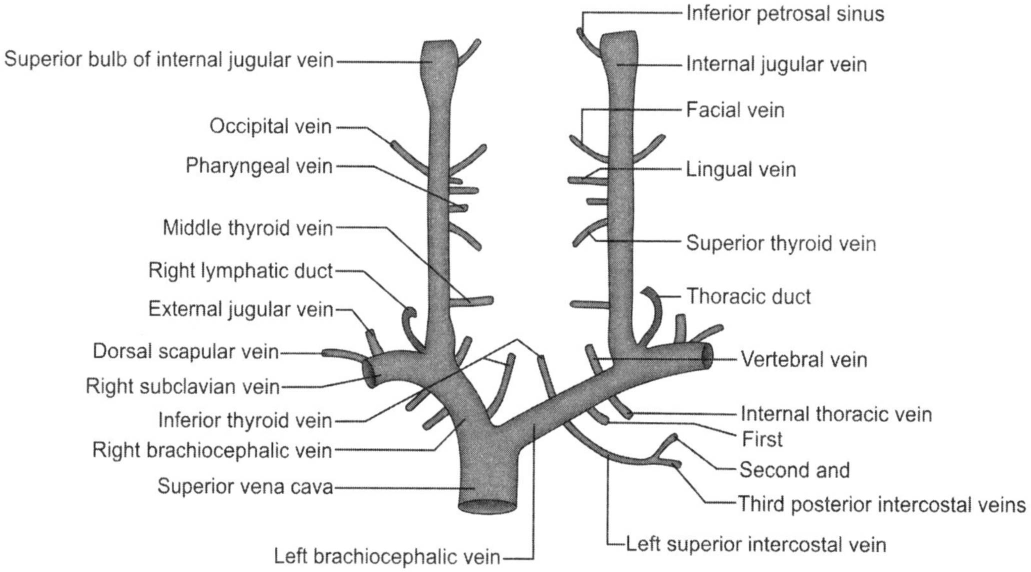
Inferior petrosal sinus
Superior bulb of internal jugular vein
Internal jugular vein
Facial vein
Occipital vein
Pharyngeal vein
Lingual vein
Middle thyroid vein
Superior thyroid vein
Right lymphatic duct
Thoracic duct
External jugular vein
Dorsal scapular vein
Vertebral vein
Right subclavian vein
Internal thoracic vein
Inferior thyroid vein
First
Right brachiocephalic vein
Second and
Superior vena cava
Third posterior intercostal veins
Left superior intercostal vein
Left brachiocephalic vein

Fig. 11.5: Brachiocephalic vein

- Right brachiocephalic vein is shorter than the left.
- The two brachiocephalic veins unites at the right 1st costal cartilage to form the superior vena cava.

Tributaries

Tributaries of brachiocephalic vein are described in Table 11.1.

Table 11.1: Tributaries of brachiocephalic vein

Right brachiocephalic	*Left brachiocepalic*
• Vertebral • Internal thoracic • Inferior thyroid • First posterior intercostals	• Vertebral • Internal thoracic • Inferior thyroid • First posterior intercostal • Left superior intercostal • Thymic and pericardial veins

NERVES OF THE NECK

Cervical Part of Sympathetic Trunk

- Cervical part of left and right sympathetic trunk are situated one on each side of the cervical part of vertebral column.
- This part of trunk is formed by fibers from segments T1 to T4 of spinal cord.

Relations

Anterior
I. Internal and common carotid artery
II. Carotid sheath
III. Inferior thyroid artery.

Nerve	*Features*	*Branches*	*Clinical anatomy*
• **Glossopharyngeal (IX Cranial nerve)**	• Nerve of third branchial arch. • Motor to stylopharyngeus. • Sensory to pharynx, tonsil, posterior 1/3rd of tongue, carotid body and carotid sinus. • Secretomotor to parotid gland	• Tympanic • Carotid • Pharyngeal • Muscular • Tonsillar • Lingual	• Taste sensibility is lost in IX nerve lesion • Phayngitis may cause referred pain in ear

Contd...

Contd...

Nerve	*Features*	*Branches*	*Clinical anatomy*
• **Vagus (X Cranial nerve)**	• So called because of extensive (vague) course through the head, neck, thorax and abdomen. • Two ganglion i. Superior: Rounded and lies in the jugular foramen ii. Inferior: Cylindrical and lies near base of the skull	• In jugular foramen: – Maningeal – Auricular • In neck: – Pharyngeal – Carotid – Superior laryngeal – Right recurrent laryngeal – Cardiac	• Paralysis of vagus nerve produces: – Nasal regurgitation – Nasal twang – Hoarseness of voice – Dysphagia. • Irritation of the auricular branch causes persistent cough and vomiting.
• **Accessory (XI Nerve)**	• It has two roots (Cranial, spinal) • Spinal root has more independent course	• Muscular branches – To sternocleidomastoid along with C2 and C3 nerves. – Supplies trapezius along with C3 and C4 nerves. • Communicating branches Communicates with cervical spinal nerves: – C2, deep to sternomastoid – C2, C3, in posterior triangle. – C3, C4, deep to trapezius.	• Lesions of accessory nerve are accompanied by lesions of glossopharyngeal and vagus nerve because of their close approximity. • Irritation of this nerve produce torticollis, or wry neck.
• **Hypoglossal (XII Cranial nerve)**	• Supplies the muscles of the tongue	• Hypoglossal nerve proper. • Hypoglossal nerve containing fibers of nerve C1: – Meningeal branch – Descending branch – Branches to thyrohyoid and geniohyoid muscles.	• Lesion of hypoglossal nerve produce paralysis of tongue on same side. • On protrusion, the tongue deviates to side paralyzed.

Posterior I. Prevertebral fascia
II. Transverse processes of lower 6 cervical vertebrae.

Ganglia

Three ganglia (Theoretically eight ganglia)

i. Superior
ii. Middle
iii. Inferior.

Clinical and Applied Anatomy

Figure 11.6 shows cervical part of sympathetic truck.

Horner's Syndrome

- Injury to cervical sympathetic trunk produces Horner's syndrome.
- It is characterized by:
  - Ptosis, i.e. drooping of eyelids.
  - Miosis, i.e. constriction of pupil.
  - Anhidrosis, i.e. loss of sweating on that side of face.
  - Enophthalmos, i.e. retraction of the eyeball.
  - Loss of ciliospinal reflex (i.e. pinching the skin on nape of the neck, doesnot produce dilatation of the pupil).

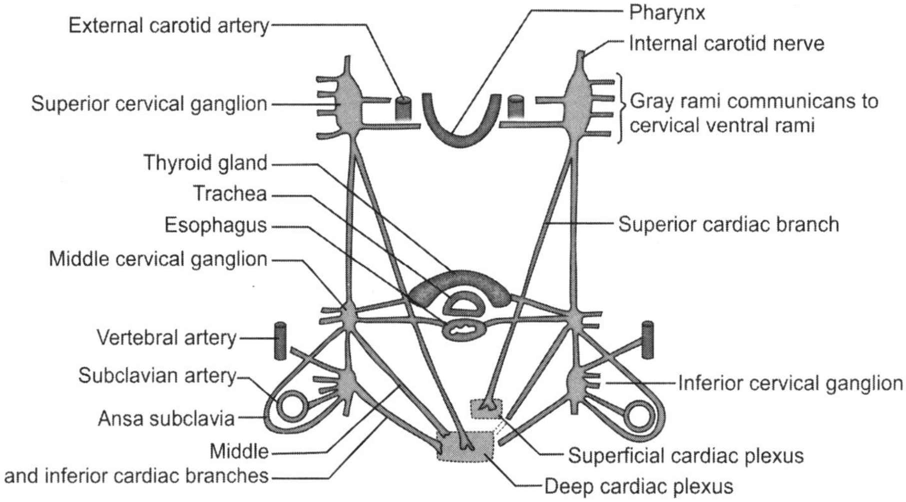
External carotid artery
Superior cervical ganglion
Thyroid gland
Trachea
Esophagus
Middle cervical ganglion
Vertebral artery
Subclavian artery
Ansa subclavia
Middle
and inferior cardiac branches
Pharynx
Internal carotid nerve
Gray rami communicans to
cervical ventral rami
Superior cardiac branch
Inferior cervical ganglion
Superficial cardiac plexus
Deep cardiac plexus

Fig. 11.6: Cervical part of sympathetic truck

Ganglia	*Size and shape*	*Situation and formation*	*Branches*
• **Superior cervical ganglion**	• Largest • Spindle shaped • 2.5 cm long	• Lies below the skull opposite the 2nd and 3rd cervical vertebrae behind the carotid sheath. • Formed by fusion of upper four cervical ganglia	• Gray rami communicans pass to ventral rami of the upper four cervical nerves. • Internal carotid nerve • External carotid nerve. • Pharyngeal nerve • Cardiac nerve
• **Middle cervical ganglion**	• Very small • Divided into 2 to 3 small parts	• Lies in the lower part of the neck infront of C6 above inferior thyroid artery behind the carotid sheath. • Formed by fusion of 5 and 6th cervical ganglion. • Connected with the inferior cervical ganglion directly and also through a loop that winds round the subclavian artery, this loop is known as Ansa subclavia.	• Gray rami communicans are given to the ventral rami of the V and VI cervical nerves. • Thyroid branch • Tracheal branch • Esophageal branch. • Cardiac branch.
• **Inferior cervical ganglion**	• Star-shaped, hence called stellate ganglion	• Lies between the transverse process of C7 and neck of 1st rib, behind the vertebral artery.	• Gray rami communicans are given to ventral rami of nerves C7 and C8. • Subclavian branch • Vertebral branch • Cardiac branch.

- Horner's syndrome can also be caused by lesion within the central nervous system anywhere at or above the first thoracic segment of the spinal cord involving sympathetic fibers.

CERVICAL PLEXUS

- It supplies the skin and muscles of neck.
- It also gives rise to the phrenic nerve, which supplies the diaphragm.

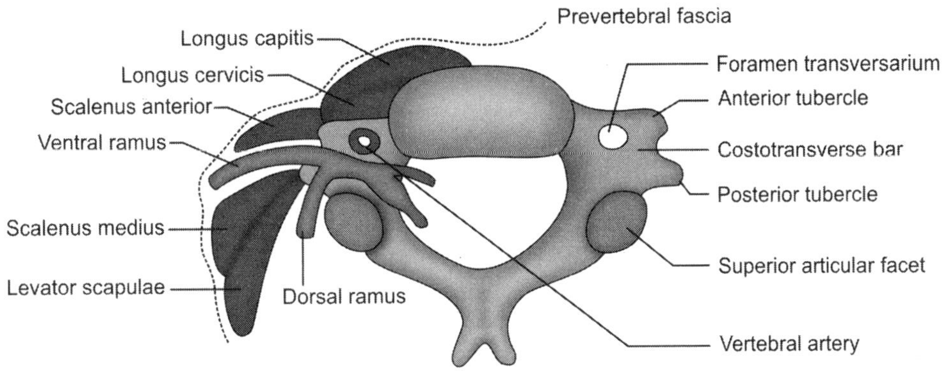
Prevertebral fascia
Longus capitis
Longus cervicis
Scalenus anterior
Ventral ramus
Scalenus medius
Levator scapulae
Dorsal ramus
Foramen transversarium
Anterior tubercle
Costotransverse bar
Posterior tubercle
Superior articular facet
Vertebral artery

Fig. 11.7: Position and relation of cervical plexus

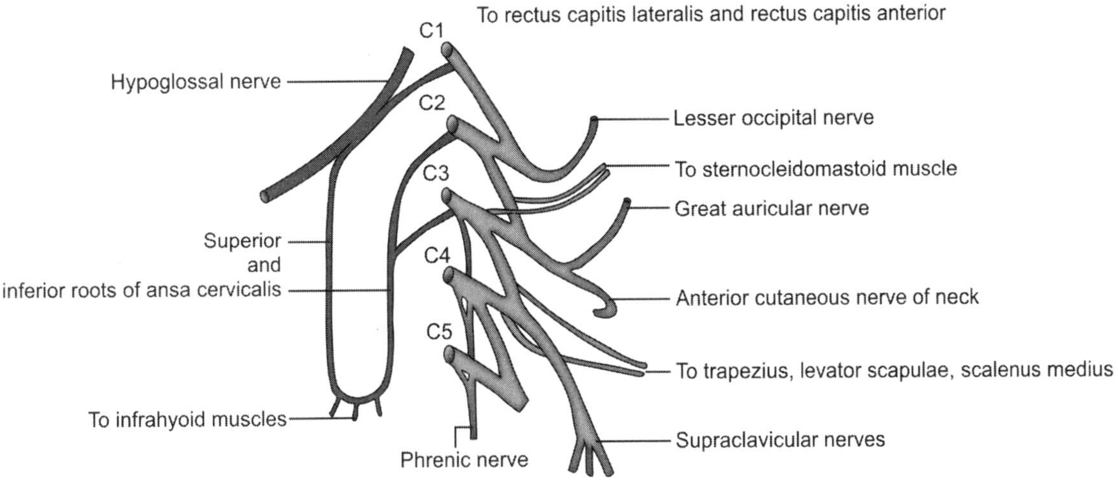
C1
To rectus capitis lateralis and rectus capitis anterior
Hypoglossal nerve
C2
Lesser occipital nerve
C3
To sternocleidomastoid muscle
Great auricular nerve
Superior
and
inferior roots of ansa cervicalis
C4
Anterior cutaneous nerve of neck
C5
To trapezius, levator scapulae, scalenus medius
To infrahyoid muscles
Supraclavicular nerves
Phrenic nerve

Fig. 11.8: Branches of cervical plexus

Formation

- Rami emerges between anterior and posterior tubercles of the cervical transverse processes.
- Cervical plexus is formed by ventral rami of upper four cervical nerves.

Position and Relations (Fig. 11.7)

Posterior	• Levator scapulae • Scalenus medius
Anterior	• Prevertebral fascia • Internal jugular vein • Sternocleidomastoid.

Branches (Fig. 11.8)

Superficial/Cutaneous Branches

- Lesser occipital (C2)
- Great auricular (C2, C3)
- Transverse/Anterior cutaneous nerve of neck (C2, C3)
- Supraclavicular (C3, C4).

Deep Branches

a. Communicating branches

i. Gray rami pass from superior cervical ganglion to the roots of C1-C4 nerve.

ii. Branch from C1 joins the hypoglossal nerve.
iii. Branch from C2 to sternocleidomastoid.
iv. Branch from C3 and C4 to trapezius.

Muscular Branches

a. ***Direct branches*** (Muscles supplied solely by cervical plexus)
   i. Rectus capitis anterior from C1
   ii. Rectus captis lateral is from C1,C2.
   iii. Longus capitis from C1,C3.
   iv. Lower root of ansa cervicalis from C2,C3.
b. ***Indirect branches*** (Supplied by cervical plexus along with brachial plexus):
   i. Sternocleidomastoid from C2 along with accessory nerve.
   ii. Trapezius from C3 and C4 along with accessory nerve.
   iii. Levator scapulae from C3 and C4, C5 along with dorsal scapular nerve.
   iv. Phrenic nerve from C3, C4 and C5.
   v. Longus colli from C3-C8.
   vi. Scalenus medius from C3-C8
   vii. Scalenus anterior from C4-C6
   viii. Scalenus posterior from C6-C8.

CERVICAL PLEURA (FIG. 11.9)

- It covers the apex of the lung
- It rises into the root of the neck, about 5 cm above the 1st costal cartilage and 2.5 cm above the medial 1/3rd of the clavicle
- Pleural dome is strengthened on its outer surface by the suprapleural membrane so that the root of the neck is not puffed up and down during respiration.

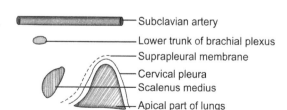

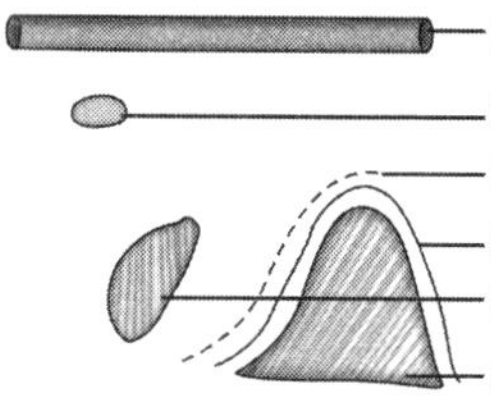
Subclavian artery
Lower trunk of brachial plexus
Suprapleural membrane
Cervical pleura
Scalenus medius
Apical part of lungs

Fig. 11.9: Cervical pleura

Relations

Anterior	I.	Subclavian artery and its branches.
	II.	Scalenus anterior.
Posterior	I.	Sympathetic trunk.
	II.	1st Posterior intercostal vein
	III.	Superior intercostal artery.
	IV.	First thoracic nerve.
Lateral	I.	Scalenus medius.
	II.	Lower trunk of brachial plexus.
Medial	I.	Vertebral bodies.
	II.	Esophagus
	III.	Trachea
	IV.	Left recurrent laryngeal nerve
	V.	Thoracic duct
	VI.	Large arteries and veins of the neck.

STYLOID APPARATUS

- Styloid process with its attached structure is known as styloid apparatus.
- It is of diverse origin.

Structures attached to styloid process are (five attachment resemble the reins of a chariot):
- Stylohyoid muscle
- Styloglossus muscle
- Stylopharyngeus muscles
- Stylomandibular ligament
- Stylohyoid ligament.

Styloid Process

- Long, slender and pointed bony process projecting downwards, forwards and slightly medially from the temporal bone.
- Descends between external and internal carotid arteries to reach the side of pharynx.
- Interposed between parotid gland (laterally) and internal jugular vein (medially).

Attachments of Styloid Process (Figs 11.10A and B)

- Styloglossus muscle
  - Arise from styloid process and stylohyoid ligament.
  - Inserted into side of the tongue.

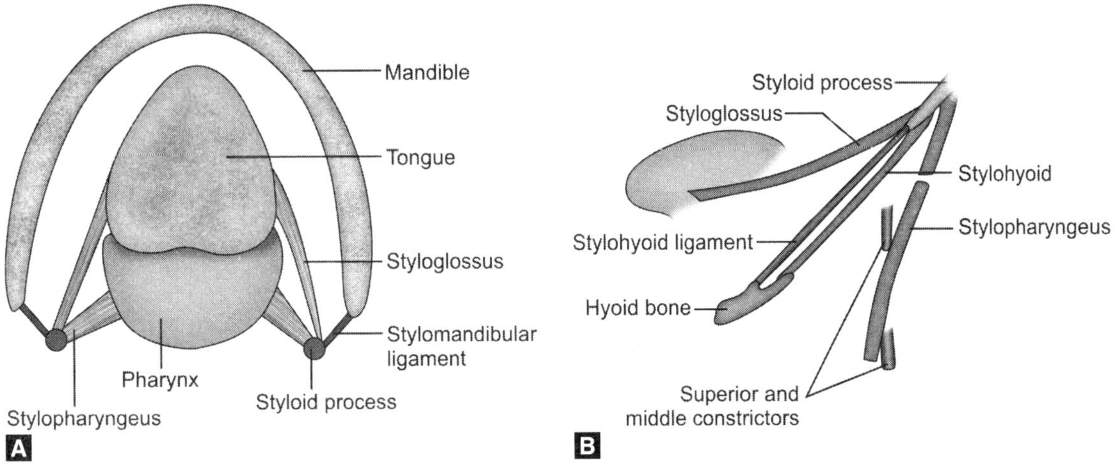

Mandible
Tongue
Styloglossus
Stylomandibular ligament
Pharynx
Styloid process
Stylopharyngeus
A
Styloid process
Styloglossus
Stylohyoid
Stylopharyngeus
Stylohyoid ligament
Hyoid bone
Superior and middle constrictors
B

Figs 11.10A and B: Attachment of styloid process

- Nerve supply—hypoglossal nerve.
- Actions—it palls the tongue upwards and backwards.

- Stylopharyngeus muscle
  - Arise from base of the styloid process.
  - Inserted into lamma of thyroid cartilage and lateral aspect of epiglottis.
  - Nerve supply—glossopharyngeal nerve.
  - Actions—helps to lift the larynx during swallowing and phonation.
- Stylomandibular ligament
  - Arise from tip of styloid process.
  - Inserted into the angle of mandible.
- Stylohyoid ligament
  - Arise from tip of the styloid process.
  - Inserted into lesser cornu of the hyoid bone.
- Stylohyoid muscle
  - Arise from posterior surface of styloid process.
  - Inserted into junction of body and greater cornu of hyoid bone.
  - Nerve supply—facial nerve.
  - Actions:
    - Pulls hyoid bone upwards and backwards.
    - With other hyoid muscles, it fixes the hyoid bone.

PREVIOUS YEAR QUESTIONS

1. Briefly describe cervical part of sympathetic chain.
2. Write a short note on Horner's syndrome.
3. Write short note on styloid process.
4. Write a note on styloid apparatus.
5. Draw a labeled diagram of cervical plexus.
6. Write short note on vertebral artery.

MULTIPLE CHOICE QUESTIONS

1. Hypoglossal nerve is:
   a. Purely sensory
   b. Purely motor
   c. Mixed
   d. Spinal nerve
2. All the cranial nerves provide innervation for the structures in the head and neck except are that additionally supplies thorax and abdomen:
   a. Glossopharyngeal
   b. Spinal accessory
   c. Vagus
   d. Hypoglossal
3. Cranial nerve which are part of parasympathetic cord via:
   a. III, IV, V, VII
   b. III, VII, VIII, IX

c. III, VII, IX, X
d. VII, IX, X, XI

4. When a patient is asked to say "Ah", if the uvula is drawn towards the left, the cranial nerve likely to be damaged is:
a. Vagus
b. Right accessory
c. Left accessory
d. Hypoglossal

5. Horner's syndrome is produced due to the pressure on:
a. Stellate ganglion
b. Spinal cord
c. Parasympathetic ganglion
d. Ciliac ganglion

6. The muscle of tongue which is not supplied by hypoglossal nerve:
a. Hypoglossus
b. Styloglossus
c. Genioglossus
d. Palatoglossus

7. Largest ganglion in the neck is:
a. Superior ganglion
b. Middle ganglion
c. Stellate ganglion
d. 2nd thoracic ganglion

8. Gag reflex is lost due to paralysis of:
a. V nerve
b. VII nerve
c. IX nerve
d. XII nerve

9. Which of the following is supplied by glossopharyngeal nerve:
a. Stylopharyngeous
b. Palatopharyngeus
c. Geniohyoid
d. Genioglossus

10. VII, IX, X cranial nerve ends in:
a. Nucleus tractus solitarius
b. Nucleus ambiguous
c. Dorsal nucleus of vagus
d. Long tract of trigeminal nerve

11. True about subclavian artery
a. Principal artery of upper limb
b Right subclavian artery is a branch of branchiocephalic artery
c. Left subclavian artery is a branch of arch of aorta
d. Internal thoracic, vertebral and thyrocervical trunk are branches of subclavian artery.
e. All of the above.

12. Vertebral artery is a branch of:
a. Subclavian artery
b. Internal carotid artery
c. External carotid artery
d. Superficial temporal artery

Answers

1. (b) 2. (c) 3. (c) 4. (b) 5. (a) 6. (d) 7. (a) 8. (c) 9. (a) 10. (a)
11. (e) 12. (a)

12 Cervical Viscera and Glands of the Neck

THYROID GLAND

Thyroid is an endocrine gland situated in the front and sides of the lower part of the neck opposite to C5-T1 vertebrae (Fig. 12.1).

Anatomical Features

Gland consists of two lobes that connects by an isthmus.

Lateral Lobes

- One right and one left lobe
- Each extends from middle of thyroid cartilage above to the 5th tracheal ring below
- Each lobe is pyramidal in shape.
- Presents with following features:
  - Apex: Directed upwards, towards the oblique line of thyroid cartilage
  - Base: Extends to 4 or 5th tracheal ring.
  - Three surfaces:
    1. Anterolateral
    2. Posterolateral
    3. Medial.
  - Two borders
    1. Anterior: Lies between anterolateral and medial surfaces.
    2. Posterior: Lies between posterolateral and medial surfaces.

Dimensions of gland – Length – 5 cm
– Breadth – 3 cm
– Thickness – 2 cm

Figure 12.2 shows relations of thyroid gland.

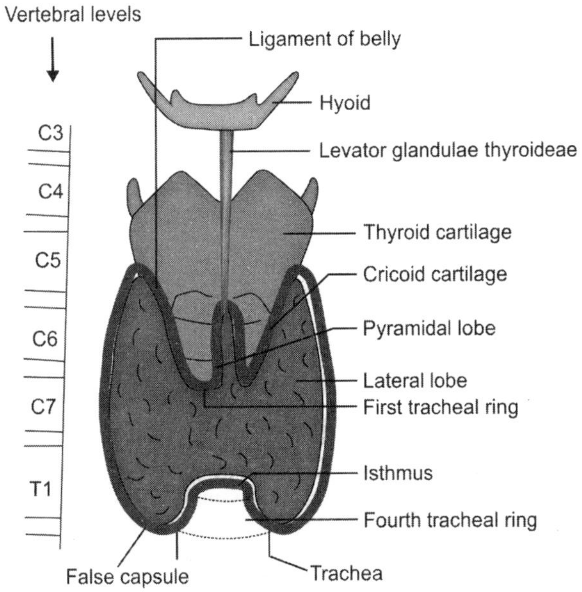
Vertebral levels
C3
C4
C5
C6
C7
T1
Ligament of belly
Hyoid
Levator glandulae thyroideae
Thyroid cartilage
Cricoid cartilage
Pyramidal lobe
Lateral lobe
First tracheal ring
Isthmus
Fourth tracheal ring
False capsule
Trachea

Fig. 12.1: Situation of thyroid gland

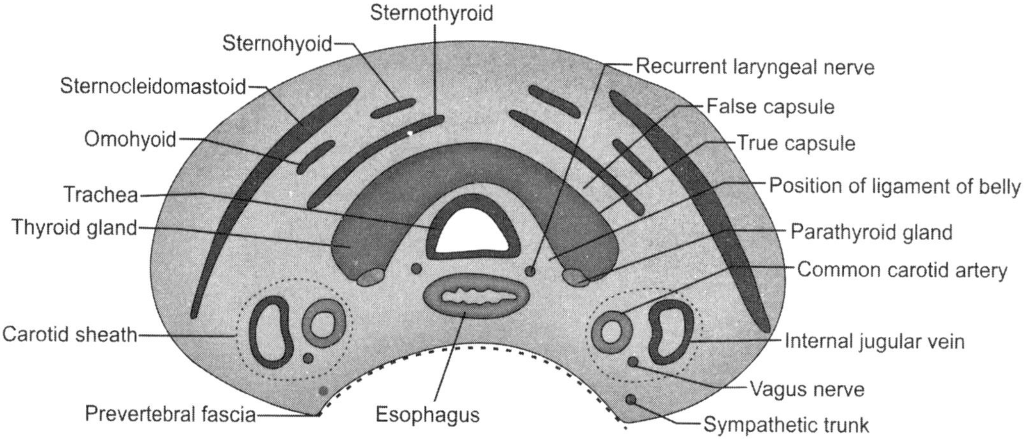
Sternothyroid
Sternohyoid
Sternocleidomastoid
Omohyoid
Trachea
Thyroid gland
Carotid sheath
Prevertebral fascia
Esophagus
Recurrent laryngeal nerve
False capsule
True capsule
Position of ligament of belly
Parathyroid gland
Common carotid artery
Internal jugular vein
Vagus nerve
Sympathetic trunk

Fig. 12.2: Relations of thyroid gland

Isthmus

- It overlies the 2nd, 3rd and 4th tracheal rings.
- Joins the two lateral lobes together.
- Dimensions—1.25 cm × 1.25 cm
- It has anterior and posterior surface and upper and lower border.

Pyramidal Lobe (Inconstant)

It projects upward from the isthmus usually on left side.

Relations of Lateral Lobes

- **Apex**
  - Medial - Inferior constrictor muscle
  - Lateral - Sternothyroid
  - Superficial - Superior thyroid artery
  - Deep - External laryngeal nerve
- **Base**
  - Loop of inferior thyroid artery and vein
  - Recurrent laryngeal nerve
- **Anterolateral surface**
  - Strap muscles (sternothyroid, sternohyoid and superior belly of omohyoid).
  - Sternocleidomastoid
- **Medial/Deep surface**
  - Trachea and esophagus
  - Inferior constrictor and cricothyroid muscles
  - External and recurrent laryngeal nerves
  - Cricoid and thyroid cartilage
- **Posterolateral surface**
  - Carotid sheath and its content
- **Anterior border:** Descending branch of superior thyroid artery
- **Posterior border**
  - Anastomosis between superior and inferior thyroid arteries
  - Parathyroid glands
  - Thoracic duct.

Capsules of Thyroid Gland

True Capsule

- The peripheral condensation of connective tissue of the gland forms its true capsule.
- Dense capillary plexus lies deep to it.

False Capsule

- Derived from the pretracheal fascia which splits to enclose gland.
- Fascia extends upwards to be attached on hyoid bone and thyroid cartilage. Below it merges with fibrous pericardium.
- On medial surface of thyroid lobe it thickens to form the suspensory ligament of berry which connects the lobe to cricoid cartilage.
- In between the two capsules are present parathyroid glands.

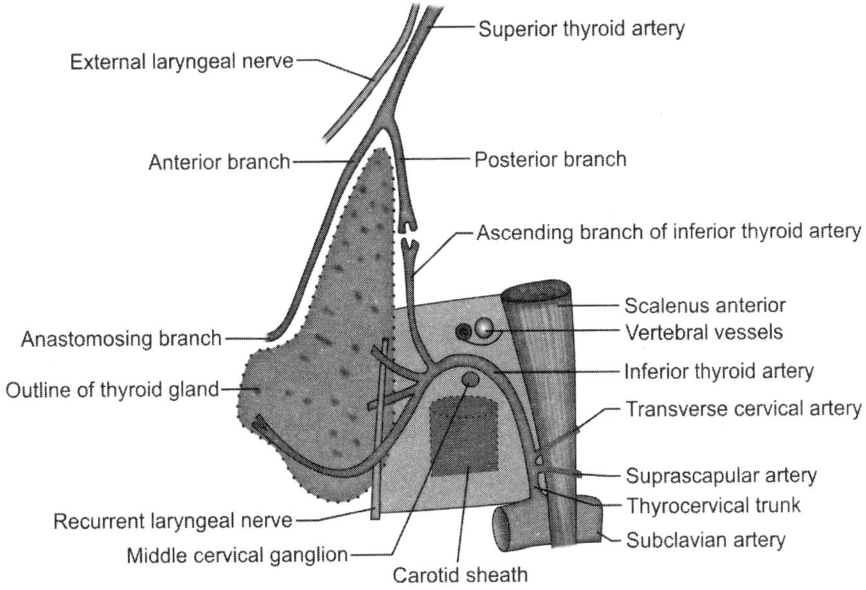
Superior thyroid artery
External laryngeal nerve
Anterior branch
Posterior branch
Ascending branch of inferior thyroid artery
Scalenus anterior
Vertebral vessels
Anastomosing branch
Inferior thyroid artery
Outline of thyroid gland
Transverse cervical artery
Suprascapular artery
Thyrocervical trunk
Recurrent laryngeal nerve
Subclavian artery
Middle cervical ganglion
Carotid sheath

Fig. 12.3: Arterial supply of thyroid gland

Arterial Supply (Fig. 12.3)

Superior Thyroid Artery

- A branch from external carotid artery
- It divides into anterior and posterior branches
- It supplies upper 1/3rd of the lobe and upper half of the isthmus.

Inferior Thyroid Artery

- A branch of thyrocervical trunk from the first part of subclavion artery.
- It supplies lower 2/3rd of the lobe and lower ½ of the isthmus.

Thyroidea Ima Artery (Present in 30% Cases)

- Branch of bachiocephalic trunk.
- May occasionally arise directly from the arch of aorta.
- It enters the isthmus from below.

Accessory Thyroid Arteries

Branches from tracheal and esophageal arteries.

Venous Drainage

- Superior thyroid vein: Middle thyroid vein drains into internal jugular vein
- Inferior thyroid veins: Drains into left brachiocephalic vein.

Lymphatic Drainage

- Upper part drains into prelaryngeal and jugulodigastric lymph nodes.
- Lower part drains into pretracheal lymph nodes.

Nerve Supply

- Parasympathetic: Vagus nerve
- Sympathetic: Periarterial plexus of nerve.

Functions

- Produces two thyroid hormones T3 and T4 which are required for normal growth and development of the body.
- It also produces calcitonin, which has role in calcium metabolism.

Clinical and Applied Anatomy

- Thyroid gland moves up and down with deglution because it is enclosed in pretracheal fascia.
- Enlargement of thyroid gland is known as goiter.
  - Occurs due to iodine deficiency.
  - If large it tends to press trachea and esophagus, which results in dyspnea, dysphagia, dysphonea.
- During thyroidectomy, following care must be taken:
  - Superior thyroid artery is ligated as near as possible to the upper pole to avoid injury to the external laryngeal nerve.
  - Inferior thyroid artery should be ligated away from the lower pole to avoid injury to recurrent laryngeal nerve.
- Congenital anomalies
  - Isthmus may be absent.
  - One of the lobes may be absent.
  - Persistence of thyroglossal duct—results in formation of thyroglossal cyst and fistula.

PARATHYROID GLANDS (FIG. 12.4)

- These are endocrine glands situated in close relation to the thyroid gland and hence they are named so
- They are four in number
  - Two superior
  - Two inferior
- **Size and shape**
  - Lentiform in shape
  - Resemble the size of a split pea.
  - Measures around 6 mm × 4 mm × 2 mm.
- **Superior parathyroids**
  - On each side, one superior gland is present near the middle of posterior border of thyroid gland.
  - Develop from 4th pharyngeal pouch.
- **Inferior parathyroids**
  - On each side, one inferior gland lies near lower pole along posterior border of thyroid gland.
  - Develop from 3rd pharyngeal pouch.
- **Arterial supply**
  - Superior: From anastomosis between superior and inferior thyroid arteries.
  - Inferior: From inferior thyroid arteries.

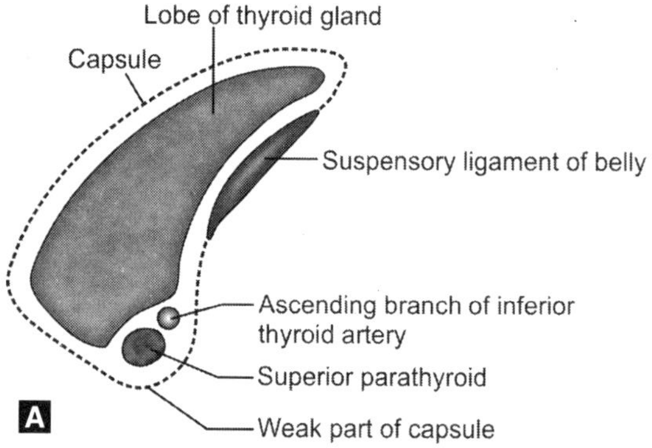
Lobe of thyroid gland
Capsule
Suspensory ligament of belly
Ascending branch of inferior thyroid artery
Superior parathyroid
Weak part of capsule
A

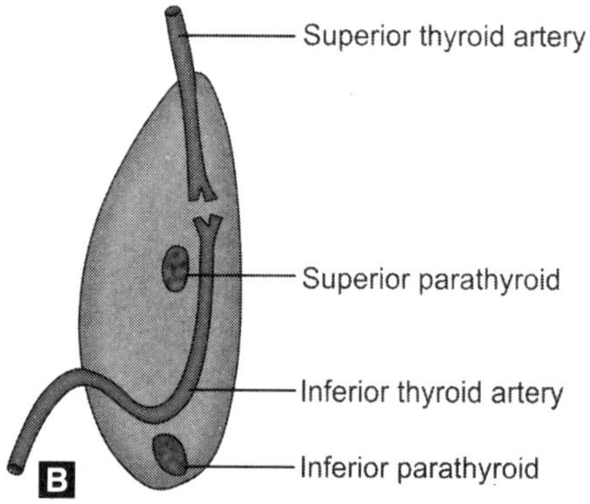
Superior thyroid artery
Superior parathyroid
Inferior thyroid artery
Inferior parathyroid
B

Figs 12.4A and B: Situation of parathyroid gland

- **Nerve supply**
  - Superior and middle cervical sympathetic ganglia.
- **Function**
  - Secrete parathormone which maintains the calcium balance of body.
- **Clinical or applied anatomy**
  - Parathyroids are closely related to thyroid gland and during thyroidectomy they can be removed as a lymph node by mistake.
  - Tumors of parathyroid lead to excessive secretion of parathormone (Hyperparathyroidism).

TRACHEA

- It is a wide membrane—cartilaginous tube that extends downwards from the larynx.
- It lies mainly in neck and partly in thorax.

- It is made of 16 to 20 C-shaped rings of hyaline cartilage connected posteriorly by fibroelastic tissue.
- The gap between two rings is occupied by muscular fibers.

Extent

- Upper end: Begins from cricoid cartilage opposite to C6 vertebra and enters the superior mediastinum.
- Lower end: Ends by dividing into right and left bronchi, opposite to sternal angle (T4 level).
- Measurement: Length = 10 to 11 cm, Breadth = 12 mm.

Relations

- Anterior
  - Skin, superficial and deep fascia.
  - Jugular venous arch.
  - Isthmus of thyroid gland.
  - Superior and inferior thyroid veins.
  - Sternohyoid and sternothyroid of both sides.
- Posterior
  - Esophagus
  - Bodies of C6 and C7 vertebrae.
- Lateral (on each side)
  - Lobes of thyroid gland.
  - Common carotid arteries.
  - Inferior thyroid arteries.
  - Recurrent laryngeal nerve.

Blood Supply

- Subclavian arteries.
- Inferior and superior thyroid arteries.

Nerve Supply

- Parasympathetic, via vagus
- Sympathetic

Function

Acts as a passage for air, hence it is called as **wind pipe**.

ESOPHAGUS

It is a muscular tube like structure which originate from the lower end of pharynx.

Extent

- Upper end: From cricoid cartilage opposite C6 vertebrae and passes through thorax in front of vertebral column.
- Lower end: Enters abdomen via opening in diaphragm and ends opposite T11 vertebra by opening into stomach.
- Measurements: Length 25 cm (5 cm lies in neck).

Relations

- Anterior
  - Trachea
  - Recurrent laryngeal nerve.
- Posterior
  - Prevertebral fascia.
  - Bodies of C6 and C7 vertebrae.
- Lateral (on each side)
  - Lobe of thyroid gland.
  - Common carotid artery
  - Thoracic duct.

Blood Supply

- Thyrocervical trunk branches
- Subclavien artery branches
- Esophageal branches of aorta
- Gastric branches.

Function

Acts as a passage for food, hence named as **food pipe**.

Nerve Supply

- Parasympathetic—from vagus
- Sympathetic—from periarterial plexus.

PREVIOUS YEAR QUESTIONS

1. Describe thyroid gland under following heads:
   a. Relations.
   b. History
   c. Development.
2. Describe anatomy of thyroid gland.

MULTIPLE CHOICE QUESTIONS

1. Esophagus commences at the following level:
   a. Lower end of aricoid
   b. C5 vertebra

c. 10 cm from incisior teeth
d. C7 vertebra

2. Failure of descent of thyroid anlage can be seen in tongue.
   a. In anterior 2/3rd of dorsal aspect.
   b. In posterior 1/3rd of dorsal aspect.
   c. Near the base of tongue close to foramen cecum.
   d. In anterior 2/3rd of inferior surface.
3. Thyroid gland develops from:
   a. Thyroglossal duct
   b. Rathke's pouch
   b. Notochordal process
   d. Embryonal dise
4. From which pharyngeal pouches, do the parathyroid glands develops:
   a. I and IInd
   b. IInd and IIIrd
   c. IIIrd and IVth
   d. IV and Vth
5. Cartilage lining trachea is:
   a. Elastic
   b. White fibrocartilage
   c. Hyaline
   d. Cellular
6. Which of the following is not a cartilage:
   a. Cricoid
   b. Thyroid
   c. Epiglottis
   d. Hyoid
7. Thyroid gland's false capsule is derived from which layer:
   a. Prevertebral
   b. Investing
   c. Pretracheal
   d. All of the above

Answers

1. (a) 2. (c) 3. (a) 4. (c) 5. (c) 6. (d) 7. (c)

13 Prevertebral and Paravertebral Region

PREVERTEBRAL MUSCLES

The following muscles are included in the group:
1. Longus colli
2. Longus capitis
3. Rectus capitis anterior
4. Rectus capitis lateralis.

General Features of Prevertebral Muscles (Fig. 13.1 and Table 13.1)

1. Lie in front of vertebral column
2. Are covered anteriorly by a thick prevertebral fascia.
3. Form the posterior boundary of retropharyngeal space.
4. Extend from the base of the skull to the superior mediastinum.
5. Weak flexors of head and neck.
6. Supplied by ventral rami of C1 and C2 nerves except longus colli which is supplied by C2-C6 nerves.

Scalenovertebral Triangle

It is a triangular space present at root of neck of either side.

Boundaries

- Medial: Lower oblique part of longus colli
- Apex: Scaleneus anterior
- Base: 1st part of subclavian artery
- Floor: Neck of 1st rib.

Contents

- 1st part of vertebral artery and accompanying vein
- Cervical part of sympathetic trunk.

PARAVERTEBRAL MUSCLES

The paravertebral muscles are (Fig. 13.2 and Table 13.2):
- Scalenus anterior

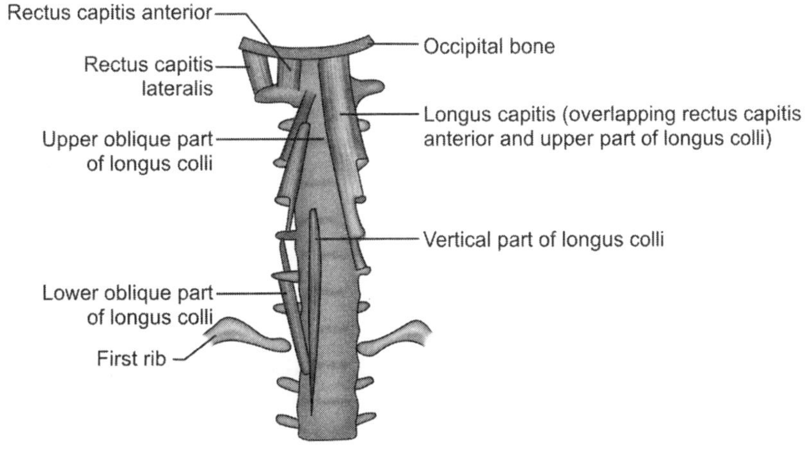

Rectus capitis anterior
Rectus capitis lateralis
Upper oblique part of longus colli
Lower oblique part of longus colli
First rib
Occipital bone
Longus capitis (overlapping rectus capitis anterior and upper part of longus colli)
Vertical part of longus colli

Fig. 13.1: Prevertebral muscles

Table 13.1: Features of prevertebral muscles

Muscle	*Features*	*Origin*	*Insertion*
Longus colli (Cervicis)	• Covers the anterior aspect of upper 10 vertebrae • Three parts: i. Superior oblique part ii. Middle vertical part iii. Inferior oblique part	Anterior tubercle of C3 to C5 Bodies of C5-T3 vertebrae Bodies of T1-T3 vertebrae	Anterior tubercle of anterior arch of atlas. Bodies of C2-C4. Anterior tubercles of C5-C6 vertebrae.
Longus capitis	• Strap like muscle which appears to be continuous with scalenus anterior. • Overlaps the longus colli	Anterior tubercle of transverse process of C3-C6 vertebrae	Basilar part of occipital bone, along side the pharyngeal tubercle.
Rectus capitis anterior	• Very short and flat • Lies deep to longus capitis	Lateral mass of atlas and adjoining root of transverse process	Basilar part of occipital bone, in front of the occipital condyle.
Rectus capitis lateralis		Upper surface of transverse process of atlas	Jugular process of occipital bone.

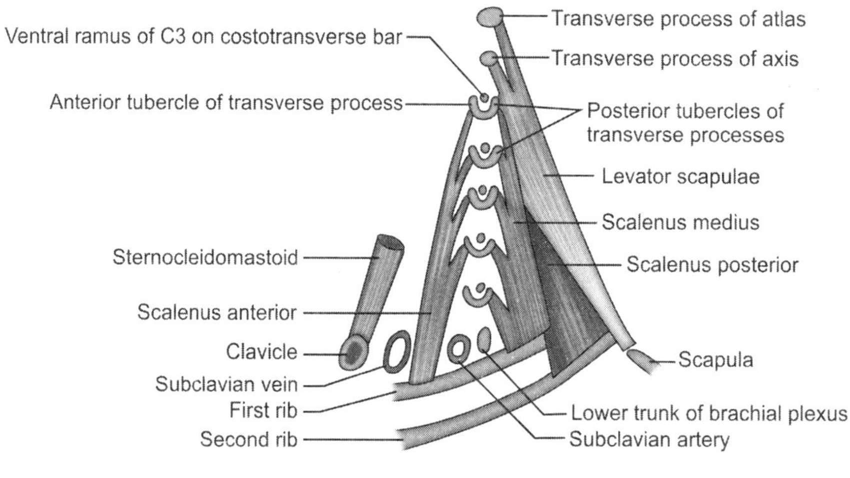
Transverse process of atlas
Ventral ramus of C3 on costotransverse bar
Transverse process of axis
Anterior tubercle of transverse process
Posterior tubercles of transverse processes
Levator scapulae
Scalenus medius
Sternocleidomastoid
Scalenus posterior
Scalenus anterior
Clavicle
Scapula
Subclavian vein
First rib
Second rib
Lower trunk of brachial plexus
Subclavian artery

Fig. 13.2: Paravertebral muscles

- Scalenus medius
- Scalenus posterior.

General Features

- Scalenus medius is the largest of all three scalene muscles.
- Scalenus posterior is the smallest.
- Scalenus anterior is the '**key muscle**' of the paravertebral region.
- They extend from the transverse process of cervical vertebrae to the 1st two ribs.
- Actions:
  - Elevate the ribs as in inspiration.
  - Bends the cervical part of vertebral column laterally to ipsilateral side.

PREVIOUS YEAR QUESTIONS

1. Write a sort note on scalenus anterior muscle.

Table 13.2: Features of paravertebral muscles

Muscle	*Origin*	*Insertion*	*Nerve supply*	*Actions*
• **Scalenus anterior**	• Anterior tubercle of transverse process of C3-C-6 vertebrae	• Scalene tubercle and adjoining ridge on 1st rib	• Ventral rami of C4-C6	• Anterolateral flexion of spine. • Rotates cervical spine to opposite side. • Elevates 1st rib during inspiration • Stabilize the neck.
• **Scalenus medius**	• Posterior tubercle of C3-C7 vertebrae. • Transverse process of axis.	• Superior surface of 1st rib behind the groove for subclavian artery.	• Ventral rami of C3-C8.	• Lateral flexion of cervical spine • Elevation of 1st rib. • Stabilize the neck
• **Scalenus posterior**	• Posterior tubercles of transverse processes of C4-C6	• 2nd rib behind the tubercle for the serratus anterior	• Ventral rami of C6-C8.	• Lateral flexion of cervical spine. • Elevation of 2nd rib. • Stabilizes neck.

MULTIPLE CHOICE QUESTIONS

1. All of the following forms the boundaries of scalenovertebral triangle except:
   a. Longus colli – lower oblique part
   b. 1st part of subclavian artery
   c. Scalenus medium muscle
   d. Neck of 1st rib
2. Which one is the prevertebral muscle:
   a. Rectus capitis anterior
   b. Scalenus anterior
   c. Scalenus medius
   d. Scalenus posterior
3. Which is the key muscle of paravertebral region:
   a. Scalenus posterior
   b. Scalenus medius
   c. Scalenus anterior
   d. Longus colli

Answers

1. (c) 2. (a) 3. (c)

14 Lymphoid Tissue of Head and Neck

LYMPH NODES OF HEAD AND NECK

- Head and neck has 300 lymph nodes out of a total of 800 present in the body.
- Entire lymph from head and neck drains ultimately into the deep cervical nodes either directly or through the peripheral nodes (Fig. 14.1).

DEEP CERVICAL LYMPH NODES

- These nodes the along and around the internal jugular vein deep to the sternocleidomastoid.
- Divided into two groups by the intermediate tendon of omohyoid.

Superior Group

- Lies above the mylohyoid muscle.
- These nodes are present in a triangle formed by the internal jugular vein, posterior belly of digastric and facial vein and are known as Jugulodigastric nodes.

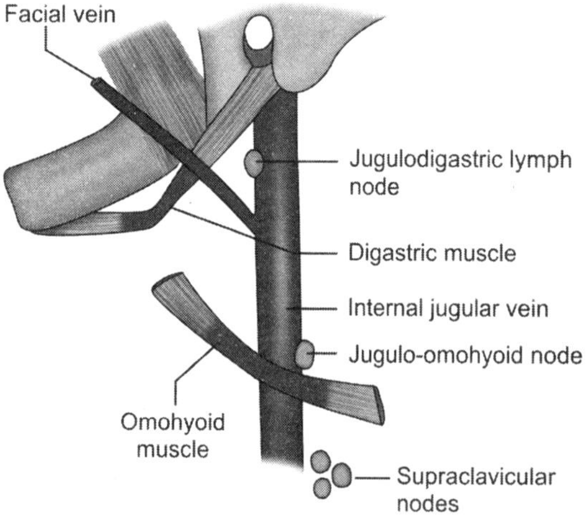

Facial vein
Jugulodigastric lymph node
Digastric muscle
Internal jugular vein
Jugulo-omohyoid node
Omohyoid muscle
Supraclavicular nodes

Fig. 14.1: Lymph nodes of head and neck

- Receives lymph primarily from palatine tonsils, hence named node of tonsil.
- Drains into the inferior group.

Inferior Group

- Lie along the internal jugular vein below the omohyoid.
- One lymph node is found over the intermediate tendon of omohyoid as it cross the vein.
- It is named as jugulo-omohyoid node.
- This node receives lymph primarily from the tongue, hence named as node of tongue.
- Few nodes lie along the brachial plexus and subclavian vessels in the supraclavicular triangle and in front of scalenus anterior.

Afferent from

- Superficial cervical lymph nodes.
- Lymph nodes related to viscera of head and neck:
  - Pretracheal and paratracheal nodes.
  - Prelaryngeal nodes.
  - Retropharyngeal nodes.
  - Lingual nodes.
- Palatine tonsils
- Tongue
- Larynx above the vocal folds.

Efferent Channels

Lymph from deep cervical lymph nodes forms the right and left jugular lymph trunks (Table 14.1).

Table 14.1: Occipitofrontalis (Front part)

Right side	*Left side*
Lymph trunk joins at the junction of the subclavian and internal jugular vein either directly or via the right lymphatic duct	Jugular trunk joins with the terminal part of thoracic duct

Table 14.2: Features of superficial cervical and deep cervical lymphnodes

S.No.	Drains Into	Parts
Superficial cervical lymph nodes		
1.	Submental lymph node	Chin Central part of lower lip Tip of tongue
2.	Submandibular lymph node	Central part of forehead Nose and paranasal sinuses Upper lip Outer part of lower lip Anterior 2/3rd of tongue Floor of mouth
3.	Parotid lymph nodes	TMJ Parotid gland Temple External acoustic meatus Eyelid and orbits
4.	Postauricular nodes	Part of scalp Margin of auricle
5.	Buccal lymph nodes	Part of cheek Lower eyelid
6.	Occipital lymph nodes	Posterior part of scalp
7.	Retroauricular or Mastoid nodes	Auricle and adjoining scalp External acoustic meatus
Deep cervical lymph node		
1.	Prelaryngeal and Pretracheal	Larynx Trachea Isthmus of thyroid
2.	Paratracheal nodes	Esophagus Tracea Larynx
3.	Retropharyngeal nodes	Pharynx Soft palate Posterior part of hard palate Nose

SUPERFICIAL CERVICAL LYMPH NODES

- Arranged in circular fashion like a collar.
- Lies at the junction of base of skull with neck.

Features of superficial cervical and deep cervical lymph nodes are depicted in Table 14.2.

WALDEYER'S LYMPHATIC RING

Introduction

It consists of submucosal collection of lymphoid tissue around the commencement of air and food passages arranged in a ring like pattern (Fig. 14.2).

Contents

From posterior to anterior it is made up of:

- Pharyngeal/Nasopharyngeal tonsil
- Tubal tonsils
- Palatine tonsils
- Lingual tonsil

Functions

Prevent invasion of microorganism into the air and food passages.

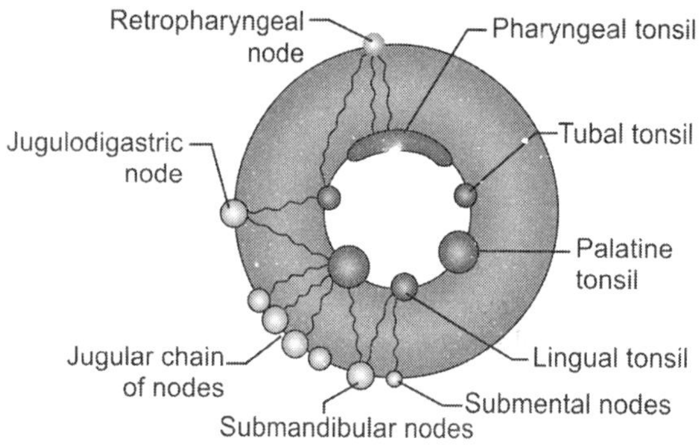
Retropharyngeal node
Pharyngeal tonsil
Jugulodigastric node
Tubal tonsil
Palatine tonsil
Lingual tonsil
Jugular chain of nodes
Submental nodes
Submandibular nodes

Fig. 14.2: Waldeyer's lymphatic ring

Drainage

Lymph drains into superficial and deep cervical group of lymph node, which forms the external ring of Waldeyer.

Clinical and Applied Anatomy

Same as palatine tonsil.

Palatine Tonsil

- It is a collection of lymphoid tissue situated in the tonsilar fossa (Fig. 14.3).
- One on each side, in the lateral wall of oropharynx.
- It is a almond shaped.
- The tonsillar fossa is triangular shaped and is formed by
  - Anterior wall - Palatoglossal arch
  - Posterior wall - Palatopharyngeal arch
  - Apex - Meeting of both arches
  - Base - Posterior 1/3rd of tongue
  - Floor - Superior constrictor and palatopharyngeus muscles.

Development

Refer Chapter 29 Embryology.

External features

- Medial surface is covered by stratified squamous epithelium and presents with 12-15 crypts, largest of these are called intratonsillar cleft.
- Lateral surface is covered by fibrous capsule formed by the condensation of pharyngobasilar fascia.
- Upper pole—related to soft palate.
- Lower pole—related to posterior 1/3rd of tongue.

Arterial Supply (Fig. 14.4)

- Tonsillar branch of facial artery—Principal artery
- Dorsalis linguae, branch of lingual artery.
- Ascending palatine, branch of external carotid artery.
- Ascending pharyngeal, branch of external carotid artery.
- Greater palatine, branch of maxillary artery.

Venous Drainage

Pharyngeal plexus of veins through the paratonsillar vein.

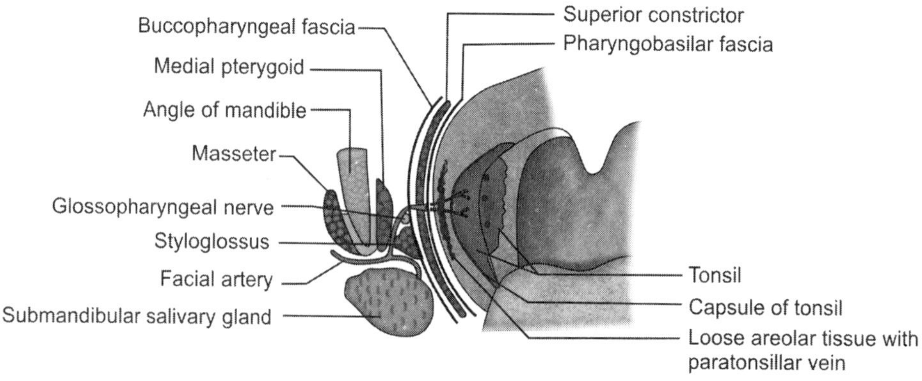
Buccopharyngeal fascia
Medial pterygoid
Angle of mandible
Masseter
Glossopharyngeal nerve
Styloglossus
Facial artery
Submandibular salivary gland
Superior constrictor
Pharyngobasilar fascia
Tonsil
Capsule of tonsil
Loose areolar tissue with paratonsillar vein

Fig. 14.3: Relations of palatine tonsil

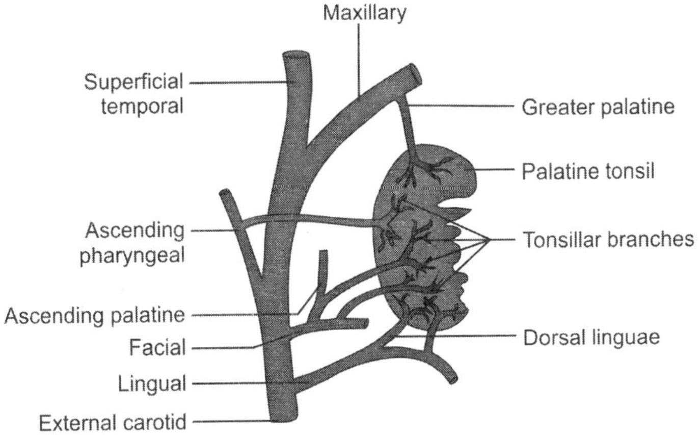
Maxillary
Superficial temporal
Greater palatine
Palatine tonsil
Ascending pharyngeal
Tonsillar branches
Ascending palatine
Facial
Dorsal linguae
Lingual
External carotid

Fig. 14.4: Arterial supply of palatine tonsil

Lymphatic Drainage

Jugulodigastric lymph nodes.

Nerve Supply

Glossopharyngeal nerve.

Clinical and Applied Anatomy

1. Enlargement of lymph node present on the scalenus anterior is known as **Virchow's node**. It is enlarged in patient with advanced cancer.
2. Tonsils are known to increase in size in childhood due to repeated infection causing **"Tonsilitis"**. **Tonsiliectomy** is necessary if they enlarge so much that they block the passage or there is tonsillar abscess.

THYMUS

- It is an important lymphoid organ.
- Situated in anterior and superior mediastinum of thorax.
- It is well developed at birth, continues to grow up to puberty.
- Then undergoes gradual atrophy and replacement by fat.

Anatomical Features

- Bilobed structure.
- Made up of two pyramidal lobes of unequal size which are connected together by areolar tissue.
- Each lobe developes from endoderm of 3rd pharyngeal pouch.
- Weight:
  - 10-15 g of the birth.
  - 30-40 g at puberty.
  - 10 g after mid adult life.

Blood Supply

- Branches from internal thoracic and inferior thyroid arteries.
- Veins drains into left branchiocephalic, internal thoracic and inferior thyroid veins.

Nerve Supply

- Vasomotor nerve from stellate ganglion.
- Capsule is supplied by phrenic nerve and by descendens cervicalis.

Functions

- Controls lymphopoieses
- Control development of peripheral lymphoid tissues of the body.
- Medullary epithelial cells of thymus secrete
  - Lymphopoietin.
  - Competence – inducing factor.

Applied and Clinical Anatomy

1. Thymic hyperplasia or tumors are often associated with myasthenia gravis, characterized by excessive fatiguability of voluntary muscles.

2. Tumors of thymus may press on trachea, esophagus and large veins of neck causing hoarseness, cough, dysphagia and cyanosis.

PREVIOUS YEAR QUESTIONS

1. Describe the palatine tonsil under the following heads:
   a. Development
   b. Histology
   c. Blood supply.
2. Write a note on gross and applied anatomy of tonsils.
3. Write in brief on cervical lymph node.
4. Write a note on Waldeyer's ring with applied anatomy.
5. Enumerate only structures forming bed of tonsil.

MULTIPLE CHOICE QUESTIONS

1. Waldeyer's lymphatic ring is formed by:
   a. Palatine tonsils
   b. Pharyngeal tonsils
   c. Lingual and tubal tonsils
   d. All of the above
2. Lining epithelium of tonsils is:
   a. Simple squamous
   b. Stratified squamous
   c. Pseudostratified
   d. Transitional
3. Blood supply of tonsil is:
   a. Lingual artery
   b. Superior thyroid artery
   c. Facial artery
   d. Pharyngeal artery
4. Main nerve supply of palatine tonsil is:
   a. Lesser palatine
   b. Greater palatine
   c. Glossopharyngeal
   d. Facial
5. Lymph from tonsils drain into the:
   a. Jugulo-omohyoid node
   b. Jugulodigastric node
   c. Submental node
   d. Upper cervical node

Answers

1. (d) 2. (b) 3. (c) 4. (c) 5. (b)

15 Joints of Head and Neck

ATLANTO–OCCIPITAL JOINTS

The first cervical vertebra, atlas articulates with the occipital condyles present on either side of the foramen magnum to form atlanto-occipital joints (Fig. 15.1).

Type

Ellipsoid variety of synovial joint.

Articular Surfaces

Upper: Condyles of occipital bone of skull (Convex).
Lower: Superior articular facets in lateral mass of atlas vertebrae (Concave).

Ligaments

- Fibrous capsule (Capsular ligament)
  - Surrounds the joint and is attached to the margins of articular surfaces.
  - Thick posterolaterally and thin posteromedially.
  - Synovial membrane lines it internally.
- Accessory ligaments
  - Anterior – atlanto-occipital membrane.
  - Posterior – atlanto-occipital membrane.

Nerve Supply

Branch from C1 nerve.

Movements (Table 15.1)

Table 15.1: Movements of joints

Movement	*Axis*	*Muscle involved*
Flexion	Transverse	• Longus capitus • Rectus capitis anterior
Extension	Transverse	• Rectus capitis posterior major and minor • Semispinalis capitis • Splenius capitis • Upper part of trapezius
Lateral flexion (slight)	Anteroposterior	• Rectus capitis lateralis

Clinical and Applied Anatomy

- The line of gravity of weight of the head (about 7 Ibs) passes in front of joints and hence it tends to fall forwards with gravity.
- Erect position of head is maintained by the traction caused by the extensor muscles.

ATLANTOAXIAL JOINTS

The atlas (1st cervical vertebra) and axis (2nd cervical vertebrae) form 3 joints namely:

- Median atlantoaxial joints – One, central joint.
- Lateral atlantoaxial joints – Two, central joint.

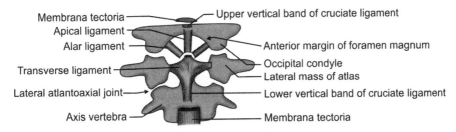

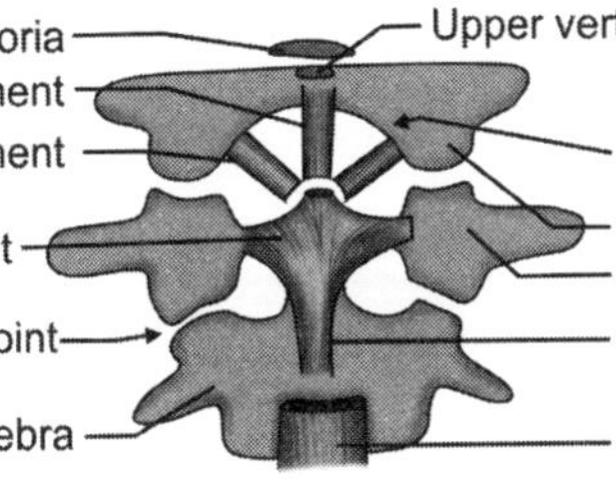
Membrana tectoria
Upper vertical band of cruciate ligament
Apical ligament
Alar ligament
Anterior margin of foramen magnum
Transverse ligament
Occipital condyle
Lateral mass of atlas
Lateral atlantoaxial joint
Lower vertical band of cruciate ligament
Axis vertebra
Membrana tectoria

Fig. 15.1: Ligaments of atlanto-occipital joint

Median Atlantoaxial Joints

Type

Pivot variety of synovial joint.

Articular Surfaces

- Oval articular facet on dens (odontoid process of axis)
- Oval facet on posterior surface atlas.

Ligaments

Fibrous capsule:
- Loose capsule is attached around margins of articular facets.

Transverse ligament of atlas:
- Attached on each side to medial surface of lateral mass of atlas.
- Fibers:
  i. Upwards to basiocciput → Form cruceform ligaments.
  ii. Downwards to body of axis ↑.
- Prevents backward dislocation of neck of dens.
- Dens divides the joint into two parts
  i. Anterior
  ii. Posterior
- Ligaments connecting axis with occipital base.
  - Apical ligament of dens
  - Cruciform ligament
  - Alar ligament
  - Membrana tectoria.

Lateral Atlantoaxial Joints

Type

Plane variety of synovial joints.

Articular Surfaces

- **Upper:** Inferior articular facet of atlas (concave)
- **Lower:** Superior articular facet of axis (convex)

Ligaments

Capsule
- Attached to margins of articular surfaces.
- Supported by anterior longitudinal ligament and ligamentum flavum posteriorly.

Nerve Supply

Atlantoaxial joints are supplied by rami of C2 nerves.

Movements

- Side to side movement of head is produced by rotation of the atlas along with cranium around the dens of the axis.
- Muscles involved in the movement of head to one side are:
  - On same side
    - Obliques capitis inferior
    - Rectus capitis posterior major
    - Splenius capitis
  - On opposite side – Sternocleidomastoid.

PREVIOUS YEAR QUESTION

1. Write a short note on atlantoaxial joint.

MULTIPLE CHOICE QUESTIONS

1. Atlas (C1) vertebra is identified by:
   a. Ring shaped
   b. No body
   c. No spine
   d. All of the above
2. The joint between the atlas and axis is:
   a. Synovial
   b. Closely related to the 1st cervical nerve
   c. Allow rotation of head
   d. Supported by the alar ligament
3. Atlantoaxial joint is:
   a. Pivot b. Synovial
   c. Saddle d. Hinge

Answers

1. (d) 2. (c) 3. (a)

16 Oral Cavity

ORAL CAVITY

- It is the first part of digestive tract
- It is divided into two parts–
  - Oral cavity proper
  - Vestibule

Oral Cavity Proper (Fig. 16.1)

- Largest part of oral cavity

Boundaries

- Anterior–Alveolar arches with teeth and gums on each side.
- Posterior–Palatoglossal arch
- Roof–Hard and soft palate
- Floor–Two mylohyoid muscles and other soft tissue.

Contents–Tongue

Communications

Posterior–with pharynx through isthmus of fauces (oropharyngeal isthmus).

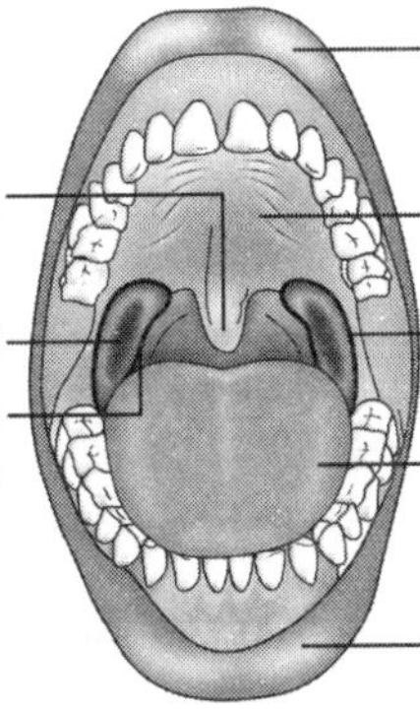

Upper lip
Uvula
Palate
Palatine tonsil
Palatoglossal arch
Palatopharyngeal arch
Tongue
Lower lip

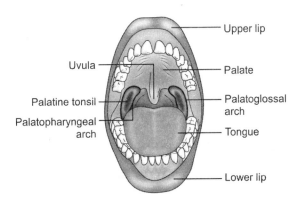

Fig. 16.1: Oral cavity proper

Sublingual Regions

- It is region below anterior part of tongue and above the floor of oral cavity.
- Features
  - Lower surface of tongue is connected to floor of mouth by frenulum linguae.
  - On each side of lower end of frenulum, there is an elevation called sublingual papillae for the opening of submandibular duct.

Vestibule (Fig. 16.2)

- It is a narrow space that lies outside the teeth and gums and inside the lips and cheeks.
- When the mouth is open, it communicates with the oral cavity proper.

Openings in the Vestibule of the Mouth

- Opening of parotid duct: Duct opens into the lateral wall of vestibule opposite the upper second molar teeth.
- Opening of labial and buccal mucous glands.
- Openings of 4/5 molar glands (mucous) situated on the buccopharyngeal fascia.

LIPS AND CHEEKS

Lips

- Lips are a part of mobile musculofibrous folds that surround the opening of the mouth.
- Upper and lower lip meet laterally on each side at an angle called, angle of mouth.
- The lips are lined externally by skin and internally by mucous membrane.
- Structure
  - Largely composed of orbicularis oris muscle
  - Contains labial glands and blood vessels

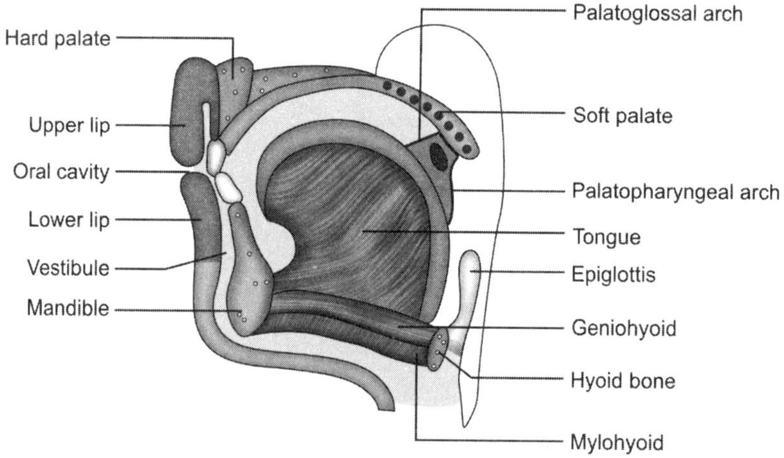
Hard palate
Upper lip
Oral cavity
Lower lip
Vestibule
Mandible
Palatoglossal arch
Soft palate
Palatopharyngeal arch
Tongue
Epiglottis
Geniohyoid
Hyoid bone
Mylohyoid

Fig. 16.2: Vestibule of oral cavity

- Covered by the skin with hair follicles, sebaceous and sweat gland externally and non-keratinized squamous epithelium internally.

Cheeks

- Cheeks are fleshy flaps which lie over maxilla and mandible.
- Form a large part of face.
- Each cheek is continuous in front with the lip.
- Junction between the two (lip and cheek) is marked by nasolabial sulcus.

SULCUS

Structures

- Composed of buccinater muscle, which is covered by **buccopharyngeal fascia.**
- Contains buccal glands, blood vessels and nerves.
- Buccal pad of fat, overlies the buccopharyngeal fascia.

Layers of Cheek

- Skin
- Superficial fascia containing muscles.
- Buccal pad of fat.
- Buccopharyngeal fascia.
- Submucosa, containing buccal gland.
- Mucous membrane.

(Buccal pad of fat to Mucous membrane: Pierced by parotid duct)

Teeth

- Teeth are mineralized structures projecting from the jaws.
- Teeth form part of the masticatory apparatus and fixed to the jaws.
- In human, teeth are replaced only once (diphyodont).
- The teeth of first set (dentition) are known as **Milk or decidous teeth**, and the second set, as **permanent teeth.**
  - Decidous teeth – 20 in number.
  - Permanent – 32 in number.

Anatomical Features – three part (Fig. 16.3)

- **Crown:** Projecting above or below the gum.
- **Root:** Embedded in the jaw beneath the gum.
- **Neck:** Between crown and root and surrounded by the gum.

Gomphosis

- It is a peg and socket joint.
  - It is restricted to the fixation of teeth in their alveolar sockets.
  - It is restricted to the fixation of teeth in their alveolar sockets in mandible and maxillae.
  - Periodontal ligament fibers connect tooth with alveolar bone.

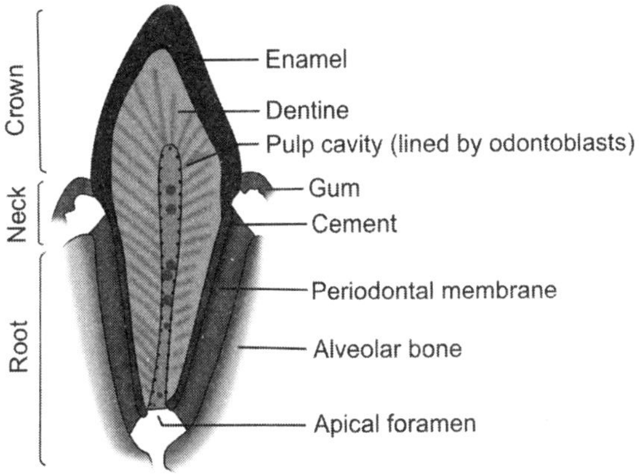
Crown
Neck
Root
Enamel
Dentine
Pulp cavity (lined by odontoblasts)
Gum
Cement
Periodontal membrane
Alveolar bone
Apical foramen

Fig. 16.3: Parts of tooth

Structure of a Tooth

Each tooth is composed of:

- **Pulp cavity:** Inner soft tissue core containing blood vessels, nerves and lymphatics in a specialized connective tissue called Pulp. Pulp is covered by a layer of odontoblasts.
- **Dentine:** It is calcified material surrounding pulp cavity produced by odontoblasts.
- **Enamel:** It consists of densely calcified material covering the crown of tooth. It is the hardest substance in the body.
- **Cementum:** Resembles bone in structure, covering over the neck and root of tooth.
- **Periodontal ligament:** Present between cementum and tooth socket. It holds the tooth in the socket.

Nerve Supply

- Upper teeth: Superior dental plexus of nerves (maxillary division of C2 nerve/Trigeminal nerve).
- Lower teeth: Inferior alveolar nerve (mandibular division of C5 nerve/Trigeminal nerve).

Blood Supply

- Upper teeth – Maxillary artery.
- Lower teeth – Inferior alveolar artery.

Function

- To incise and grind the food material during mastication.
- To provide beauty to the face and means for facial expression.

Types of teeth: Four groups:

1. Incisors – 4 in each jaw
2. Canines – 2 in each jaw
3. Premolar – 4 in each jaw
4. Molar – 6 in each jaw

Eruption of Teeth

Eruption of decidous teeth (Table 16.1)

Table 16.1: Eruption of decidous teeth

Teeth	*Eruption*
Central incisors (A)	6-7 months
Lateral incisors (B)	8-9 months
Canines (C)	18 months
First molar (D)	12 months
Second molar (E)	24 months

Eruption of permanent teeth (Table 16.2)

Table 16.2: Eruption of permanent teeth

Teeth	*Time of eruption*
First molar	6 years
Central incisor	7 years
Lateral incisor	8 years
First premolar	9 years
Second premolar	10 years
Canines	11 years
Second molars	12 years
Third molar (Wisdom tooth)	17-25 years

Development of Teeth

Refer to chapter 29, Embryology.

Gums/Gingivae

- Gums are the soft tissues which envelop the alveolar processes of the upper and lower jaws and surrounds the neck of tooth.
- Composed of dense fibrous tissue covered by stratified squamous epithelium.
- Gums has two parts
  - Free part
  - Attached part

- Nerve supply
  - Upper gums
    - By superior alveolar nerves.
    - By greater palatine or nasopalatine nerve.
  - Lower gums
    - By buccal branch of mandibular nerve and lingual nerve
- Lymphatics
  - Upper – Submandibular nodes
  - Lower – Submandibular nodes.

HARD PALATE

- Forms anterior 2/3rd of the palate.
- Forms partition between nasal and oval cavity.
- Anterior 3/4th – by palatine processes of maxilla.
- Posterior 1/4th – by horizontal plates of palatine bone.

Margins

Anterolateral margins: Continuous with alveolar arches and gums.
Posterior margins: Attached to soft palate.

Surface

Superior surface: Floor of nose.
Inferior surface: Roof of oral cavity.

- Nerve supply
  - Greater palatine
  - Nasopalatine Pterygopalatine ganglion.
- Blood supply
  - Arterial – Greater palatine.
  - Vein – Pterygoid plexus of vein.
- Lymphatic drainage: Upper deep cervical nodes and retropharyngeal nodes.

SOFT PALATE

- It is mobile muscular fold suspended from the posterior border of the hard palate like a curtain.
- It separates nasopharynx from oropharynx.
- Features
  - ***Anterior surface:*** Concave, marked by median raphe.
  - ***Posterior surface:*** Convex, continuous with floor of nasal cavity.
  - ***Superior border:*** Attached to posterior border of hard palate.
  - ***Inferior border:*** Free, forms anterior boundary of pharyngeal isthmus containing uvula.
  - ***On each side:*** From the base of uvula, 2 curved folds of mucous membrane extend laterally and downwards, that are:
    - Palatoglossal fold
    - Palatopharyngeal fold.

Figure 16.4 shows relations of soft palate.

Functions

1. Separates oropharynx from nasopharynx during swallowing.
2. Isolates the oral cavity from oropharynx during chewing.
3. Helps to modify the quality of voice.

Nerve Supply

1. **Motor supply:** Cranial part of accessory nerve via pharyngeal plexus except tensor palati which is supplied by nerve to medial pterygold.
2. **Sensory supply**
   - Greater and lesser palatine nerves
   - Sphenopalatine nerves
   - Glossopharyngeal nerves.

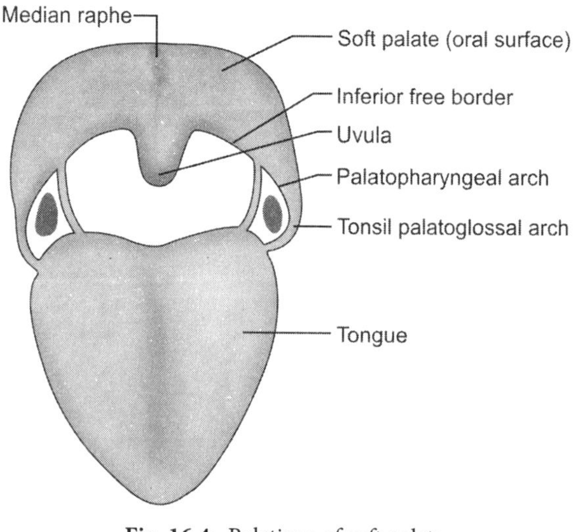
Median raphe
Soft palate (oral surface)
Inferior free border
Uvula
Palatopharyngeal arch
Tonsil palatoglossal arch
Tongue

Fig. 16.4: Relations of soft palate

3. **Secretomotor supply to palatine glands**
   - ***Preganglionic fibers:*** Run in facial nerve and nerve of pterygold canal.
   - ***Postganglionic fibers:*** Run in greater and lesser palatine nerve.

Arterial Supply

- ***Supply***
  - Greater palatine artery, branch of maxillary artery.
  - Ascending palatine artery, branch of facial artery.
  - Palatine branch of ascending pharyngeal artery.
- ***Venous drainage***
  - Pharyngeal plexus via paratonsillar veins.
- ***Lymphatic drainage***
  - Retropharyngeal nodes.
  - Deep cervical lymph nodes.
- ***Muscles of the soft palate (Fig. 16.5 and Table 16.3)***

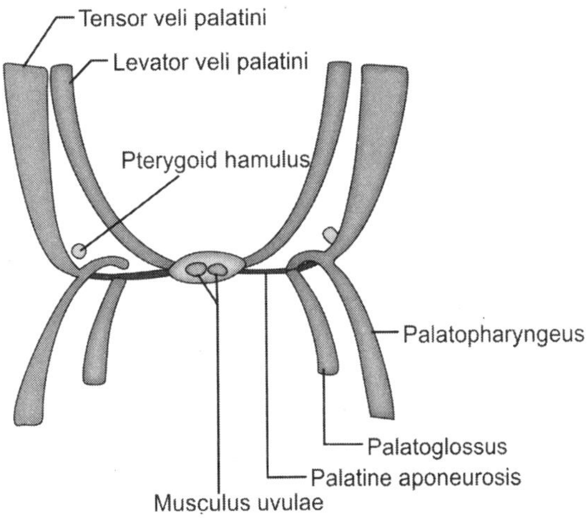
Tensor veli palatini
Levator veli palatini
Pterygoid hamulus
Palatopharyngeus
Palatoglossus
Palatine aponeurosis
Musculus uvulae

Fig. 16.5: Muscles of soft palate

PREVIOUS YEAR QUESTIONS

1. Write a note on palate.
2. Write a short note on vestibule of mouth.
3. Write short note on gums.
4. Briefly describe innervations of teeth of upper and lower jaw and add a note on eruption of decidous and permanent teeth.
5. Enumerate muscles of soft palate and give their nerve supply.
6. Write external features of various teeth and basic internal structure of canine tooth.

Table 16.3: Muscles of the soft palate

Muscle	*Origin*	*Insertion*	*Actions*
Tensor palati	• Auditory tube • Greater wing of sphenoid	• Posterior part of hard palate • Hard palate behind the palatine crest	• Tightens soft palate • Helps in opening the auditory tube
Levator palati	• Auditory tube • Petrous temporal bone	Upper surface of the palatine aponeurosis	• Elevate soft palate • Helps in opening the auditory tube
Musculus uvulae	• Posterior nasal spine • Palatine aponeurosis	Mucous membrane of the uvula	Pulls uvula forwards to its own side
Palatoglossus	Palatine aponeurosis	Side of tongue	• Pulls up the roof of tongue • Approximates the palatoglossal arches to close the oropharyngeal isthmus
Palatopharyngeus	• Anterior fasiculus – hard palate • Posterior fasiculus – palatine aponeurosis	• Median fibrous raphe of pharyngeal wall • Laming of thyroid cartilage	Raises wall of pharynx and larynx during swallowing

7. Describe parts, structure, and time of eruption, development and clinical anatomy of teeth.
8. Write short note on baby teeth.

MULTIPLE CHOICE QUESTIONS

1. Soft palate is made up of:
   a. Palatoglossus and palatopharyngeus
   b. Uvula
   c. Mucous membrane and muscles
   d. All
2. The place where the hard palate is continuous with soft palate posteriorly is overlapped by:
   a. Alveolar periosteum
   b. Periosteum
   c. Mucoperiosteum
   d. Aponeurosis
3. Lymph from lower lip – middle part drains directly into:
   a. Submandibular nodes
   b. Submental node
   c. Sublingual nodes
   d. Preauricular node
4. Eruption sequence of decideous teeth:
   a. A, B, D, C, E
   b. A, B, C, D, E
   c. A, B, E, D, C
   d. A, D, B, C, E
5. Upper gums on labial aspect is supplied by:
   a. Posterior, middle, anterior superior alveolar nerve
   b. Anterior palatine
   c. Greater palatine
   d. Buccal branch of mandibular nerve.
6. Lower jaw teeth are supplied by:
   a. Superior alveolar
   b. Inferior alveolar
   c. Buccal
   d. Mental

Answers

1. (d) 2. (d) 3. (b) 4. (a) 5. (a) 6. (b)

17 Tongue

Tongue is a mobile muscular organ present in the oral cavity.

FUNCTIONS OF TONGUE

1. Speech
2. Taste
3. Mastication
4. Deglutition

Development

(See chapter 29, Embryology)

Anatomical Features

Tongue consists of two parts:
- Oral part – Anterior 2/3rd
- Pharyngeal part – Posterior 1/3rd
  - Conical in shape
  - Presents following features

Tip

Anterior end of the tongue and lies in contact with the incisor teeth.

Base

Formed by the posterior 1/3rd of tongue. Connected to the epiglottis by 3 folds of mucous membrane.
- Median glossoepiglottic fold.
- Right lateral glossoepiglottic fold.
- Left lateral glossoepiglottic fold.
  On either side of median fold is present a depression called vallecula.

Root

Part of tongue attachéd to the floor of mouth.

Two Lateral Margin

Present on either side of tongue.
Two surfaces:
1. Dorsal
2. Ventral / Inferior

DORSAL SURFACE OF TONGUE

- Convex on all sides.
- Divided into two by an inverted 'V' shaped sulcus, known as sulcus terminalis.
- Apex of sulcus is directed backward and is marked by a shallow depression called foramen cecum.
- Foramen cecum represents the site of embryological origin of thyroid gland.
- Two parts.
  a. **Presulcal / Oral part**
     - Constitute anterior 2/3rd of dorsal surface.
     - Numerous papillae of different types are present.
  b. **Postsulcul / Pharyngeal part**
     - Large number of lymphoid follicles known as lingual tonsil are present.
     - No papillae are present.

Dorsal surface of tangue as shown in Fig. 17.1.

Papillae of Tongue

Five Types

1. **Vallate – Largest** in diameter
   - 8-12 in number
   - Situated in front of sulcus terminalis.
2. **Fungiform**
   - Numerous rounded reddish elevation.
   - Present near the tip and margins of the tongue.

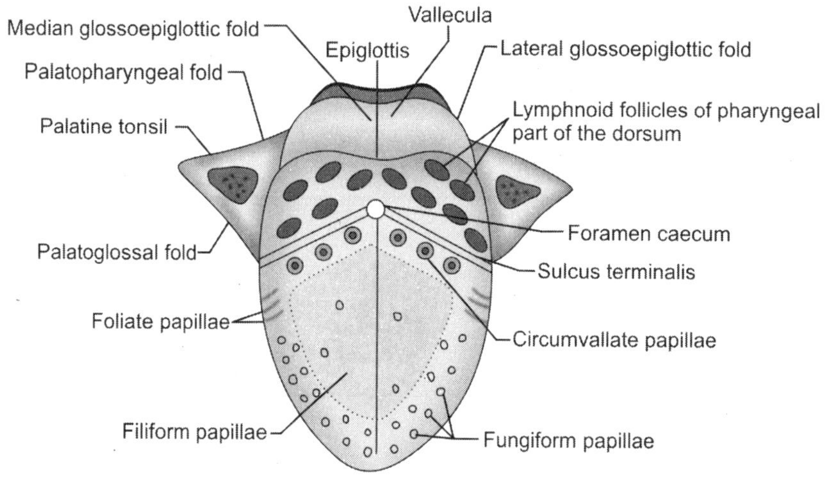
Median glossoepiglottic fold
Vallecula
Epiglottis
Lateral glossoepiglottic fold
Palatopharyngeal fold
Palatine tonsil
Lymphnoid follicles of pharyngeal part of the dorsum
Foramen caecum
Palatoglossal fold
Sulcus terminalis
Foliate papillae
Circumvallate papillae
Filiform papillae
Fungiform papillae

Fig. 17.1: Dorsal surface of tongue

3. **Filiform**
   - Most numerous
   - Covers most of the presulcul area
   - Impart a velvety appearance
4. **Foliaite -**
   - Present on the margin of tongue in front of sulcus terminalis.
5. **Papillae simplex**
   - These are not surface projection and can be seen in microscope.

Taste Buds

- All papillae except filiform contains taste bud.
- Present at following site
  - Anterior 2/3rd of dorsum of tongue.
  - Inferior surface of soft palate.
  - Palatoglossal arch
  - Posterior surface of epiglottis
  - Posterior wall of oropharynx.

Four types of taste sensation:

1. Salt
2. Sweet
3. Sour
4. Bitter

VENTRAL / INFERIOR SURFACE OF TONGUE

Does not contain papillae (Fig. 17.2)

Features

- Frenulum linguae
- Lingual veins
- Plica fimbriata
- Sublingual papilla.

MUSCLES OF TONGUE

- Tongue is divided into two symmetrical halves by a median fibrous septum.
- Each halves contains –
  - Four intrinsic muscle (alter the shape)
  - Four extrinsic muscle (alter the position).

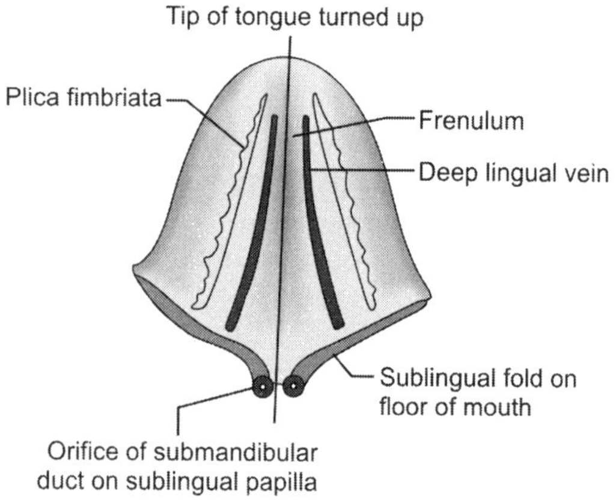
Tip of tongue turned up
Plica fimbriata
Frenulum
Deep lingual vein
Sublingual fold on floor of mouth
Orifice of submandibular duct on sublingual papilla

Fig. 17.2: Ventral surface of tongue

Table 17.1: Intrinsic muscles of tongue			
Intrinsic muscle	*Origin*	*Insertion*	*Action*
• **Superior longitudinal**	Median septum	Margin of tongue	• Shorten the tongue • Make the dorsum concave
• **Inferior longitudinal**	Posterior sides of the tongue	Medial septum	• Shorten the tongue • Make the dorsum convex
• **Transverse linguae**	Median septum	Margins of tongue	• Decrease the width of tongue and elongate it
• **Verticalis linguae**	Lamina propria of dorsum of tongue	Sides of tongue	• Increases the width and flattens it

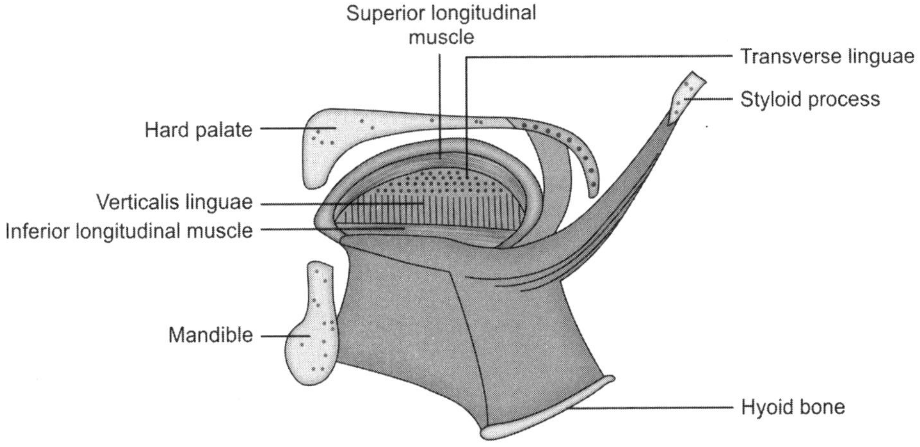
Superior longitudinal muscle
Transverse linguae
Styloid process
Hard palate
Verticalis linguae
Inferior longitudinal muscle
Mandible
Hyoid bone

Fig. 17.3: Intrinsic muscles of tongue

Table 17.2: Extrinsic muscles of tongue			
Extrinsic muscle	*Origin*	*Insertion*	*Action*
• **Hyoglossus quadrilateral shape**	Greater cornua of hyoid bone Body of hyoid	Sides of tongue between styloglossus and inferior longitudinal muscles	• Depresses the sides of the tongue • Makes the dorsal surface convex
• **Genioglossus (Bulk of tongue) – Fan shaped**	Superior genial tubercles or spine	Throughout the tongue from apex of root Body to hyoid	• Protrude tongue tip • Make the dorsum concave • Prevents the tongue from falling back
• **Styloglossus – Elongated**	Tip of styloid process. Stylomandibular ligament	Along the entire length of side of tongue	• Draw the tongue upwards and backwards • Antagonist to genioglossus
• **Palatoglossus Slender**	Oral surface of palatine aponeurosis	Side of tongue at the junction of its oral and pharyngeal part	• Pulls up the curve of tongue • Approximates the palatoglossal arches to decrease width of oropharyngeal isthmus

Intrinsic Muscle

See Table 17.1 and Figure 17.3.

Extrinsic Muscle

See Table 17.2 and Figure 17.4.

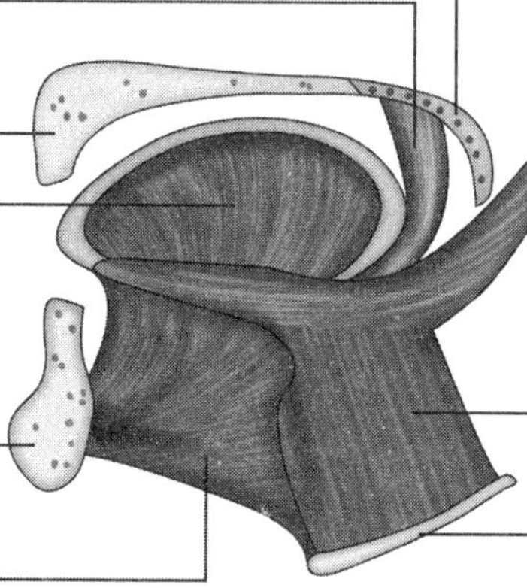
Palatoglossus
Soft palate
Styloid process
Hard palate
Styloglossus
Genioglossus
Mandible
Hyoglossus
Hyoid bone
Genioglossus

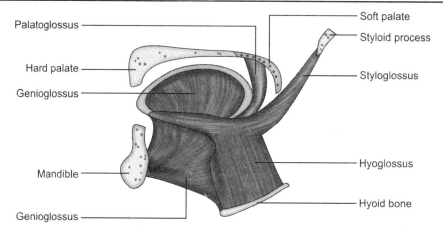

Fig. 17.4: Extrinsic muscles of tongue

NERVE SUPPLY

Motor Supply

Somatomotor

- *Hypoglossal nerve:* Supplies all extrinsic and intrinsic muscles except palatoglossus muscle.
- Cranial part of accessory nerve through pharyngeal plexus.

Secretomotor to Lingual Glands

- *Preganglionic fibers* : Arise in superior salivatory nucleus pass through submandibular ganglion via facial nerve, chorda tympani and lingual nerve.
- *Postganglionic fibers* : Conveyed via lingual nerve.

Vasomotor

- Derived from the sympathetic plexus around lingual artery.

Sensory Supply

- *Lingual nerve:* Receives general sensation from anterior 2/3rd of tongue.
- *Chorda tympani:* Receives taste sensation from anterior 2/3rd except form vallate papillae.
- *Glossopharyngeal nerve:* Conveys all sensation from posterior 1/3rd of tongue.
- *Internal laryngeal branch of superior laryngeal nerve:* Convey taste sensation.

ARTERIAL SUPPLY

1. Lingual artery, branch of external carotid artery – Chief artery.
2. Ascending palatine
3. Tonsillar artery.

Venous Drainage

1. Superficial veins.
2. Deep vein of tongue – Principle vein.

Lymphatic Drainage (Fig. 17.5)

Grouped into three:

1. Tip and inferior surface of tongue—submental lymph nodes.
2. Anterior 2/3rd of dorsum of tongue—submandibular lymph nodes, and then to deep cervical lymph nodes.
3. Posterior 1/3rd of dorsum of tongue—upper deep cervical lymph nodes

Clinical and Applied Anatomy

Congenital anomalies of tongue can be:

a. Aglossia
b. Bifid tongue

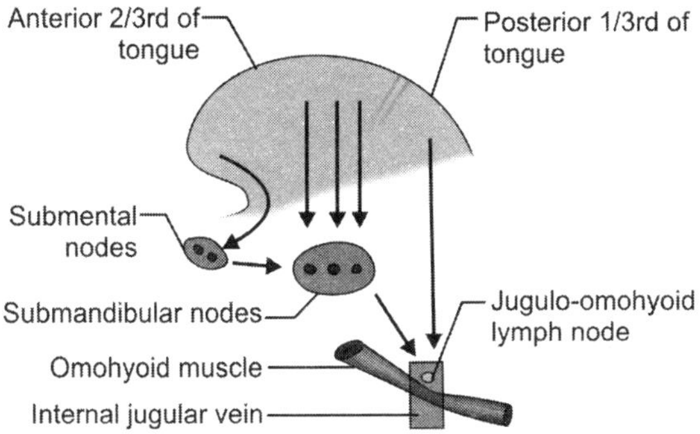
Anterior 2/3rd of tongue
Posterior 1/3rd of tongue
Submental nodes
Submandibular nodes
Jugulo-omohyoid lymph node
Omohyoid muscle
Internal jugular vein

Fig. 17.5: Lymphatic drainage of tongue

c. Lingual thyroid
d. Tongue tie.

PREVIOUS YEAR QUESTIONS

1. Describe tongue under following heads:
   a. Musculature
   b. Development
   c. Histology of anterior 2/3rd of tongue.
2. Write sensory, gustatory and motor nerve supply of tongue.
3. Write short note on.
4. Describe tongue under following headings.
   a. Innervations
   b. Blood supply
   c. Lymphatic drainage

MULTIPLE CHOICE QUESTIONS

1. Which cranial nerve carries the taste sensations from posterior 1/3rd of tongue:
   a. Glossopharyngeal
   b. Facial nerve
   c. Trigeminal nerve
   d. Vagus
2. Taste sensation from anterior 2/3rd of tongue is carried by:
   a. Hypoglossal nerve
   b. Chorda tympani nerve
   c. Glossopharyngeal nerve
   d. Vagus nerve
3. Lymphatic vessels of tongue drain primarily into the:
   a. Deep cervical nodes
   b. Parotid nodes
   c. Submental nodes
   d. Submandibular nodes
4. Taste buds are predominantly located in which papillae:
   a. Circumvallate
   b. Filiform
   c. Fungiform
   d. Foliate
5. The papillae present on margins of tongue:
   a. Fungiform
   b. Filiform
   c. Vallate
   d. Foliate
6. Muscles of tongue are supplied by:
   a. Glossopharyngeal nerve
   b. Lingual nerve
   c. Chorda tympani
   d. Hypoglossal nerve
7. Main arterial supply to the tongue is:
   a. Ascending palatine artery
   b. Ascending pharyngeal artery
   c. Lingual artery
   d. Facial artery
8. Hypoglossal nerve supplies to all the following muscle except:
   a. Palatoglossus
   b. Genioglossus
   c. Hyoglossus
   d. Styloglossus
9. Safety muscle of tongue is:
   a. Hyoglossus
   b. Genioglossus
   c. Palatoglossus
   d. Styloglossus
10. Palsy of right genioglossus causes:
    a. Deviation of tongue to right
    b. Deviation of tongue to left
    c. Deviation of soft palate to right
    d. Deviation of soft palate to left

Answers

1. (a) 2. (b) 3. (a) 4. (a) 5. (a) 6. (d) 7. (c) 8. (a) 9. (b) 10 (a)

18 Nose and Paranasal Sinuses

NOSE

- Most proximal part of upper respiratory system
- Lined by respiratory and olfactory epithelium
- It consists of external nose and nasal cavity.

External Nose

Forms a pyramidal projection in the middle of the face.

Features

Type or apex: Lower free end of nose

Root: Forehead

Dorsum: Rounded border between top and root of nose.

Nostrils / Nares: Two piriform shaped appertures present at broad lower part of nose.

Nerve Supply

External nasal, infratrochlear and infraorbital nerve.

Skeleton of External Nose

Formed by bones and cartilages:

- *Bony framework*
  - Two nasal bone – forming bridge of nose.
  - Frontal process of maxillae.
- *Cartilaginous framework* – 5 main cartilage
  - Two lateral alar cartilages or superior nasal cartilage
    1. One upper
    2. One lower.
  - A single median septal cartilage.
  - Two major alar cartilage/Inferior nasal cartilage.

Nasal Cavity

- Extends from nostrils in front of the posterior nasal apperture behind
- Subdivided into two parts by nasal septum
- Each nasal cavity presents with following boundaries.

Boundaries

Roof

- Very narrow
- Formed by cribriform plate of ethmoid bones
- Anterior part – formed by nasal bones
- Posterior part – formed by anterior sphenoid bones
- Lined by olfactory epithelium.

Floor

- Horizontal
- Formed by upper surface of hard palate.

Medial wall / Nasal septum

- Formed by various bones and cartilages
- It is osseocartilagenous partition between two halves of nasal cavity
- Lined by mucous membrane.

Nasal cavity of nasal septum and nasal septum of arterial supply are shown in Figures 18.1 and 18.2 and Tables 18.1 and 18.2.

Arterial Supply

1. Septal branch of anterior ethmoid artery–Ophthalmic artery.
2. Septal branch of sphenopalatine artery–Maxillary artery.

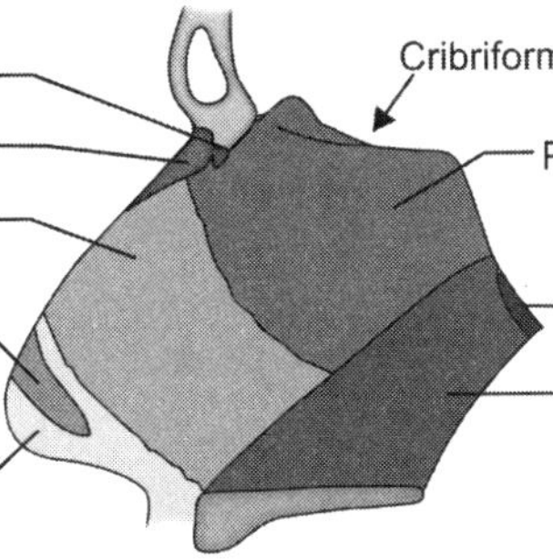
Nasal spine of frontal bone
Nasal crest of nasal bone
Septal cartilage
Septal process of inferior nasal cartilage
Columella
Cribriform plate of ethmoid
Perpendicular plate of ethmoid
Rostrum of sphenoid
Vomer

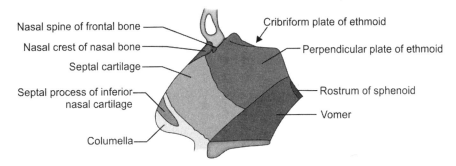

Fig. 18.1: Nasal septum of nasal cavity

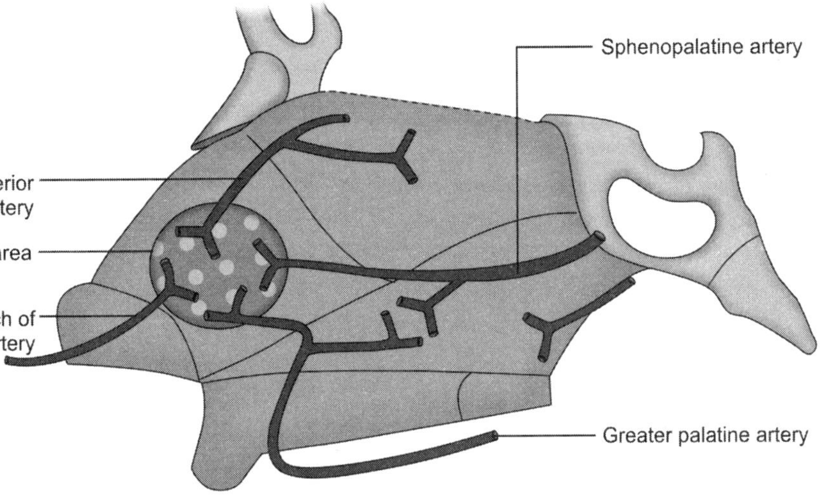
Sphenopalatine artery
Anterior ethmoidal artery
Little's area
Septal branch of superior labial artery
Greater palatine artery

Fig. 18.2: Arterial supply of nasal septum

Table 18.1: Nasal cavity of nasal septum

Bony part	*Cartilaginous part*
• Vomer • Perpendicular plate of ethmoid • Nasal spine of frontal bone • Nasal crest of nasal bone • Sphenoidal crest / Rostrum • Palatine processes of maxilla • Horizontal plates of palatine bones	• Septal cartilage • Septal process of inferior nasal cartilage • Jacobson's cartilage.

Table 18.2: Nasal sepfum of arterial supply

Bony part	*Cartilaginous part*
Anteriorly • Nasal • Frontal process of maxilla • Lacrimal bone • Superior and middle conchae with Labyrinth of ethmoid • Inferior nasal conchae **Posteriorly** • Perpendicular plates of palatine • Medial pterygoid plate of sphenoid	• Superior/lateral nasal cartilage • Inferior/major nasal cartilage • 3 or 4 tiny alar cartilage
Lined by mucous membrane	Lined by skin

3. Septal branch of greater palatine artery.
4. Septal branch of superior labial artery–Facial artery.

Venous Drainage

- Veins form plexes in Litte's area
- Plexus drains anteriorly into facial vein
- Posteriorly into plerygoid venous plexus.

Nerve Supply

- Olfactory nerves – 5-20 in number of and supply olfactory zone
- Internal nasal branch of anterior ethmoidal nerve – Anterosuperior part.
- Medial posterior superior alveolar nerve – Intermediate part.
- Nasopalatine nerve – Supply posterior part.
- Nasal branch of greater palatine nerve – Supply posterior part.
- Anterior superior alveolar – Antero inferior part.
- External nasal nerve, from anterior ethmoid – Lower mobile part.

Clinical and Applied Anatomy

Kesselbach's Plexus

- Little's area on the septum is a common site of bleeding or epistaxis.
- Pathological deviation of nasal septum is responsible for repeated attacks of common cold, allergic rhinitis, sinusitis, etc. It requires surgical correction.

Lateral Wall of Nasal Cavity

- Irregular
- Present with three shelf—Life bony projection called conchae.
- Conchae increase the surface area of nose for effective air—conditioning of inspired air.
- It is also formed by bones and cartilages.

Subdivision of Lateral Wall

- Anterior part: Presents vestibule, lined by skin containing hairs called as **vibrissae**.
- Middle part: Known as **atrium of middle meatus**
- Posterior part: Presents conchae and meatus (space separating conchae).

Features of Lateral Wall

1. **Conchae:** Three curved bony projections directed downwards and medially from the lateral wall.
   a. Superior conchae – smallest – Part of ethmoidal labyrinth
   b. Middle conchae – Maximum no. of openings – Part of ethmoidal labyrinth
   c. Inferior concha – largest – Independent bone
2. **Meatuses:** Passages present beneath the overhanging conchae:
   a. Inferior meatus
      i. Largest
      ii. Lies below inferior nasal conchae.
   b. Middle meatus
      i. Lies below middle nasal conchae
      ii. Features.
         - Ethmoidal bulla (rounded elevation)
         - Hiatus semilunaris (semicircular sulcus below ethmoidal bulla).
         - Infundibulum (short passage at the anterior end of middle meatus).
   c. Superior meatus
      i. Smalles
      ii. Lies below superior concha.
3. Sphenoethmoidal recess:
   – Triangular depression, above and behind superior concha.
4. Atrium of middle meatus:
   – Shallow depression present in front of the middle meatus and above vestibule of nose.

Openings in the Lateral Wall of Nose (Table 18.3 and Fig. 18.3)

Table 18.3: Openings in the lateral wall of nose

Site	*Openings*
Sphenoethmoidal recess	Sphenoidal air sinus
Superior meatus	Posterior ethmoidal air sinuses
Middle meatus	Middle ethmoidal air sinuses Frontal air sinus Anterior ethmoidal air sinus Maxillary air sinus
Inferior meatus	Nasolacrimal duct

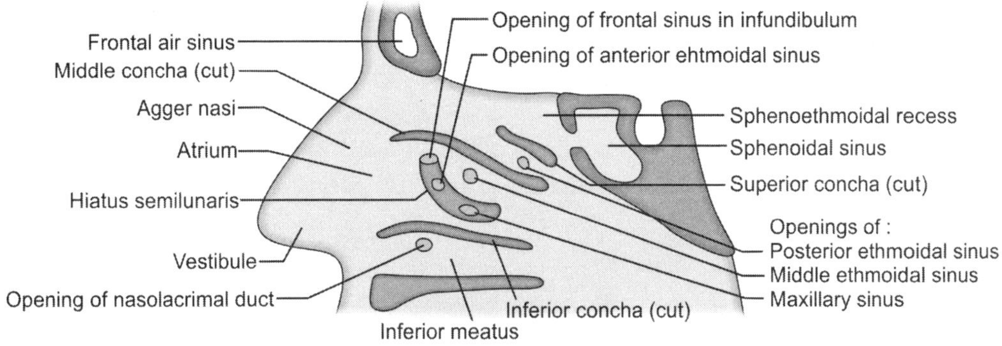
Frontal air sinus
Middle concha (cut)
Agger nasi
Atrium
Hiatus semilunaris
Vestibule
Opening of nasolacrimal duct
Opening of frontal sinus in infundibulum
Opening of anterior ehtmoidal sinus
Sphenoethmoidal recess
Sphenoidal sinus
Superior concha (cut)
Openings of :
Posterior ethmoidal sinus
Middle ethmoidal sinus
Maxillary sinus
Inferior concha (cut)
Inferior meatus

Fig. 18.3: Openings in the lateral wall of nose

Arterial Supply of Lateral Wall (Fig. 18.4)

1. Anterior ethmoidal artery—Anterosuperior quadrant.
2. Branches of facial artery—Anteroinferior quadrant.
3. Sphenopalatine artery—Posterosuperior quadrant.
4. Greater palatine artery—Posteroinferior quadrant.

Venous Supply

Veins form a plexus which drains:

1. Anteriorly—facial vein.

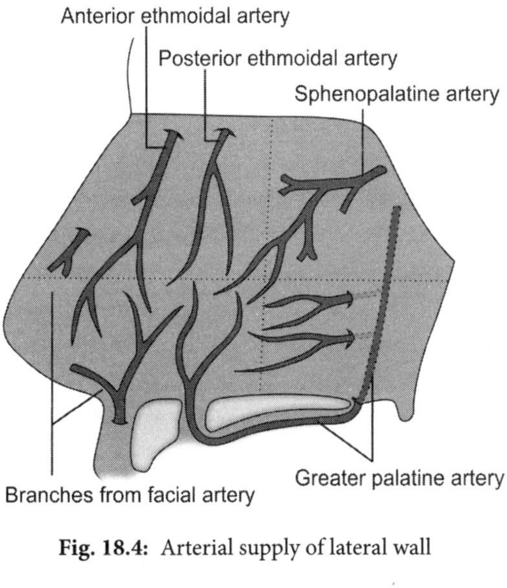
Anterior ethmoidal artery
Posterior ethmoidal artery
Sphenopalatine artery
Branches from facial artery
Greater palatine artery

Fig. 18.4: Arterial supply of lateral wall

2. Middle—pterygoid plexus.
3. Posterior—Pharyngeal plexus.

Nerve Supply

1. General sensory nerves - From trigeminal nerve
   - Anterior ethmoid nerve - Anterosuperior quadrant.
   - Anterior superior alveolar nerve - Anteroinferior quadrant.
   - Posterior superior lateral nasal branch - Posterior superior quadrant.
   - Greater palatine nerve - Posterioinferior quadrant.
2. Special sensory nerves or olfactory nerve- Supplies upper part of lateral wall just below cribriform plate.

Lymphatic Drainage

- Anterior half: Submandibular node
- Posterior half: Retropharyngeal and Upper deep cervical nodes.

Clinical or Applied Anatomy

- Common cold/Rhinitis is the commonest infection of nose.
- Paranasal air sinuses may get infected, maxillary sinusitis is the commonest.

PARANASAL SINUSES (FIG. 18.5)

- These are all filled spaces within the bones around nasal cavity.

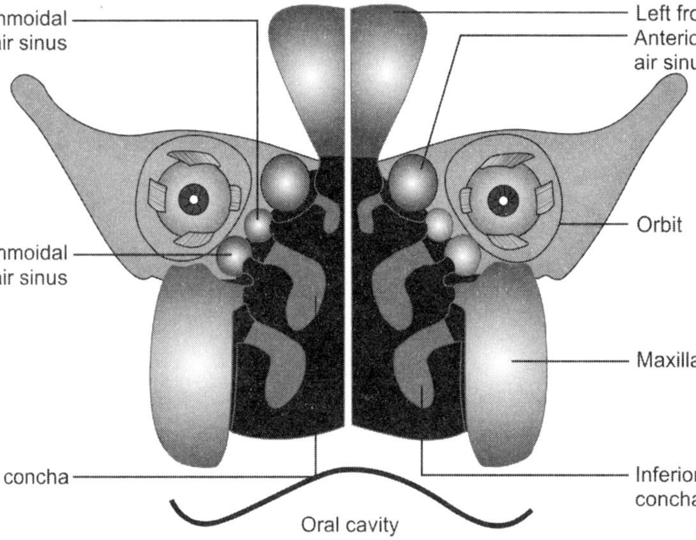
Posterior ethmoidal air sinus
Left frontal air sinus
Anterior ethmoidal air sinus
Orbit
Middle ethmoidal air sinus
Maxillary air sinus
Middle nasal concha
Inferior nasal concha
Oral cavity

Fig. 18.5: Paranasal sinuses

- Lined by mucous membrane, consisting of ciliated columnar epithelium.
- They communicate with nasal cavity through narrow channels.

Functions

1. Add humidity to inspired air.
2. Adjust temperature of inspired air.
3. Make the skull lighter.
4. Add resonance to the voice.

- All paranasal sinuses are arranged in pairs except ethmoidal sinuses which are arranged in three groups.
- Paranasal sinuses are:
  - Frontal
  - Ethmoidal
  - Maxillary
  - Sphenoidal.

Maxillary Sinus/Antrum of Highmore (Fig. 18.6)

- Largest air sinus
- Present in the body of maxilla
- One on either side of the nasal cavity
- It drains into hiatus semilunaris of middle meatus
- Measurements

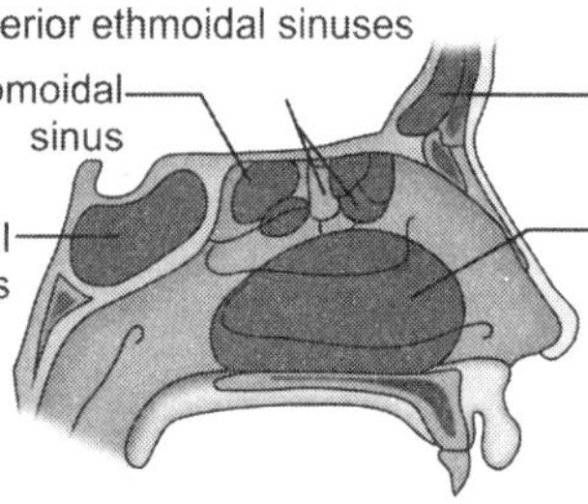
Anterior ethmoidal sinuses
Posterior ethomoidal sinus
Frontal air sinus
Sphenoidal sinus
Maxillary sinus

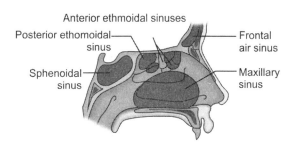

Fig. 18.6: Maxillary sinus

  - Vertical – 3.5 cm
  - Transverse – 2.5 cm
  - Anteroposterior – 3.25 cm.

Parts of maxillary sinus and their relations

Pyramidal in shape:

- *Roof:* Floor of orbit
- *Floor:* Alveolar process of maxilla
- *Base:* Nasal surface of body of maxilla
- *Apex:* Extends into zygomatic process of maxilla
- *Anterior wall:* Related to infraorbital plexus of nerves
- *Posterior wall:* Forms anterior boundaries of infratemporal fossa.

Arterial Supply

Anterior, middle and posterior superior alveolar arteries—Branch of maxillary artery.

Venous Drainage

i. Facial vein
ii. Pterygoid plexus of vein.

Lymphatic Drainage

Submandibular lymph nodes.

Nerve Supply

1. Anterior, middle and posterior superior alveolar nerve—Branch of maxillary nerve.
2. Infraorbital nerve.

Clinical and Applied Anatomy

- Maxillary sinus is the commonest site of infection, known as maxillary sinusitis.
- Sources of infection
  - Infection in the nose
  - Caries of upper molar teeth
- Surgical drainage is performed in two ways
  - Antral puncture
  - Caldwell-Luc operation.

PREVIOUS YEAR QUESTIONS

1. Write a note on maxillary sinus.
2. Write a short note on para nasal air sinuses.
3. Draw a labeled diagram of lateral wall of nose showing various openings.
4. Write a short note on lateral wall of nose.

Other Parnasal Sinuses (Table 18.4)

Table 18.4: Features of paranasal sinuses

Sinus	*Features*	*Blood supply*	*Nerve supply*
Ethmoidal	• Made up of number of air cells present within labyrinth of ethmoid bone. • Located between upper part of lateral wall of nose and orbit • Divided into three groups – – Anterior group drains into middle meatus – Middle group drains into middle meatus – Posterior group – Superior meatus	• Anterior and • Posterior ethmoidal vessels	• Anterior and • Posterior ethmoidal nerve • Orbital branch of pterygopalatine ganglion
Sphenoidal	• Present in pair as right and left • Lies within body of sphenoid bone • Seperated from each other by nasal septum • Drains into sphenoethmoidal recess of nasal cavity	**Arterial –** • Posterior ethmoid artery. • Internal carotid artery. **Vein** • Cavernous sinus	• Posterior ethmoidal nerve • Orbital branch of plerygopalatine nerve
Frontal	• Lies in frontal bone deep to subciliary arch, drains into middle meatus • Triangular in shape • Divided as right and left sinus of uniqual size	Supraorbital vessels	Supraorbital nerve

5. Enumerate paranasal air sinuses. What are the functions of it? Name the nerve supplying them. Add a note on their applied anatomy.
6. Write a short note on nasal septum and its nerve and blood supply.

MULTIPLE CHOICE QUESTIONS

1. First sinus developed is:
   a. Maxillary
   b. Frontal
   c. Sphenoidal
   d. Ethmoidal.
2. The frontal paranasal sinus drains into the:
   a. Superior meatus
   b. Middle meatus
   c. Inferior meatus
   d. Spenoethmoidal recess.
3. Sphenoidal air sinus is supplied by which nerve:
   a. Posterior ethmoidal
   b. Posterior superior
   c. Sphenoidal
   d. Infratemporal.
4. Nasolacrimal duct opens into:
   a. Superior meatus
   b. Middle meatus
   c. Inferior meatus
   d. None.
5. Middle conchae of nose are a part of:
   a. Nasal bone
   b. Ethmoid
   c. Vomer
   d. Maxilla.
6. Nerve supply of nasal septum is from:
   a. Facial
   b. Ophthalmic
   c. Maxillary
   d. Ascending palatine.
7. Inferior concha is an extension of:
   a. Ethmoid bone
   b. Vomer
   c. Nasal septum
   d. Independent bone.
8. All are paranasal sinuses except:
   a. Maxillary
   b. Sphenoidal
   c. Covernous
   d. Ethmoidal.

Answers

1. (a) 2. (b) 3. (a) 4. (c) 5. (b) 6. (c) 7. (d) 8. (c)

19 Pharynx

DEFINITION

Pharynx is a musculo facial tube extending from the base of skull to the esophagus.

- It is situated behind the nose, mouth and larynx with which it communicates.
- It acts as a common channel for both deglutition and respiration.

Measurements

Length	–	12-14 cm
Width	–	Upper part 3.5 cm
	–	Lower part 1.5 cm

Boundaries

Superior	–	Base of skull
Inferior	–	Continuous with esophagus at the level of C6 vertebra and cricoid cartilage
Posterior	–	Prevertebral fascia
Anterior	–	Communicates with nasal cavity, oral cavity and larynx.

Each side:

a. It is attached to:
   - Medial pterygoid plate
   - Pterygomandibular raphe
   - Mandible
   - Tongue
   - Hyoid bone
   - Thyroid and cricoid cartilage

b. Communicates with middle ear cavity through the auditory tube.

c. Related to:
   - Styloid apparatus
   - Carotid arteries and cranial nerve

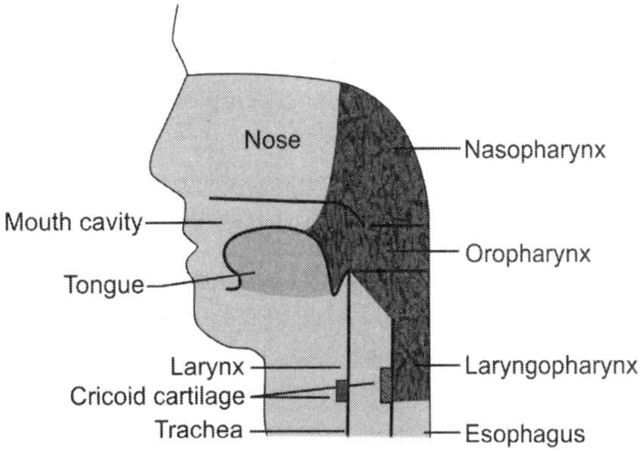
Nose
Nasopharynx
Mouth cavity
Oropharynx
Tongue
Larynx
Laryngopharynx
Cricoid cartilage
Trachea
Esophagus

Fig. 19.1: Parts of pharynx

SUBDIVISIONS/PARTS OF PHARYNX

Divides into (Fig. 19.1):

a. Nasal part – Nasopharynx
b. Oral part – Oropharynx
c. Laryngeal part – Laryngopharynx

Nasopharynx

- Situated behind nose and above soft palate.
- Resembles nose both structurally and functionally as
  - Respiratory function
  - No food enters it normally
  - Walls are rigid and noncollapsable
  - Lined by ciliated epithelium
  - Supplied by pharyngeal branch of pterygopalatine ganglion

(Other parts of pharynx are supplied by IX and X cranial nerve).

Features

- Superiorly limited by body of sphenoid and basi-occiput.
  - Anteriorly communicates with nasal cavity through posterior nasal aperture.
  - Inferiorly, communicates with oral cavity through pharyngeal isthmus.
  - Two structures lie in this part. These are:
    - *Nasopharyngeal tonsil.*
      Collection of lymphoid tissue beneath the mucous membrane of the posterior wall.
    - Orifice of pharyngotympanic tube/Auditory/Eustachian Tube
      1. Tubular opening lies 1.2 cm behind the level of inferior concha.
      2. Upper and posterior margins of this opening are bounded by a tubal elevation known as Tubal tonsil.
      3. Two mucosal fold extending this elevation, as
         a. Salpingopharyngeal fold
         b. Salpingopalatine fold

There is a deep depression behind tubal elevation which is known as pharyngeal recess/fossa of Rosenmuller.

Clinical and Applied Anatomy

- Nasopharyngeal tonsils are more prominent in children.
- Enlargement of it is usually due to repeated upper respiratory tract infection known as Adenoids.

Oropharynx

- Extends from palate above to the tip of epiglottis below.
- Anteriorly, communicates with the oral cavity through oropharyngeal isthmus.
- Inferiorly, continues with laryngopharynx at the epiglottis.
- Posteriorly, lies over C2-C3 vertebrae and separated from them by retropharyngeal space.

Oropharyngeal Isthmus

Boundaries

- Above - Soft palate
- Below – Dorsal surface of posterior 1/3rd of tongue
- Lateral – Palatoglossal arch

It is closed during deglutition to prevent regurgitation of food from pharynx into the mouth.

Features

Lateral wall of oropharynx on each side presents with:

- Tonsillar fossa
- Palatoglossal arch
- Palatopharyngeal arch

Laryngopharynx

- It extends from upper border of epiglottis to lower end of pharynx.
- Continues as esophagus at the level of C6 vertebrae.

Relations

- *Anterior:* Communicates with laryngeal cavity through the laryngeal inlet.
- *Inferior:* Esophagus at pharyngo esophagus junction.
- *Posterior:* Overlies the body of C4, C5 and C6 vertebrae seperated by retropharyngeal space.

Features

- Laryngeal inlet
  - Opening into larynx
  - It closes during deglutition to prevent entry of food into laryngeal cavity.
- Piriform fossa
  - It is a recess produced due to inward bulging of lamina of thyroid cartilage on each side.
- Internal laryngeal nerve and superior laryngeal vessel
  - Pierce the thyrohyoid membrane to reach the medial wall.

Clinical and Applied Anatomy

- Piriform fossa is a depressed area where occasionally the ingested food particles can get stuck.
- Adequate care should be given during removal to prevent damage of internal laryngeal nerve.

STRUCTURE OF PHARYNX

Wall of pharynx consists of five layer from within outwards.

- Mucosa: Stratified squamous epithelium except nasopharynx.
- Submucosa: Thick and fibrous.
- Pharyngobasilar fascia/Pharyngeal aponeurosis:
  - It is a fibrous sheet internal to the pharyngeal muscles.
  - Thickest at two parts:
    - Upper part: Where it fills the gap between upper border of superior constrictor and base of skull.
    - Lower part: Where it forms the pharyngeal raphe.
- Muscular coat:
  - Consists of striated muscles.
  - Arranged in outer circular and inner longitudinal layers.
    - Outer circular – Two constrictor muscles.
    - Inner longitudinal
      - Stylopharyngeus
      - Palatopharyngeus
      - Salpingopharygeus.
- Buccopharyngeal fascia (Fig. 19.2):
  - Covers outer surface of constrictor muscle.
  - Extends anteriorly across the pterygomandibular raphe to cover the buccinator muscle.
  - Between buccopharyngeal fascia and muscular coat, the pharyngeal plexus of nerve and vessels are present.

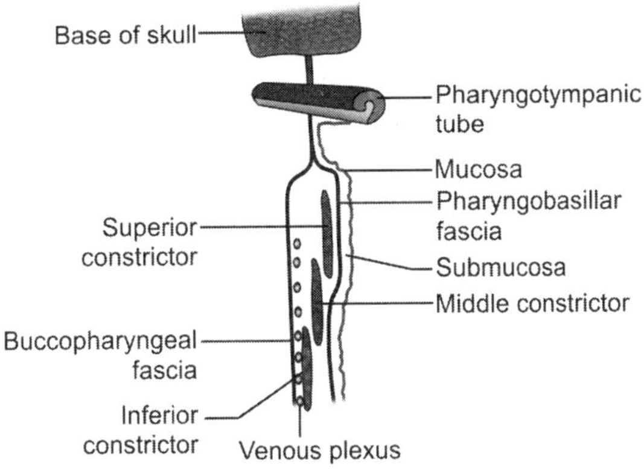
Base of skull
Pharyngotympanic tube
Mucosa
Pharyngobasillar fascia
Submucosa
Middle constrictor
Superior constrictor
Buccopharyngeal fascia
Inferior constrictor
Venous plexus

Fig. 19.2: Buccopharyngeal fascia with its relations

CONSTRICTOR MUSCLES OF PHARYNX

- Forms the main bulk of muscular coat of pharyngeal wall (Table 19.1).
- They arise from posterior openings of nose, mouth and pharynx.
- Inserted into median fibrous raphe.
- This raphe extend from base of skull (pharyngeal tubercle) to esophagus.

Arrangement

- Inferior constrictor muscle overlaps middle constrictor, which in turn overlap superior constrictor muscle.
- **Functions:** Aid in deglutition by coordinated contraction.
- **Nerve supply:**
  - Pharyngeal branches of cranial root of accessory nerve carried by vagus nerve.
  - Inferior constrictor is in addition supplied by:
    - External laryngeal
    - Recurrent laryngeal nerve

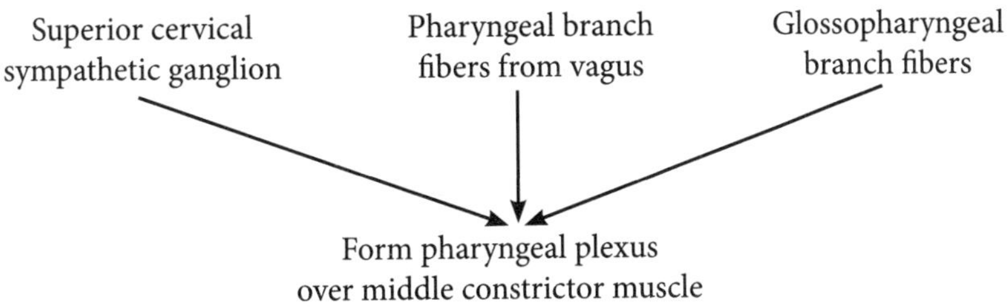
Superior cervical sympathetic ganglion
Pharyngeal branch fibers from vagus
Glossopharyngeal branch fibers
Form pharyngeal plexus over middle constrictor muscle

Table 19.1: Muscles of pharynx

Muscle	*Origin*	*Insertion*
Superior	• Pterygoid humulus • Pterygomandibular raphe • Mandible at upper end of mylohyoid line • Side of posterior part of tongue	i. Median fibrous raphe ii. Pharyngeal tubercle on base of skull
Middle	• Stylohyoid ligament • Lesser cornu of hyoid • Greater cornu of hyoid	Median fibrous raphe
Inferior a. Thyropharyngeus b. Cricopharyngeus	• Lamina of thyroid cartilage • Tendon between inferior thyroid tubercle and cricoid cartilage • Cricoid cartilage	Median fibrous raphe Median fibrous raphe

LONGITUDINAL MUSCLES OF PHARYNX (TABLE 19.2)

Table 19.2: Longitudinal muscles of pharynx

Muscle	*Origin*	*Insertion*	*Nerve supply*
Stylopharyngeus	Base of Styloid process	Posterior border of lamina of thyroid cartilage	Glossopharyngeal nerve via pharyngeal plexus
Palatopharyngeus	Anterior fasciculi and posterior fasciculi from palatine aponeurosis	Posterior border of lamina of thyroid cartilage	Cranial root of accessory nerve (XI) via pharyngeal plexus
Salpingopharyngeus	Tubal elevation of nasopharynx	Posterior border of lamina of thyroid cartilage	Cranial root of accessory (XI) nerve via pharyngeal plexus

Action of Longitudinal Muscles

- Elevate larynx during swallowing
- Shortern pharynx during swallowing
- Palatopharyngeus sphincter closes pharyngeal isthmus

Passavant's Ridge

- Some fibers of palatopharyngeus sweep horizontally backwards forming 'U' – shaped loop within the pharyngeal wall.
- This raised area is called as Passavant's ridge.
- This 'U' shaped muscle loop acts as palato – pharyngeal sphincter.

Structures passing between constrictors of pharynx (Table 19.3)

Table 19.3: Structures passing between constrictors of pharynx

Base of skull (Sinus of Morgagni)
↕ 1. Auditory tube 2. Levator palate muscle 3. Ascending palatine artery 4. Palatine branch of ascending pharyngeal artery
Superior Constrictors
↕ 1. Stylopharyngeus muscle 2. Glossopharyngeal nerve
Middle Constrictors
↕ 1. Internal laryngeal nerve 2. Superior laryngeal vessles
Esophagus

Nerve Supply of Pharynx

Motor – All pharyngeal muscle are supplied by cranial root of accessory nerve except **stylopharyngeus** which is supplied by glossopharyngeal nerve.

Sensory

a. *Nasopharynx:* Pharyngeal branch of pterygopalatine ganglion.
b. *Oropharynx:* Glossopharyngeal nerve.
c. *Laryngopharynx:* Internal laryngeal nerve.

Blood Supply

Arteries

1. Ascending pharyngeal branch – External carotid artery
2. Ascending palatine and tonsilar – Facial artery
3. Dorsal lingual – Lingual artery
4. Greater palatine
5. Pharyngeal
6. Pterygoid

(4–6) From maxillary artery

Veins

Form a plexus, receiving blood from pharynx, soft palate and drains into internal jugular and facial vein.

Lymphatic Drainage

1. Retropharyngeal lymph nodes
2. Deep cervical lymph nodes

DEGLUTITION / SWALLOWING

- Deglutition is a process by which the food is transferred from the mouth to the stomach.
- It consists of three successive stages:
  1. First stage (in mouth) – Voluntary
  2. Second stage (in pharynx) – Involuntary
  3. Third stage (in oesophagus) – Involuntary

Deglutition Process

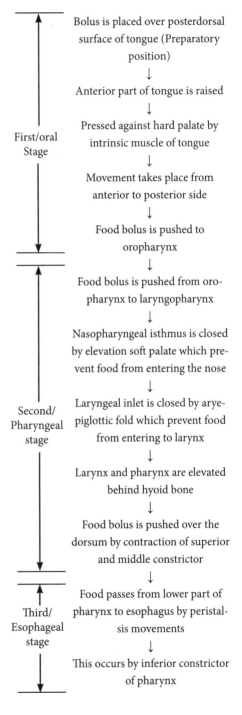

First/oral Stage

Bolus is placed over posterdorsal surface of tongue (Preparatory position)
↓
Anterior part of tongue is raised
↓
Pressed against hard palate by intrinsic muscle of tongue
↓
Movement takes place from anterior to posterior side
↓
Food bolus is pushed to oropharynx
↓

Second/Pharyngeal stage

Food bolus is pushed from oropharynx to laryngopharynx
↓
Nasopharyngeal isthmus is closed by elevation soft palate which prevent food from entering the nose
↓
Laryngeal inlet is closed by aryepiglottic fold which prevent food from entering to larynx
↓
Larynx and pharynx are elevated behind hyoid bone
↓
Food bolus is pushed over the dorsum by contraction of superior and middle constrictor
↓

Third/Esophageal stage

Food passes from lower part of pharynx to esophagus by peristalsis movements
↓
This occurs by inferior constrictor of pharynx

Clinical and Applied Anatomy

- A potential gap is present posteriorly in the pharynx between thyropharyngeus and cricopharyngeus muscles.
- It is called pharyngeal dimple or Killien's dehiscence.
- Weakest part of the pharynx.
- Formation of a pharyngeal pouch may occur in this region.

AUDITORY TUBE/EUSTACHIAN TUBE (FIG. 19.3)

- Also known as **pharyngotympanic tube.**
- It is an osseo-cartilagenous channel which connects the lateral wall of nasopharynx with the middle ear (tympanum).
- It maintains the equilibrium of air pressure on either side of tympanic membrane.
- It is 4 cm long.
- Directed downwards, forwards and medially.

Features

Tube comprises of two parts:

1. **Osseous or bony part**
   a. Form lateral 1/3rd of tube.
   b. Extends from tympanic cavity towards the anterior border of petrous temporal.
2. **Cartilaginuous part**
   a. Form anterior 2/3rd of tube.
   b. Lies in sulcus tubae.
   c. Form by articulation of petrous temporal and greater wing of sphenoid.
   d. Made up of triangular plate of elastic fibrocartilage.

Blood Supply

Artery

- Ascending pharyngeal artery
- Middle meningeal artery
- Artery of pterygoid canal

Veins

- Pharyngeal and
- Pterygoid plexuses of veins

Lymphatic Drainage

Retropharyngeal nodes

Never Supply

1. *At ostium*: By pharyngeal branch of pterygo-palatine ganglion.
2. *Cartilagenous part:* Nervus spinosus
3. *Bony part*: By tympanic plexus formed by glospharyngeal nerve.

Function

- Tube provides communication of middle ear cavity with the exterior.

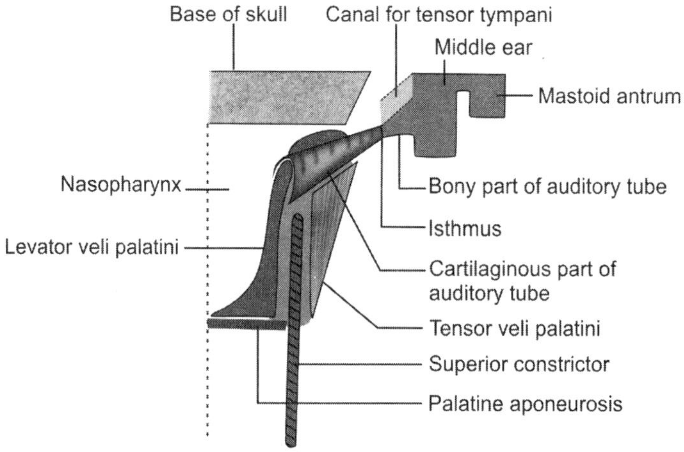
Base of skull
Canal for tensor tympani
Middle ear
Mastoid antrum
Nasopharynx
Levator veli palatini
Bony part of auditory tube
Isthmus
Cartilaginous part of auditory tube
Tensor veli palatini
Superior constrictor
Palatine aponeurosis

Fig. 19.3: Relations of auditory tube

- The tube is usually closed.
- It opens during swallowing, yawning and sneezing.

Clinical and Applied Anatomy

1. Infection may pass from the throat to the middle ear through the auditory tube.
2. Inflammation of auditory tube (Eustachian Catarrh) is secondary to common cold and sore throat.

PREVIOUS YEAR QUESTIONS

1. Enumerate muscles of pharynx with their nerve supply.
2. Write a short note on constrictor muscles of pharynx.
3. Briefly describe anatomy of pharynx and add a note on mechanism of swallowing.
4. Write a note on deglutition.
5. Write a short note on auditory tube.

MULTIPLE CHOICE QUESTIONS

1. The weakest part of pharynx is:
   a. Sinus of Morgagni
   b. Between thyropharyngeus and cricopharyngeus
   c. Pyriform fossa
   d. Pharyngeal recess
2. Main motor nerve supply to the pharynx is:
   a. Vagus
   b. Accessory
   c. Glossopharyngeal
   d. Facial
3. Nasopharynx consists of all except:
   a. Pyriform recess
   b. Pharyngeal recess
   c. Pharyngeal tonsil
   d. Salpingopharyngeal fold
4. The nerve that is related to pyriform recess in pharynx:
   a. Recurrent laryngeal
   b. External laryngeal
   c. Internal laryngeal
   d. Glossopharyngeal
5. The only pharyngeal muscle innervated by glossopharyngeal nerve is:
   a. Stylopharyngeus
   b. Palatopharyngeus
   c. Superior constrictor
   d. Middle constrictor
6. 2nd State of degultition is characterized by:
   a. Elevation of larynx
   b. Momentory apnea
   c. Paristalsis of pharyngoesophageal sphincter
   d. Relaxation of pharyngeal constrictors
7. Auditory tube is supplied by:
   a. Ascending pharyngeal
   b. Middle meningeal
   c. Artery of pterygoid canal
   d. All
8. The stage of deglutition which is voluntary to nature:
   a. One
   b. Two
   c. Three
   d. Four

Answers

1. (b) 2. (b) 3. (a) 4. (c) 5. (a) 6. (a) 7. (d) 8. (a)

20 Larynx

- Larynx is that part of upper respiratory tract which is located in the neck.
- It communicates with laryngopharynx above and trachea below.
- It is the organ for production of voice or phonation.
- Acts as a sphincter at the inlet of lower respiratory passages.

SITUATION AND EXTENT

- Lies in anterior midline of neck.
- Extending from the root of tongue to trachea.
- In adult male, it lies in front of C3-C6 vertebrae.
- In children and adult female, lies at higher level.

Size

Length

1. 44 mm in males.
2. 36 mm in females.

CONSTITUTION OF LARYNX (FIG. 20.1)

- Made up of skeletal framework of cartilages.
- Cavity of larynx is lined by mucous membrane.

SKELETON OR CARTILAGES OF LARYNX

Contains nine cartilage, of which three are unpaired and three are paired.

Unpaired cartilages	*Paired cartilages*
1. Thyroid	1. Arytenoid
2. Cricoid	2. Corniculate
3. Epiglottis	3. Cuneiform

Unpaired Cartilage

Thyroid Cartilage

- This is 'V' shaped in cross section.
- It is consists of 2 quadrilateral laminae (right and left) which are fused anteriorly at an angle called thyroid angle.
- Thyroid angle is more prominent in males and responsible for a prominence in front of the neck called "Adam's apple".
- Angle measures 90° in males and 120° in females.
- Each lamina has four borders
  - Upper
  - Lower
  - Anterior
  - Posterior.

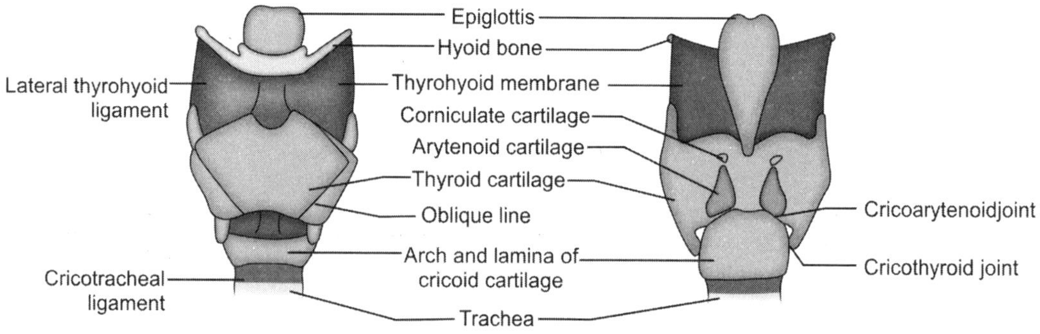
Epiglottis
Hyoid bone
Lateral thyrohyoid ligament
Thyrohyoid membrane
Corniculate cartilage
Arytenoid cartilage
Thyroid cartilage
Oblique line
Cricoarytenoidjoint
Arch and lamina of cricoid cartilage
Cricothyroid joint
Cricotracheal ligament
Trachea

Fig. 20.1: Anterior and posterior aspect of larynx

Two Surfaces
1. Outer
2. Inner.

Cricoid Cartilage

- This is shaped like a signet ring with a narrow anterior arch and a broad posterior lamina.
- It is situated at the level of C6 vertebra and completely encircles the lumen of the larynx.
- It has three surfaces
  - i. Outer
  - ii. Inner
  - iii. Posterior.

Epiglottis

- It is a leaf like structure that extends upwards behind the hyoid bone and the base of tongue.
- It has an upper and a lower end.
- It has an anterior and posterior surface with two lateral border.
- Anterior surface of epiglottis is connected with the base of lougue by a median and two lateral glossoepiglottic folds.

The depression on each side of median fold is called as **vallecula**.

Paired Cartilage

Arytenoid Cartilages

Each arytenoid cartilage is pyramidal in shape and presents as:
- Apex
- Base
- *Two processes:* Muscular and vocal
- *Three surfaces:* Anterolateral, medial, posterior

Cuneiform Cartilages

These are tiny cartilages lying in the posterior inferior part of aryepiglottic folds, above the apex of arytenoids.

Corniculate Cartilages

These are tiny rods of cartilage situated in the aryepiglottic fold anterosuperior to the coneiform cartilages.

LIGAMENTS AND MEMBRANE OF LARYNX

1. Extrinsic
   a. Thyrohyoid membrane
   b. Hyoepiglottic ligament
   c. Cricotracheal ligament.
2. Intrinsic
   a. Quadrate membrane
      i. Vestibular fold
      ii. Aryepiglottic fold
   b. Conus elasticus/Cricovocal membrane
      i. Cricothyroid ligament
      ii. Vocal fold.

CAVITY OF THE LARYNX

- It extends from the inlet of larynx to the lower border of cricoid cartilage.
- Within the laryngeal cavity, the mucous membrane presents with two fold:
  - Vestibular fold/False vocal cords – Acts as exit valve.
  - Vocal folds/True vocal cords.
- Acts as entry valve
- Speech is produced by vibrations of vocal cords.

EPITHELIAL LINING OF LARYNX

Mucous membrane is primarily ciliated pseudostratified columnar epithelium except at
1. Upper part of posterior surface of epiglottis.
2. Aryepiglottic folds covered by stratified squamous non keratinized epitheliam.
3. Vocal folds.

INTRINSIC MUSCLES OF THE LARYNX

Nerve Supply of Larynx

Motor

All intrinsic muscle are supplied by recurrent laryngeal nerve except cricothyroid which is supplied by external laryngeal nerve.

Sensory

Mucous membrane is supplied by:
- Above the vocal cords: Internal laryngeal nerve.
- Below the vocal folds: Recurrent laryngeal nerve.

Table 20.1: Intrinsic muscles of the larynx

Muscle	*Origin*	*Insertion*	*Action*
Cricothyroid–Only muscle outside larynx	Lower border and lateral surface of cricoid	Inferior cornua, Lower border of thyroid cartilage	Tensor of vocal cords
Posterior cricoarytenoid – Triangular	Posterior surface of cricoid	Muscular process of anytenoid	Abducters of vocal cords
Lateral cricoarytenoid	Upper border of arch of cricoid	Muscular process of arytenoids	Adductor of vocal cords
Transverse arytenoids	Posterior surface of one arytenoid	Posterior surface of another aytenoids	Adductor of vocal cords.
Oblique arytenoid and aryepiglotticus	Muscular process of one arytenoids	Apex of the other arytenoids	Closing inlet of larynx Adductor of vocal cord
Thyroarytenoid and thyroepiglottic	Thyroid angle, cricothyroid ligament	Anterolateral surface of arytenoids	Opening inlet of larynx Relaxor of vocal cords.

Blood Supply

- Up to vocal folds:
  - Superior laryngeal artery and vein.
- Below the vocal folds:
  - Inferior laryngeal artery and vein.

Lymphatic Drainage

- Above the vocal folds – Anterosuperior group of deep cervical.
- Below the vocal folds – Posteroinferior group of deep cervical, prelaryngeal nodes.

Clinical and Applied Anatomy

1. **Laryngeal edema** is the collection of fluid in the vestibular fold which result in blockage of glottic area and inability to breath.
2. If internal laryngeal nerve is damaged, there is anesthesia of the mucous membrane.
3. If external laryngeal nerve is damaged, there is weakness of phonation.

PREVIOUS YEAR QUESTIONS

1. Enumerate cartilages of larynx.
2. Write a note on nerve supply of larynx.

MULTIPLE CHOICE QUESTIONS

1. Larynx extends from:
   a. C2-C7 b. C1-C4
   c. C5-C6 d. C3-C6
2. Abductors of Larynx are:
   a. Posterior crico arytenoids
   b. Trenasverse arytenoids
   c. Arytenoid Cricothyroid
   d. All
3. Nerve Supply of mucosa of larynx is:
   a. External and recurrent laryngeal
   b. Internal and recurrent laryngeal
   c. External laryngeal
   d. Superior laryngeal
4. Which laryngeal cartilage is above glottis?
   a. Arytenoid
   b. Epiglottis
   c. Cricoid
   d. Thyroid
5. All of the muscles of larynx are supplied by recurrent laryngeal nerve except:
   a. Cricohyoid
   b. Cricothyroid
   c. Arytenoid
   d. Eryepiglottis
6. Damage to internal laryngeal nerve results in:
   a. Hoarseness
   b Loss of timber of voice
   c. Anesthesia of larynx
   d. Breathing diffculty

Answers

1. (d) 2. (a) 3. (b) 4. (b) 5. (b) 6. (c)

21 Ear

- Ear is the organ of hearing.
- It is also concerned with maintaining the balance of the body.
- In consists of three parts (Fig. 21.1):
  1. External ear
  2. Middle ear
  3. Internal ear

EXTERNAL EAR

It consists of two parts namely:
1. Pinna
2. External auditory meatus

Pinna or Auricle

- Shell like projection present on each side of head
- Consists of single crumpled plato of elastic fibro-crtilage closely lined by skin.
- Lowest part is soft and consists of fibrofatty tissue only and called as lobule of ear.

Features

Lateral Surface

Presents with number of elevation and depressions as:
- Concha
- Helix
- Antihelix
- Scaphoid fossa
- Cymbar concha
- Tragus
- Antitragus
- Lobule of pinna

Medial Surface/cranial Surface

Presents with few elevations as
- Eminentia cenchae
- Eminentia triangularis

Muscles of Pinna

Supplied by branches of facial nerve:
- Extrinsic muscles
  - Auricularis anterior
  - Auricularis posterior
  - Auricularis superior
- Intrinsic muscles
  - Helicis major and minor
  - Tragicus and antitragicus.

Ligaments of Pinna

1. Extrinsic ligament
2. Intrinsic ligament

Blood Supply

1. Posterior auricular branch of external carotid artery.
2. Anterior auricular branches of superficial temporal artery.
3. Branches of occipital artery.
   - Veins follow artery and drains into external jugular and superficial temporal veins.

Lymphatic Drainage

1. Parotid lymph node
2. Mastoid lymph node
3. Upper group of deep cervical lymph node.

Nerve Supply

1. Great auricular nerve
2. Lesser occipital nerve
3. Auriculotemporal nerve
4. Auricular branch of vagus nerve.

External Auditory/Acoustic Meatus

Extends from bottom of concha to tympanic membrane.

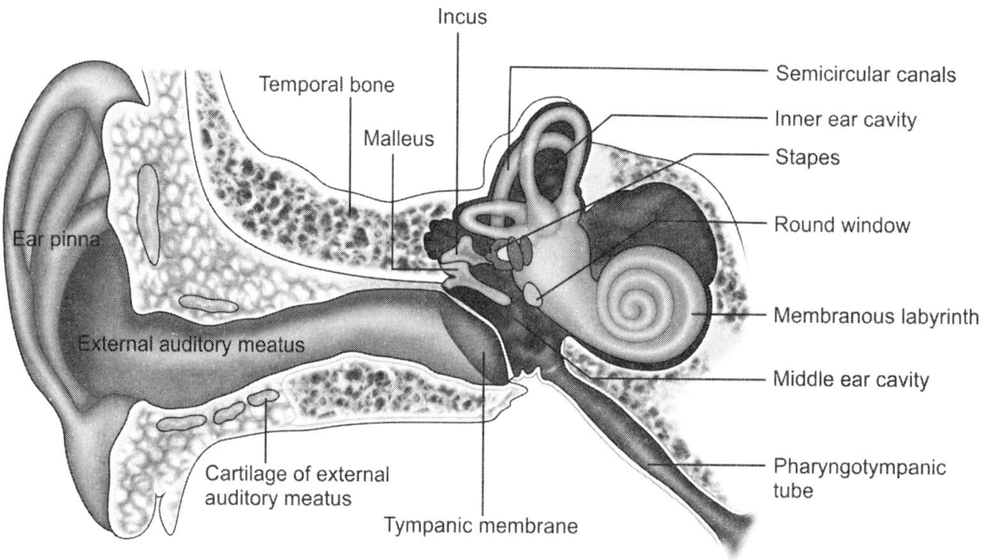
Incus
Temporal bone
Malleus
Semicircular canals
Inner ear cavity
Stapes
Round window
Ear pinna
Membranous labyrinth
External auditory meatus
Middle ear cavity
Pharyngotympanic
tube
Cartilage of external
auditory meatus
Tympanic membrane

Fig. 21.1: Parts of ear

It consists of two parts

1. Cartilaginous part
2. Bony part
   - Tympanic plate of temporal bone
   - Squamous part of temporal bone.

Blood Supply

Artery

1. Anterior auricular artery
2. Posterior auricular artery
3. Deep auricular artery.

Vein

Veins follow artery and drain into external jugular and maxillary veins.

Nerve Supply

1. Auriculotemporal nerve
2. Auricular branch of vagus nerve.

Tympanic Membrane/Ear Drum (Fig. 21.2)

- A thin transparent membrane which separates the external auditory meatus from the middle ear is known as tympanic membrane.
- Oval in outline.

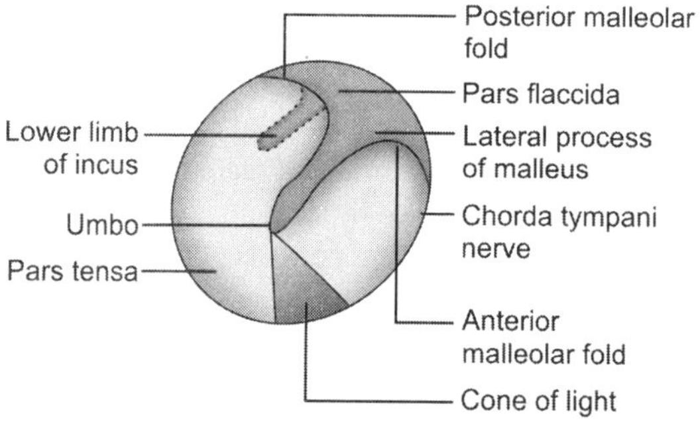
Posterior malleolar
fold
Pars flaccida
Lower limb
of incus
Lateral process
of malleus
Umbo
Chorda tympani
nerve
Pars tensa
Anterior
malleolar fold
Cone of light

Fig. 21.2: Tympanic membrane

Anatomical Features

- It is directed laterally, forward and downwards.
- Make an angle of 55° with the floor of external auditory meatus.
- It is divided into two parts by
  1. Pars tensa—greater part of membrane which is taut.
  2. Pars flacida—part of membrane, which is thin and lax.
- It has two surfaces.
  1. Lateral surface
     - Concave
     - Directed downward, forward and laterally.

2. Medial surface
   - Convex
   - Attached to the handle of malleus
   - This point of attachment is called as Umbo.

Structure

Compared to three Layers
1. Outer cutaneous—continuous with skin.
2. Middle fibrous—has loose connective tissue.
3. Inner mucus—continuous mucus lining of middle ear

Blood Supply

1. Deep auricular branch } Maxillary artery
2. Anterior tympanic branch }
3. Stylomastoid branch—posterior auricular artery:
   – Veins follow artery and drains into external jugular vein and pterygoid venous plexus.

Nerve Supply

1. Auriculotemporal nerve } Outer surface
2. Auricular branch of vagus nerve }
3. Glossopharyngeal nerve—supplies inner surface.

Clinical or Applied Anatomy

- Myringotomy means incision in tympanic membrane.
- It is usually given to drain pus collected in middle ear in acute ear infection.

MIDDLE EAR

- It is narrow, slit-like, air filled space in petrous part of temporal bone between the external ear and inner ear.
- Shape: Biconcave.
- The medial and lateral walls are close to each other in the center.

Communication

1. Anteriorly—nasopharynx through pharyngo-tympanic tube.
2. Posteriorly: mastoid antrum, through aditus to anturm.

Contents

1. Three ear ossicles—malleus, incus and stapes.
2. Two muscles—tensor tympani and stapedius
3. Two nerves—chorda tympani and tympanic plexus.
4. Vessels supplying and draining the middle ear. Strictly speaking middle ear contains only air.

Boundaries

1. Roof—formed by thin sheet of bone called tegman tympani.
2. Floor—formed by plate of petrous temporal bone.
3. Anterior wall—present with canal for bony part of pharyngotympanic tube.
4. Posterior wall—present with bony canal for facial nerve.
5. Medical wall—separates the tympanic cavity from the internal ear.
6. Lateral wall—formed by tympanic membrane
   – The portion—situated above the tympanic membrane is called as **epitympanic recess.**
   – Formed by the squamous part of temporal bone.
   – Opens posteriorly into aditus to antrum.

Ear Ossicles (Fig. 21.3)

- Malleus consists of:
  – Head lies in epitympanic part and articulates with incus
  – Neck
  – Three processes:
    - Handle
    - Anterior process
    - Lateral process
- Incus consists of:
  – Body—articulates with malleus
  – Short process
  – Long process—articulates with stapes
- Stapes
  – Resembles and stirrup
  – Consists of:
    - Head—articulate with incus
    - Neck

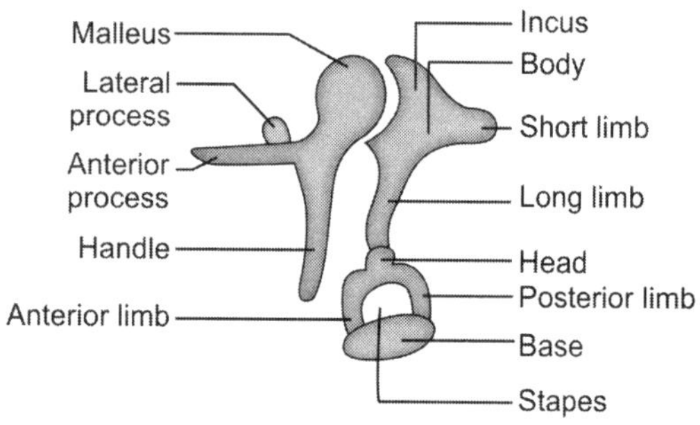
Malleus
Lateral process
Anterior process
Handle
Anterior limb
Incus
Body
Short limb
Long limb
Head
Posterior limb
Base
Stapes

Fig. 21.3: Ear ossicles

- Anterior and posterior limbs
  1. Arise from neck and diverge to attach to base
- Base/foot plate
  1. Reniform in shape
  2. Connected to fenestra vestibuli.

Muscles of Middle Ear

1. Tensor tympani
2. Stapedius

Arterial Supply

- Stylomastoid
- Anterior tympanic
- Petrosal branch
- Superior tympanic branch

(Petrosal branch and Superior tympanic branch > Middle meningeal artery)

- Branches from ascending pharyngeal artery. Internal carotid artery.

Nerve Supply

- Tympanic branch of glossopharyngeal nerve
- Superior and inferior carotico—tympanic nerve.

Clinical and Applied Anatomy

1. In children, upper respiratory tract infectious are common. Infection spreads easily from nasopharynx to middle ear via Eustachian tube.
2. Middle ear infections spread to mastoid antrum through aditus-ad-antrum.

INTERNAL EAR

Located within the petrous part of temporal bone

Structure

- Consists of membranous labyrinth (fluid filled spaces).
- Membranous labyrinth is lodged within bony cavities called **Bony labyrinth**.
- Membranous labyrinth is filled with endolymph and bony labyrinth filled with perilymph.

Bony Labyrinth

Three Parts

1. Vestibule
2. Cochlea
3. Three semicircular canals.

Membranous Labyrinth

Three Parts

1. Cochlear duct
2. Saccule and utricle
3. Three semicircular canals.

Spiral Organ of Corti

- Peripheral organ of hearing present in cochlear duct.
- It rests on the basilar membrane.
- Structures:
  - Inner and outer rod cells
  - Inner and outer hair cells
  - Supporting cells
  - Tunnel of corti
  - Membrana tectoria.
- It is innervated by bipolar neuron located in the spiral ganglion.

Arterial Supply

- Labyrinthine artery.
- Organ of corti has no blood vessels but receives oxygen via cortilymph.

Nerve Supply

- Vestibular nerve
- Cochlear nerve.

Clinical and Applied Anatomy

- Vertigo—it is a feeling of giddiness with subjective sense of rotation. It is a cardinal sign of labyrinthine dysfunction.
- Motion sickness—characterized by vertigo, headache, nausea and vomiting. It is due to excessive stimulation of utricle and saccule.

PREVIOUS YEAR QUESTIONS

1. Write a short note on tympanic membrane.
2. Write a short note on auditory ossicles.
3. Write a short note on boundaries of middle ear.
4. Draw labelled diagram of lateral wall of middle ear.

MULTIPLE CHOICE QUESTIONS

1. Contents of middle ear cavity are all except:
   a. Malleus
   b. Stapes
   c. Chorda tympani
   d. Cells of cord
2. The anterior relation of the middle ear cavity:
   a. Chorda tympani
   b. Tegmen tympani
   c. Tensor tympani
   d. Facial nerve
3. Which one is not a part of membranous labyrinth:
   a. Cochlear duct
   b. Cochlea
   c. Saccule and utricle
   d. Three semicircular canal
4. External ear cartilage is:
   a. Elastic
   b. Hyaline
   c. Fibrous
   d. All
5. Tympanic membrane separates:
   a. Middle ear from internal ear
   b. External auditory meatus from middle ear
   c. External auditory meatus from internal ear
   d. None
6. Inner surface of tympanic membrane is supplied by:
   a. Auriculotemporal
   b. Vagus
   c. Glossopharyngeal
   d. Zygomatic branch of vagus

Answers

1. (d) 2. (c) 3. (b) 4. (a) 5. (b) 6. (c)

22 Cranial Cavity

- Cranial cavity, the highest placed cavity, contains the brain, meninges and venous sinuses, etc.
- Brain is enclosed in three protective membranes called Meninges from outwards to inwards
  i. Dura mater (Outermost)
  ii. Arachnoid mater (Middle)
  iii. Pia mater (Innermost).
- Dura mater—called as pachymeninx
- Arachnoid mater
- Pia mater

  } Called as Leptomeninges

Three meninges are separated from each other by two spaces:

- Subdural space between dura and arachnoid mater
- Subarachnoid space between arachnoid and pia mater, contains cerebrospinal fluid (CSF).

DURA MATER

- Thickest and toughest of the three meninges.
- Develops from mesoderm surrounding the neural tube.
- It consist of two layers:
  i. Outer endosteal layer—serves as inner periosteum (endocranium).
  ii. Inner meningeal layer.

Folds of Meningeal Dura Mater (Fig. 22.1)

1. Falx cerebri
2. Tentorium cerebelli
3. Falx cerebelli
4. Diaphragma sellae.

Falx Cerebri

- Sickle shaped fold of dura mater
- Occupying median longitudinal fissure between two cerebral hemispheres.
- Narrow anterior end is attached to crista galli.

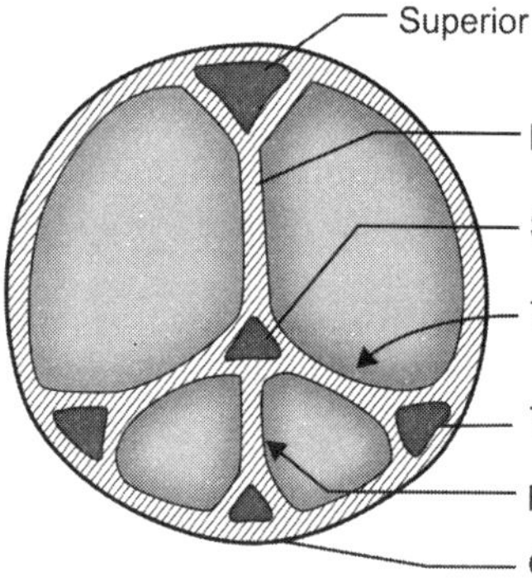
Superior sagittal sinus
Falx cerebri
Straight sinus
Tentorium cerebelli
Transverse sinus
Falx cerebelli
Occipital sinus

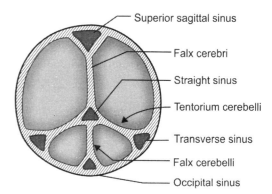

Fig. 22.1: Folds of meningeal dura mater

- Broad posterior end to tentorium cerebelli.
- Two Margin:
  - Upper—convex, attached to lips of sagittal sulcus.
  - Lower—concave, free.
- Venous sinuses enclosed in falx cerebri are:
  - Superior sagittal sinus
  - Inferior sagittal sinus
  - Straight sinus.

Tentorium Cerebelli (Fig. 22.2)

- It is tent-shaped fold of dura mater
- Forms the roof of posterior cranial fossa.
- It separates the cerebellum from occipital lobes of cerebrun.
- It has two margins:
  - Anterior free margin:
    1. 'U' shaped.
    2. Encloses tentorial notch for passage of mid-brain.
  - Outer attached margin:
    1. Convex
    2. Attached to clinoid process and lips of transverse sulcus on occipital bone.

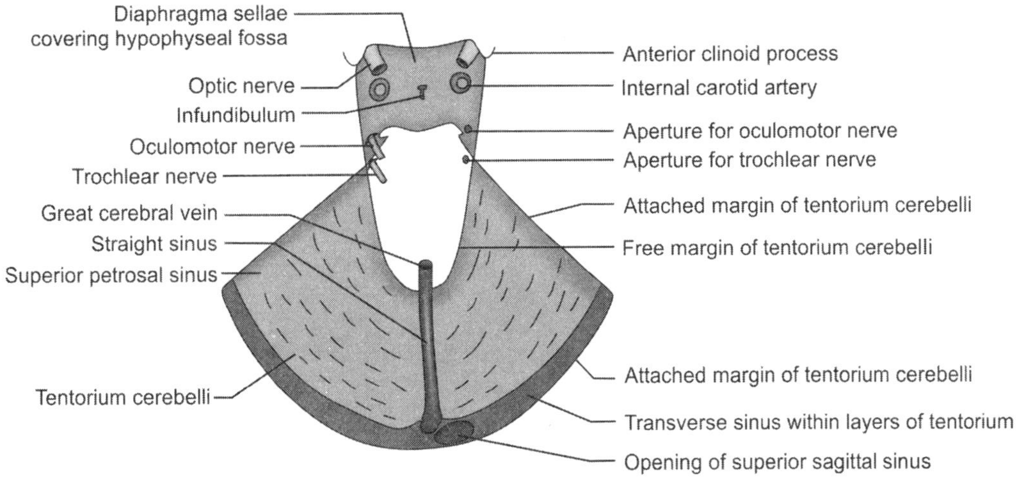
Diaphragma sellae covering hypophyseal fossa
Optic nerve
Infundibulum
Oculomotor nerve
Trochlear nerve
Great cerebral vein
Straight sinus
Superior petrosal sinus
Tentorium cerebelli
Anterior clinoid process
Internal carotid artery
Aperture for oculomotor nerve
Aperture for trochlear nerve
Attached margin of tentorium cerebelli
Free margin of tentorium cerebelli
Attached margin of tentorium cerebelli
Transverse sinus within layers of tentorium
Opening of superior sagittal sinus

Fig. 22.2: Tentorium cerebelli

- It has two surfaces:
  i. Upper surface—convex, attached to falx cerebri.
  ii. Inferior surface—concave, attaced to falx cerebelli
- Free and attached margins cross each other to enclose a triangular area, pierced by oculomotor nerve.
- Venous sinuses enclosed in tentorium cerebelli
  - Transverse sinus
  - Superior petrosal sinus
  - Straight sinus

Falx Cerebelli

- Small sickle-shaped fold of dura mater
- It has two borders:
  - Anterior—concave, free
  - Posterior—convex, attached to inferior surface of tentorium cerebelli above and internal occipital crest below.
- Venous sinuses enclosed in falx cerebelli on each side—occipital sinus.

Diaphragma Sellae

- Small circular, horizontally placed fold of dura mater
- Forms the roof of the hypophyseal fossa.
- Attached anteriorly to tubercular sellae and posteriorly to dorsum sellae.
- It has a central aperture which provides passage to stalk of hypophysis cerebri.

Arterial Supply of Dura Mater

1. Anterior ethmoidal artery
2. Posterior ethmoidal artery
3. Middle meningeal artery
4. Accessory meningeal artery
5. Meningeal branch of ascending pharyngeal artery
6. Ophthalmic artery
7. Occipital artery
8. Internal carotid artery
9. Vertebral artery.

Nerve Supply of Dura Mater

1. In anterior cranial fossa—anterior ethmoid and maxillary nerve.
2. In middle cranial fossa
   a. Maxillary nerve
   b. Mandibular nerve
   c. Trigeminal ganglion.
3. In posterior cranial fossa
   a. Recurrent branches form C1, C2, C3 spinal nerves.
   b. Meningeal branches from IX and X cranial nerve.

Functions of dura mater (intracranial dural venous sinuses) –

1. Accommodates venous sinuses.
2. Acts as protective membrane.
3. Divides cranial cavity into different compartment to provide fixity to brain.

Features

1. Lie between layers of dura mater
2. Lined by endothelium
3. Valveless
4. Receive venous blood and CSF.

Classification

Seven paired and seven unpaired sinuses (Table 22.1).

Table 22.1: Classification of paired and unpaired sinuses

Paired sinuses	*Unpaired sinuses*
• Cavernous	• Superior sagittal
• Superior petrasal	• Inferior sagittal
• Inferior petrasal	• Straight
• Transverse	• Occipital
• Sigmoid	• Anterior intracavernous
• Sphenoparietal	• Posterior intracavernous
• Petrosquamous	• Basilar venous plexus

Unpaired Sinuses

1. Superior sagittal sinus
   i. Begins at crista galli and lodges in sagittal groove.
   ii. Triangular in cross–section
   iii. Communicates with venous lacunae, the sites of drainage of diploic and meningeal veins.
   - Tributaries
     i. Superior cerebral venous
     ii. Parietal emissary veins
     iii. Small veins from nasal cavity
     iv. Veins from frontal air sinus.
   - Clinical and applied anatomy
     Spread of infection from nose, scalp and diploe to the superior sagittal sinus may cause its thrombosis.
2. Inferior sagittal sinus
   i. Small venous channel present in falx cerebri.
   ii. It ends by joining the great cerebral vein to form straight sinus.
3. Straight sinus
   i. Continuation of inferior sagittal sinus
   ii. Terminates into the left transverse sinus.

Paired Sinuses

1. Transverse sinus
   a. Right sinus is continuation of superior sagittal sinus.
   b. Left sinus is smaller and continuation of straight sinus.
   c. It ends at mastoid angle of parietal bone by continuing as sigmoid sinus.
   d. Tributaries
      i. Superior petrosal sinus
      ii. Inferior cerebral veins.
      iii. Inferior cerebellar veins.
2. Sigmoid sinus
   a. Direct continuation of transverse sinus
   b. It is sigmoid or 'S' shaped.
   c. It lodges in the 'S' shaped groove present in temporal and occipital bone.
      Tributaries
      1. Mastoid and condylar emissary veins
      2. Cerebellar veins
      3. Internal auditory veins.
3. Cavernous sinus
   a. Features
      i. 2 cm long and 1 cm wide
      ii. Situated in middle cranial fossa between two layers of dura, one on either side of body of sphenoid.
      iii. Divided into small spaces or caverns by trabeculae.
      iv. It consists of roof, floor, medial and lateral walls.

1. Roof	} formed by meningeal layer of dura mater	
2. Lateral wall		
3. Medial wall	} formed by endosteal layer of dura mater	
4. Floor		

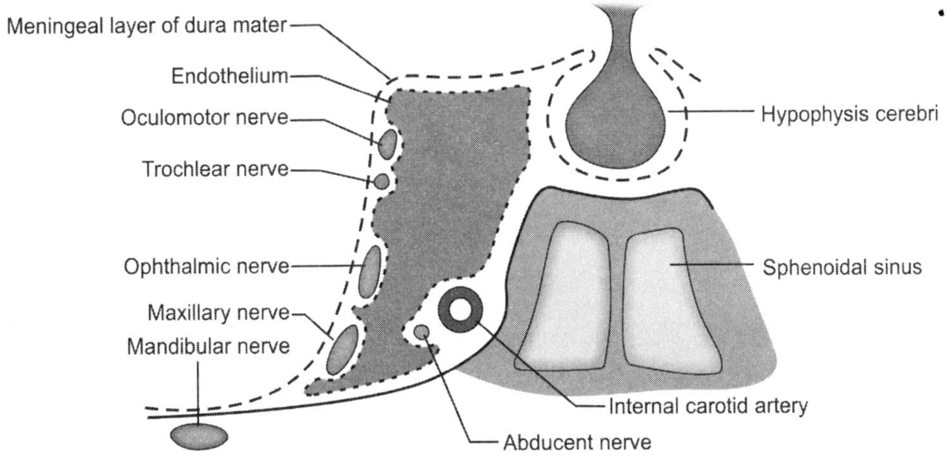
Meningeal layer of dura mater
Endothelium
Oculomotor nerve
Trochlear nerve
Ophthalmic nerve
Maxillary nerve
Mandibular nerve
Hypophysis cerebri
Sphenoidal sinus
Internal carotid artery
Abducent nerve

Fig. 22.3: Relations of cavernous sinus

b. Extent
   i. Anterior—up to medial end of superior orbital fissure.
   ii. Posterior—up to apex of petrous temporal bone.
c. Relations (Fig. 22.3)
   i. Superior
      1. Optic tract
      2. Internal carotid artery
   ii. Inferior
      1. Foramen Lacerium
      2. Junction of body and greater wing of sphenoid.
   iii. Medial
      1. Pituitary gland.
      2. Sphenoid air sinus
   iv. Lateral
      1. Temporal bone of cerebral hemisphere
      2. Trigeminal cave.
   v. Anterior
      1. Superior orbital fissure
      2. Apex of orbit
   vi. Posterior
      1. Crus cerebri of mid brain
      2. Apex of petrous temporal bone

Structures Present Within the Lateral Wall of Sinus

1. Oculomotor neve
2. Trochlear nerve
3. Ophthalmic nerve
4. Maxillary nerve

Structures Passing through the Sinus

1. Internal carotid artery
2. Abducent nerve

Tributaries of Cavernous Sinus (Fig. 22.4)

1. From orbit
   a. Superior ophthalmic vein
   b. Inferior ophthalmic vein
   c. Central vein of retina
2. From meninges
   a. Sphenoparietal sinus
   b. Anterior trunk of middle meningeal vein

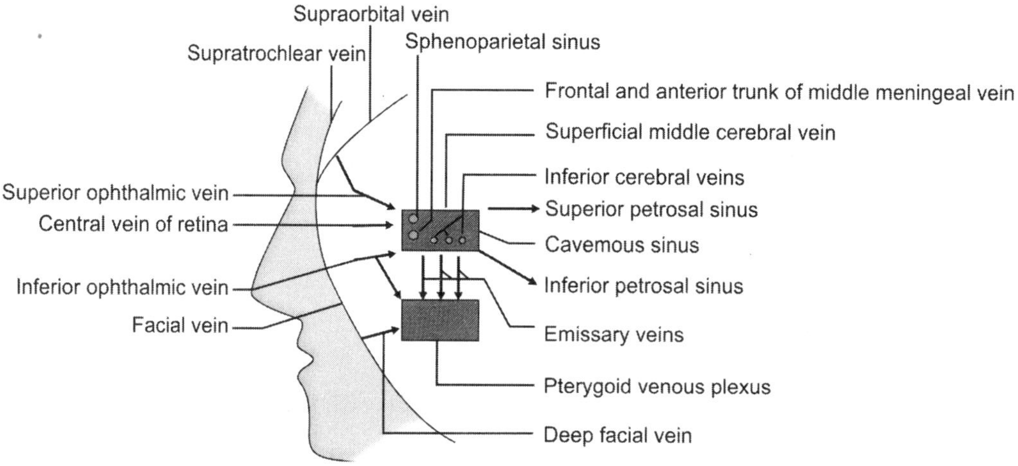

Supraorbital vein
Supratrochlear vein
Sphenoparietal sinus
Frontal and anterior trunk of middle meningeal vein
Superficial middle cerebral vein
Inferior cerebral veins
Superior petrosal sinus
Cavernous sinus
Inferior petrosal sinus
Emissary veins
Pterygoid venous plexus
Deep facial vein
Superior ophthalmic vein
Central vein of retina
Inferior ophthalmic vein
Facial vein

Fig. 22.4: Tributaries of cavernous sinus

3. From brain
   a. Superficial middle cerebral vein
   b. Inferior cerebral vein.

Communications (Table 22.2)

Table 22.2: Communication of sinuses

Communications	*Via/through*
Transverse sinus	Superior petrosal sinus
Internal jugular vein	Inferior petrosal sinus
Pterygoid venous plexus	Emissory vein
Facial vein (Via 2 routes)	• Superior ophthalmic an angular veins • Emissory vein—pterygoid venous plexus—deep facial vein
Opposite cavernous sinus	• Anterior intercavernous sinus • Posterior intercavernous sinus
Superior sagittal sinus	• Superficial middle cerebral vein • Superior anastomatic vein basilar venous plexus.
Internal vestebral venous plexus	

Clinical and Applied Anatomy

Thrombosis of cavernous sinus is due to passage of septic emboli from an infection in dangerous area of face through facial plexus of veins to deep facial veins.

- Features of cavernous sinus thrombosis (CST):
  i. Severe pain in eye and forehead.
  ii. Ophthalmoplegia.
  iii. Marked edema of eyelids with exophthalmos.

HYPOPHYSIS CEREBRI/PITUITARY GLAND

- It is a small endocrine gland.
- Situated in hypophyseal fossa on body of sphenoid.
- Suspended from the floor of 3rd ventricle of brain by a narrow stalk called Infundibulum.

Shape and Measurement/Gross Anatomy

- Oval in shape
- Size—8 mm × 12 mm
- Weight—500 mg.

Relations

- Superior—covered by diaphragma sellae, optic chiasma
- Inferior—sphenoidal air sinus
- Lateral—cavernous sinus with its contents
- Anterior to stalk—anterior intercavernous sinus
- Posterior to stalk—posterior intercavernous sinus.

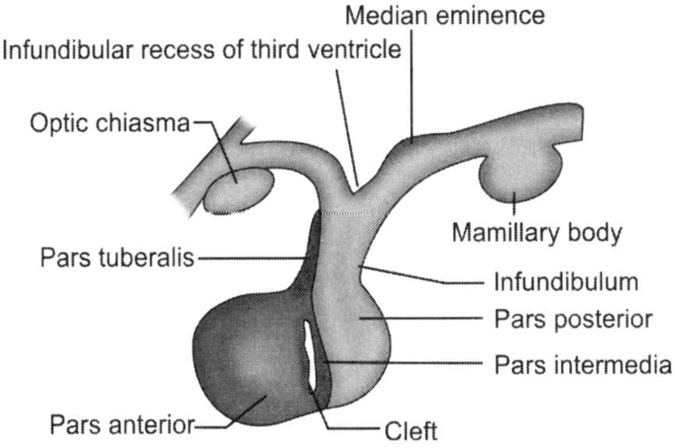
Median eminence
Infundibular recess of third ventricle
Optic chiasma
Mamillary body
Pars tuberalis
Infundibulum
Pars posterior
Pars intermedia
Pars anterior
Cleft

Fig. 22.5: Subdivisions of hypophysis cerebri

Subdivisions (Fig. 22.5)

1. Adenohypophysis
   a. Develops as an upward growth (Rathke's pouch) from stomodeum.
   b. Forms anterior lobe and consists of (Table 22.3):
      i. Pars anterior
      ii. Pars intermedius
      iii. Pars tuberalis.
2. Neurohypophysis
   a. Develops as a down growth from the floor of diencephalon.
   b. Forms posterior lobe and consists of
      i. Pars posterior
      ii. Infundibulum
      iii. Median Eminence.

Arterial Supply

1. Superior hypophyseal artery
2. Branches of internal carotid artery.
3. Inferior hypophyseal artery

Venous Drainage

Short veins drain into dural venous sinuses

Hypothalamo—Hypophyseal Portal System

Consists of two Sets of Capillary Plexuses

1. Infundibular and median eminence plexus
2. Sinusoids of pars anterior—Various part of pituitary gland and their cell types with hormone secreted (Microscopic anatomy).

Clinical and Applied Anatomy

Symptoms of pituitary tumors are divided into two groups:
1. Endocrine symptoms—due to excessive secretion of particular hormones.
2. Pressure symptoms—bitemporal hemianopia, due to pressure on the optic chiasma.

CEREBROSPINAL FLUID

Definition

Clear, colorless and odorless fluid which fills the subarachnoid space and surrounds the brain and spinal cord (Fig. 22.6).

Table 22.3: Subdivisions of hypophysis cerebri

Part	*Cell types/Nuclei*	*Hormones secreted*
Pars anterior	Acidophil cells (a-cells)	• Growth hormone • Prolactin.
	Basophil cells (b-cells)	• Adrenocorticotrophic hormone (ACTH) • Thyrotrophic hormone (TSH). • Gonadotrophic hormones. a. Follicle stimulating hormone (FSH) b. Leutinising hormone (LH)
Pars intermedia		Melanocyte stimulating hormone
Pars posterior	Supraoptic nucleus of hypothalamus Paraventricular nucleus of hypothalamus	• Vasopressin/Antidiuretic hormones. • Oxytocin

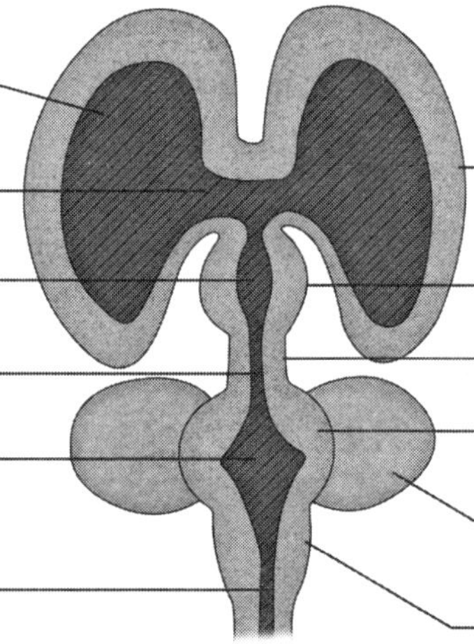
Lateral ventricle
Interventricular foramen
Third ventricle
Cerebral aqueduct
Fourth ventricle
Central canal
Cerebrum
Diencephalon
Midbrain
Pons
Cerebellum
Medulla oblongata

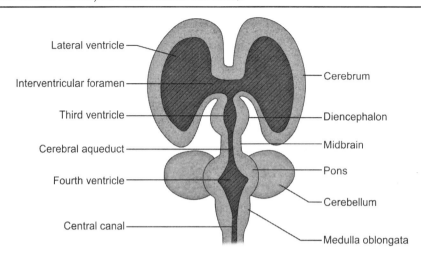

Fig. 22.6: Cerebrospinal fluid

Secretion of CSF

Secreted by choroid plexus of lateral, 3rd and 4th ventricles.

Characteristics of CSF

i. Total volume—130-150 ml.
ii. Rate of production—200 ml/hour

Formation and Circulation of CSF

Formation : Lateral ventricles

↓

Circulation : Interventricular foramina (Foramen of Monro)

↓

IIIrd Ventricle

↓

Aqueduct of sylvius/midbrain

↓

IVth ventricle

↓

Foramen of Luschka and magendie

↓

Cerebellomedullary cistem

↓

Subarachnoid space

The CSF is absorbed back into circulation via the arachnoid villi from where it enters the superior sagittal sinus.

Functions of CSF

1. Acts as a hydraulic shock absorber.
2. Provides a constant environment to neurons.
3. Helps in reduction of weight of brain.
4. Convey nutritive material to CNS.
5. Helps in removal of wasts.

Clinical and Applied Anatomy

1. CSF can be obtained by
   a. Lumbar puncture
   b. Cisternal puncture
   c. Ventricular puncture
2. Biochemical analysis of CSF is diagnostic in various diseases.
3. Obstruction to flow of CSF in ventricular system leads to hydrocephalus in children.
4. Obstruction to flow of CSF in vertebral canal produces.

Froin's syndrome or loculation syndrome

PREVIOUS YEAR QUESTIONS

1. Write a short note on Falx cerebri.
2. Enumerate paired and unpaired dural venous sinuses.
3. Mention cavernous sinus under following head with diagrams:

a. Situation
b. Boundaries
c. Contents
d. Communication
e. Tributaries.

4. Briefly describe applied anatomy of cavernous sinus.
5. Write a short note on superior sagittal sinus.
6. Describe pituitary gland under following heads:
   a. Anatomy
   b. Development
   c. Applied anatomy
7. Write a short note on tentorium cerebelli.

MULTIPLE CHOICE QUESTIONS

1. Cavernous sinus does not communicate with the:
   a. Ophthalmic vein
   b. Internal jugular vein
   c. External jugular vein
   d. Pterygoid plexus.
2. Connecting vein between facial vein and cavernous sinus is:
   a. Superior ophthalmic
   b. Inferior ophthalmic
   c. Connecting pterygoid plexus
   d. None
3. Which of the following is a paired venous sinus of dura mater:
   a. Cavernous sinus
   b. Superior petrosal
   c. Transverse
   d. All
4. Cavernous sinus communicates directly with all except:
   a. Inferior petrosal sinus
   b. Pterygoid venous plexus
   c. Veins in orbit
   d. Sigmoid and straight sinus
5. Total quantity of CSF is:
   a. 150 ml
   b. 250 ml
   c. 500 ml
   d. 750 ml
6. The transverse venous sinus continues as:
   a. Straight sinus
   b. Cavernous sinus
   c. Sigmoid sinus
   d. Ethmoidal sinus
7. All structures are related to cavernous sinus except:
   a. II or optic nerve
   b. IV nerve
   c. VI nerve
   d. Mandibular division of trigeminal nerve
8. Sella turcica lies above:
   a. Pons
   b. Frontal sinus
   c. Foramen ovale
   d. Sphenoidal sinus
9. CSF is partly absorbed by lymphatics around:
   a. I, II, VII, VIII
   b. I, II, VI, VII
   c. I, III, VII, VIII
   d. I, II, VI, VIII

Answers

1. (c) 2. (a) 3. (d) 4. (d) 5. (a) 6. (c) 7. (a) 8. (d) 9. (a)

23 Ventricular System

- There are a total of five ventricles present in central nervous system (CNS).
- In brain:
  i. Two lateral ventricles.
  ii. One 3rd ventricle.
  iii. One 4th ventricle.
- In spinal cord:
  i. Terminal ventricles.

LATERAL VENTRICLES

Definition

They are two irregular cavities situated one in each cerebral hemispere.

Features

a. C-shaped cavity lined by ependyma.
b. Filled with CSF.
c. Two lateral ventricles are separated from each other by the septum pellucidum.
d. Communicates with 3rd ventricle by interventricular foramen of Monro.

Parts of Lateral Ventricle (Fig. 23.1)

- Body
- Anterior horn
- Posterior horn
- Inferior horn—largest horn

PARTS OF LATERAL VENTRICLES WITH BOUNDARIES (TABLE 23.1)

Third Ventricles

- It is an interthalamic space
- Lined by ependyma
- Represents primitive cavity of forebrain vesicle.

Parts of Third Ventricle

Parts of third ventricle are given in Table 23.2.

FOURTH VENTRICLE

- 4th ventricle is cavity of hind brain.
- Lies between cerebellum dorsally and pons and medulla ventrally.
- Diamond-shaped.

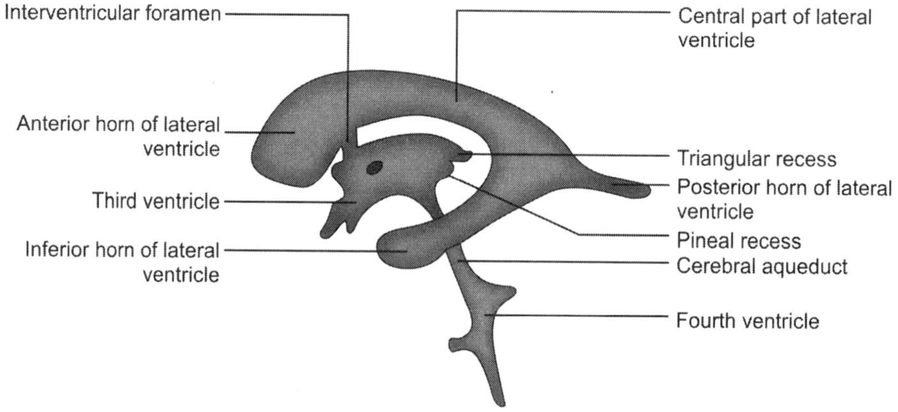
Interventricular foramen
Central part of lateral ventricle
Anterior horn of lateral ventricle
Triangular recess
Third ventricle
Posterior horn of lateral ventricle
Pineal recess
Inferior horn of lateral ventricle
Cerebral aqueduct
Fourth ventricle

Fig. 23.1: Parts of lateral ventricle

Table 23.1: Parts of lateral ventricle with boundaries

Parts	*Features*	*Roof*	*Floor*	*Medial Wall*
Body	Extends from interventricular foramen to corpus callosum – Triangular	Corpus callosum	• Caudate nucleus • Lateral part of thalamus	• Posterior part of septum of pellucidum • Body of fornix
Anterior horn	Lies of frontal lobe Roughly triangular	Body of corpus callosum	• Head of caudate nucleus laterally. • Rostrum of corpus callosum medially	Anterior part of septum pellucidum
Posterior horn	Lies in occipital lobe	Tapetum of corpus callosum	Lateral wall is formed by tapetum of corpus cllosum No floor	• Bulb of posterior horn • Calcar avis
Inferior horn	Extends into temporal lobe	• Tapetum. • Tail of caudate nucleus • Amygdaloid body	• Hippocampus • Collateral eminence	Choroid plexus

Parts of 4th Ventricle

1. Superior angle
2. Inferior angle
3. Supero-lateral boundary
4. Inferolateral boundary
5. Roof—formed by
   a. Upper part
   b. Lower part
6. Floor
   - Also known as Rhomboid fossa.
   - Formed by posterior surface of pons and upper open part of medulla oblongata.
   - Contains cranial nerve nuclei of VI, VII, X and XII nerves.

Table 23.2: Parts of third Ventricle

Parts	*Formed by*
Anterior wall	• Lamina terminalis • Anterior commissure • Diverging column of fornix
Posterior wall	• Suprapineal recess • Pineal body • Aqueduct of midbrain
Roof	• Ependyma • Tela choroidea and body of fornix • Fringes of choroid plexus
Floor	• Optic chiasma • Tuber cinereum • Infundibulum • Pair of mamillary bodies • Hypothalamus
5. Lateral walls	• Medial surface of thalamus—upper part • Hypothalamic nuclei—lower part
6. Two recess	• Triangular recess/vulva • Pineal recess

Floor of Fourth Ventricle (Fig. 23.2)

Features

1. **Median sulcus**—divides floor into two symmetrical halves.
2. **Sulcus limitans**—divides each half into medial and lateral area.
3. **Superior fovea**—depression present superiorly on sulcus limitans.
4. **Facial colliculus**—elongated Eminence at the level of superior fovea.
5. **Inferior fovea**—depression present inferiorly on sulcus limitans.
6. **Hypoglossal triangle**—inverted triangular elevation at the level of inferior fovea.
7. **Locus ceruleus**—bluish gray area of the rostral end of sulcus limitans.
8. **Vestibular area**—Present lateral to sulcus limitans.

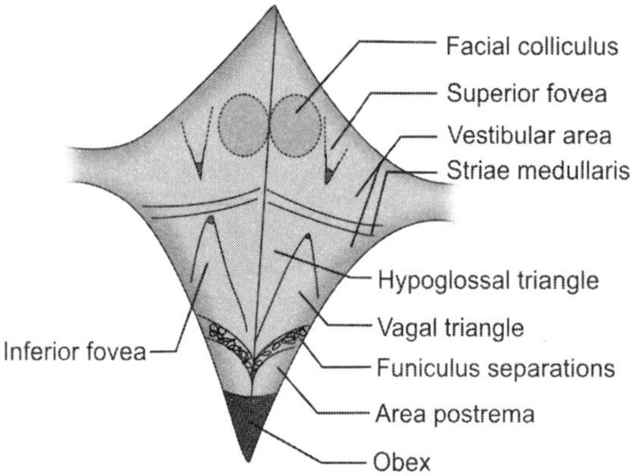
Facial colliculus
Superior fovea
Vestibular area
Striae medullaris
Hypoglossal triangle
Vagal triangle
Inferior fovea
Funiculus separations
Area postrema
Obex

Fig. 23.2: Floor of fourth ventricle

9. **Vagal triangle**—Area between vestibular area and hypoglossal triangle.
10. **Funiculus separations**—separates vagal triangle from area postrema.
11. Stria medullaris
    a. Recesses of 4th ventricle
        i. Lateral—two in number
        ii. Median dorsal
        iii. Lateral dorsal—two in number.

Clinical Applied Anatomy

Viral centers are situated in the vicinity of vagal triangle. An injury to this area is fatal.

Terminal Ventricle of Spinal Cord

Last part of central canal is dilated and forms terminal ventricle.

PREVIOUS YEAR QUESTIONS

1. Write a short note on floor of fourth ventricle with well labeled diagram.
2. Briefly describe lateral ventricle of brain.

MULTIPLE CHOICE QUESTIONS

1. There are total how many ventricles present in central nervous system (CNS):
    a. Three   b. Four
    c. Five   d. Six
2. Which is the largest horn of lateral ventricle:
    a. Body   b. Anterior horn
    c. Posterior horn   d. Inferior horn
3. All of these are true for fourth ventricle except:
    a. Cavity of hind brain
    b. Diamond shaped
    c. Communicates with 3rd ventricle by interventricular foramen
    d. Lies between cerebellum dorsally and pars and medulla ventrally.
4. Last part of central canal is formed by:
    a. Lateral ventricle   b. 3rd ventricle
    c. 4th ventricle   d. Terminal ventricle.

Answers

1. (c)   2. (d)   3. (c)   4. (d)

24 Brainstem

Brainstem consists of:
- Medulla oblongata
- Pons
- Midbrain

MEDULLA OBLONGATA (FIG. 24.1)

- Lowest part of brainstem.
- It is the caudal and ventral part of hind brain.
- Lodged in inferior cerebellar notch.
- Lies on the basi—occiput.

Extent

Extends from lower border of pons to a plane just above the first cranial nerve, where it is continuous with spinal cord.

Shape

Piriform in shape.

External Features

- Anterior median fissure
- Posterior median sulcus
- Anterolateral sulcus
- Posterolateral sulcus

Anterior fissure and sulci divide medulla into following regions:
- Anterior region
- Lateral region
- Posterior region
  a. Caudal part
  b. Rostral part

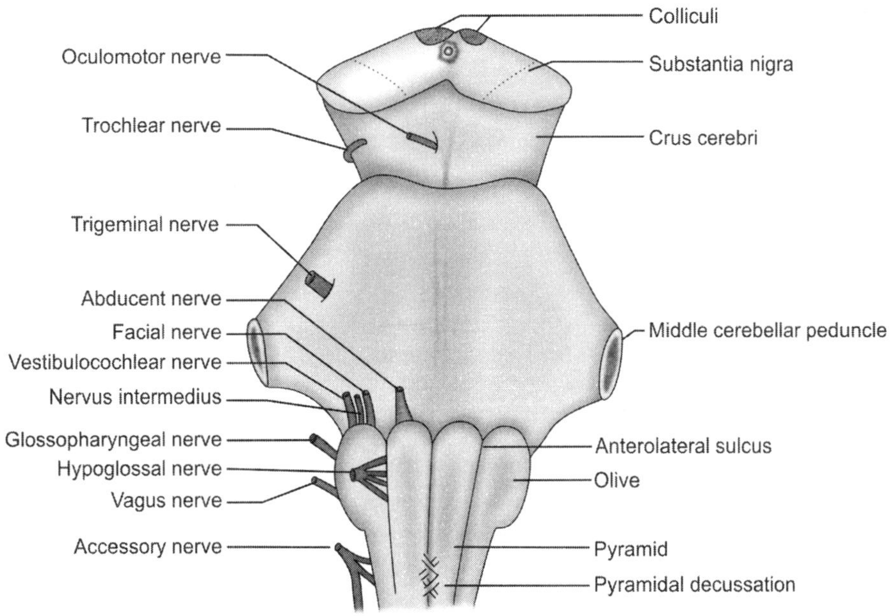
Colliculi
Oculomotor nerve
Substantia nigra
Trochlear nerve
Crus cerebri
Trigeminal nerve
Abducent nerve
Facial nerve
Middle cerebellar peduncle
Vestibulocochlear nerve
Nervus intermedius
Glossopharyngeal nerve
Anterolateral sulcus
Hypoglossal nerve
Olive
Vagus nerve
Accessory nerve
Pyramid
Pyramidal decussation

Fig. 24.1: Attachment of cranial nerve to brainstem

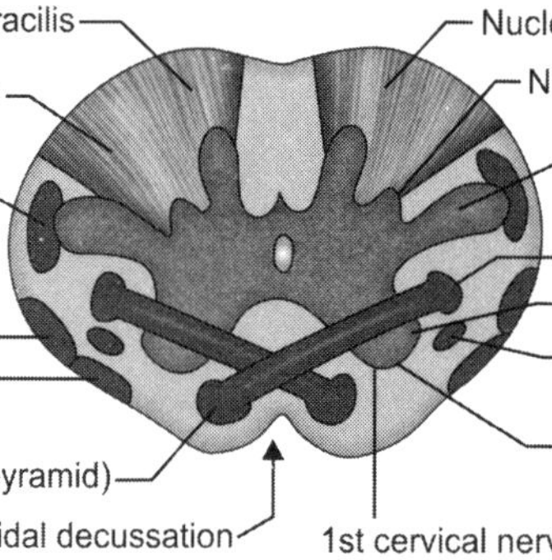
Fasciculus gracilis
Fasciculus cuneatus
Spinal tract of trigeminal nerve
Dorsal and ventral Spinocerebellar tracts
Corticospinal fibers (within pyramid)
Pyramidal decussation
1st cervical nerve nucleus
Nucleus gracilis
Nucleus cuneatus
Nucleus of spinal tract of trigeminal nerve
Lateral cortico-spinal tract
Spinal nucleus of accessory nerve
Lateral spinothalamic tract
Grey matter of anterior horn separated from central grey

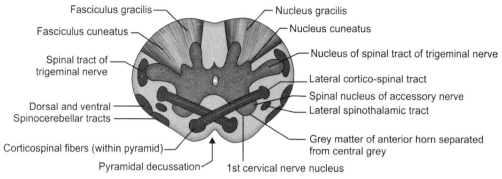

Fig. 24.2: Transverse section at the level of pyramidal decussation

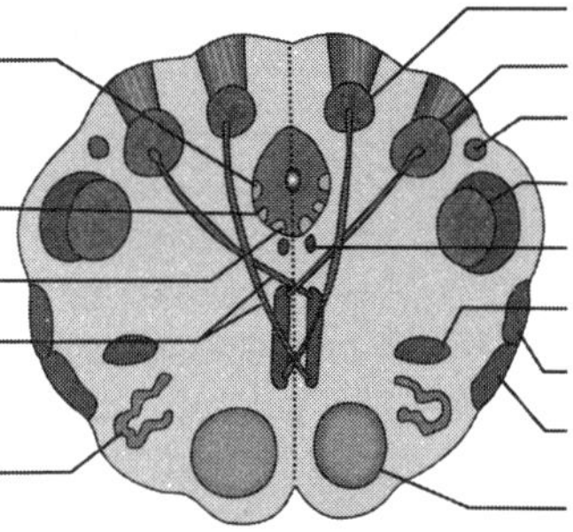
Nucleus of tractus solitarius
Dorsal nucleus of vagus
Hypoglossal nucleus
Internal arcuate fibers (sensory decussation)
Inferior olivary nucleus
Nucleus gracilis
Nucleus cuneatus
Accessory cuneate nucleus
Nucleus of spinal tract of trigeminal nerve
Medial longitudinal bundle
Lateral spinothalamic tract
Dorsal tract
Ventral spinocerebellar tracts
Pyramid

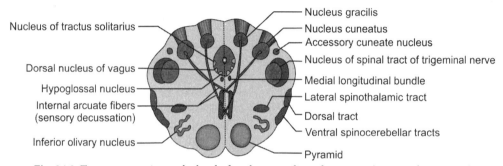

Fig. 24.3: Transverse section at the level of nucleus gracilis and cuneatus (sensory decussation)

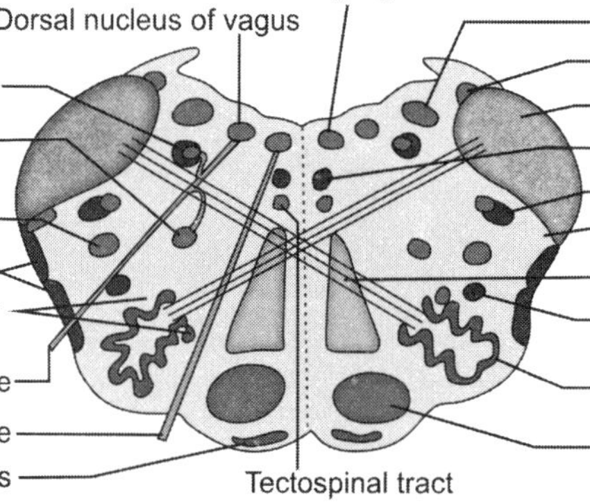
Hypoglossal nucleus
Dorsal nucleus of vagus
Nucleus of tractus solitarius
Nucleus ambiguus
Rubrospinal tract
Spinocerebellar tracts
Medial and dorsal accessory olivary nuclei
Vagus nerve
Hypoglossal nerve
Arcuate nucleus
Tectospinal tract
Vestibular nuclei
Dorsal cochlear nucleus
Inferior cerebellar peduncle
Medial longitudinal bundle
Spinal tract of trigeminal nerve
Ventral cochlear nucleus
Medial lemniscus
Lateral spinothalamic tract
Inferior olivary nucleus
Pyramid

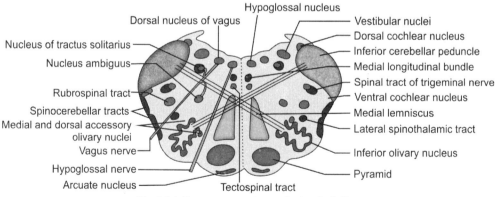

Fig. 24.4: Transverse section at the level of olive

Internal Features

It is studied in transverse section taken at three different levels:

1. Transverse section at the level of *Pyramidal decussation* (Fig. 24.2)
2. Transverse section at the level of nucleus gracilis and cuneatus (Sensory decussation) (Fig. 24.3).
3. Transverse section at the level of olive (Fig. 24.4).

PONS/METENCEPHALON

- Word 'pons' means 'bridge'
- It is the middle part of brainstem
- Connects midbrain with medulla.

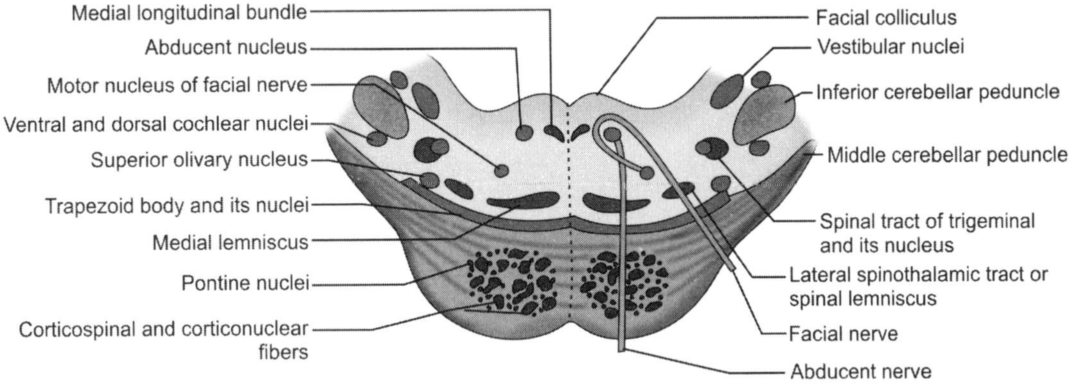
Medial longitudinal bundle
Abducent nucleus
Motor nucleus of facial nerve
Ventral and dorsal cochlear nuclei
Superior olivary nucleus
Trapezoid body and its nuclei
Medial lemniscus
Pontine nuclei
Corticospinal and corticonuclear fibers
Facial colliculus
Vestibular nuclei
Inferior cerebellar peduncle
Middle cerebellar peduncle
Spinal tract of trigeminal and its nucleus
Lateral spinothalamic tract or spinal lemniscus
Facial nerve
Abducent nerve

Fig. 24.5: Transverse section of Pons at the level of facial colliculus or lower (caudal) part

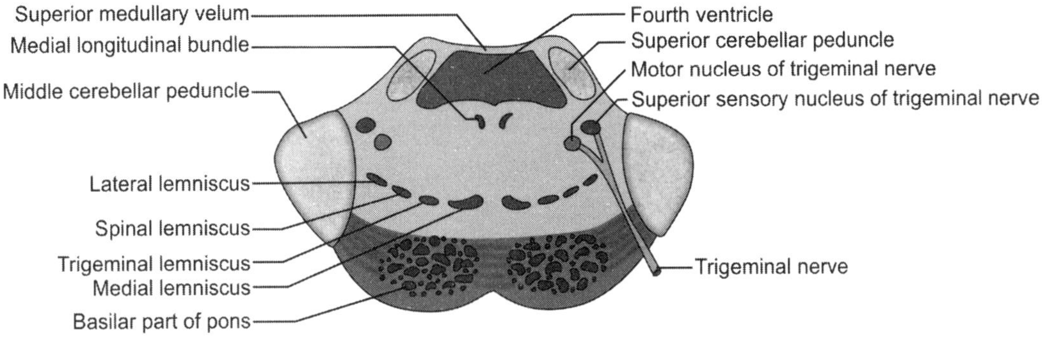
Superior medullary velum
Medial longitudinal bundle
Middle cerebellar peduncle
Lateral lemniscus
Spinal lemniscus
Trigeminal lemniscus
Medial lemniscus
Basilar part of pons
Fourth ventricle
Superior cerebellar peduncle
Motor nucleus of trigeminal nerve
Superior sensory nucleus of trigeminal nerve
Trigeminal nerve

Fig. 24.6: Transverse section of Pons at the level of rostral part or upper part

Relations

Ventral: Clivus
Dorsal: 4th ventricle and cerebellum
Lateral: Middle cerebellar peduncles.

Extent

Upper end of medulla oblongata to the cerebral peduncles of midbrain.

External Features—Two Surface

i. Ventral surface
ii. Dorsal surface.

Internal Structure

On cross section, the pons is studied in two parts:

Ventral/Basilar Part

a. Descending longitudinal fibers
   i. Coticospinal fiber
   ii. Corticonuclear fiber
   iii. Corticopontine fiber
b. Transverse fibers
c. Nuclei pontis

Tegmental part/Dorsal Part

a. Transverse section of pons at the level of facial colliculus or lower (caudal) part (Fig. 24.5)
b. Transverse section of pons at the level of rostral part or upper part (Fig. 24.6)

MID BRAIN

- Shortest segment of brainstem
- 2 cm long.
- Lies in posterior cranial fossa.

Extent

From pons to diencephalon

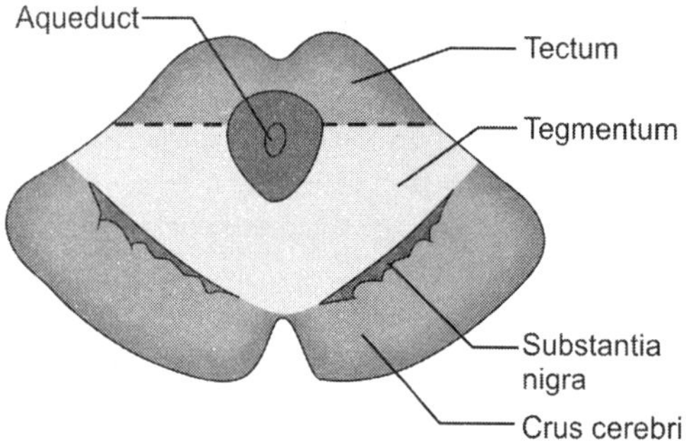
Aqueduct
Tectum
Tegmentum
Substantia nigra
Crus cerebri

Fig. 24.7: Components of cerebral peduncle

Components (Fig. 24.7)

- Midbrain can be divided into two cerebral peduncles.
- Each cerebral peduncle consists of four parts. These are:
  a. Crus cerebri
  b. Substantia nigra
  c. Tegmentum
  d. Tectum

Internal Structure

- Midbrain is situated in two transverse sections:
  1. Transverse section of midbrain at the level of inferior colliculus (Fig. 24.8).
  2. Transverse section of midbrain at the level of superior colliculus (Fig. 24.9).

PREVIOUS YEAR QUESTIONS

1. Draw a labeled diagram to show attachment of cranial nerve to brainstem.
2. Draw a labeled diagram of transverse section of midbrain at the level of superior colliculus.

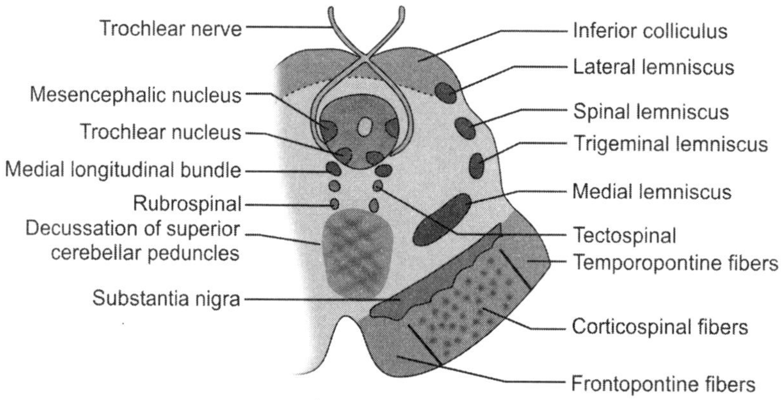
Trochlear nerve
Mesencephalic nucleus
Trochlear nucleus
Medial longitudinal bundle
Rubrospinal
Decussation of superior cerebellar peduncles
Substantia nigra
Inferior colliculus
Lateral lemniscus
Spinal lemniscus
Trigeminal lemniscus
Medial lemniscus
Tectospinal
Temporopontine fibers
Corticospinal fibers
Frontopontine fibers

Fig. 24.8: Transverse section of midbrain at the level of inferior colliculus

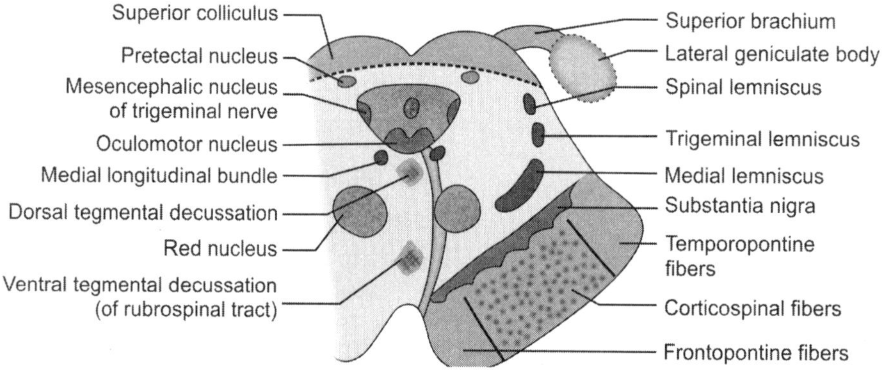
Superior colliculus
Pretectal nucleus
Mesencephalic nucleus of trigeminal nerve
Oculomotor nucleus
Medial longitudinal bundle
Dorsal tegmental decussation
Red nucleus
Ventral tegmental decussation (of rubrospinal tract)
Superior brachium
Lateral geniculate body
Spinal lemniscus
Trigeminal lemniscus
Medial lemniscus
Substantia nigra
Temporopontine fibers
Corticospinal fibers
Frontopontine fibers

Fig. 24.9: Transverse section of midbrain at the level of superior colliculus

3. Draw a labeled diagram of transverse section of open part of medulla oblongata.
4. Draw a labeled diagram of TS of medulla oblongata at pyramidal decussation.

MULTIPLE CHOICE QUESTIONS

1. Unpaired structure in brain
   a. Basilar artery
   b. Vertebral artery
   c. Middle cerebral artery
   d. Anterior cerebral artery
2. Nucleus in brain common to IX, X, XI cranial nerves
   a. Nucleus solitarius
   b. Mucleus ambiguous
   c. Nucleus dentate
   d. Red nucleus
3. Which is not a part of brainstem
   a. Medulla oblongata
   b. Pons
   c. Cerebellum
   d. Midbrain
4. Which is the shortest segment of brainstem
   a. Midbrain
   b. Pons
   c. Medulla oblongata
   d. Diencephalon
5. Which of the following connects midbrain with medulla
   a. Cerebellum
   b. Cerebral hemisphere
   c. Diencephalon
   d. Metencephalon

Answers

1. (a)   2. (b)   3. (c)   4. (a)   5. (d)

25 Cerebellum

- Cerebellum/little brain is the largest part of hind-brain.
- Situated in the posterior cranial fossa behind the pons and medulla, separated by 4th ventricle.
- It is an infratentorial structure that coordinates voluntary movements of the body.

ANATOMICAL FEATURES

- Cerebellum is made up of medullary core and 4 pairs of nuclei.
- Medullary care is made up of white matter and surrounded by cortical gray matter.
- Oval in shape.
- Consists of 2 cerebellar hemisphere that are united by each other through median vermis.

SURFACES

- Superior surface—convex.
- Inferior surface—shows a deep median notch called. **Vallecula**, which separates the right and left hemisphere.

LOBES

- *Anterior lobe:* Lies in anterior part, separated from the middle lobe by the fissura prima.
- *Middle/Posterior lobe:* Largest, limited in front by fissura prima and by posterolateral fissure.
- Flocculonodular lobe:
  - Smallest
  - Lies on inferior surface.

PARTS OF CEREBELLUM

Cerebellum is subdivided into numerous small parts by following fissures (Fig. 25.1):

a. Horizontal fissure

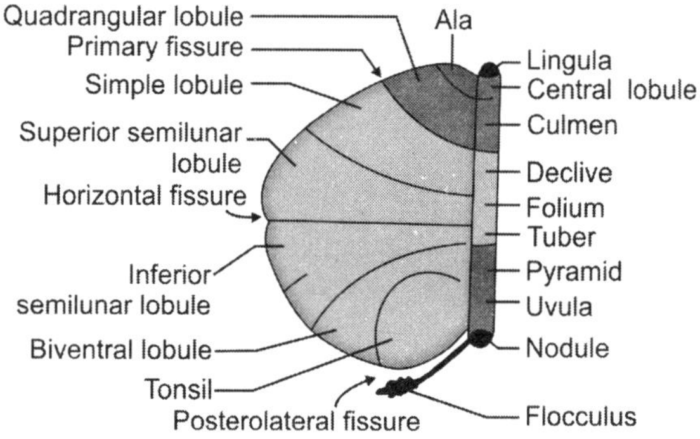

Quadrangular lobule
Primary fissure
Simple lobule
Superior semilunar lobule
Horizontal fissure
Inferior semilunar lobule
Biventral lobule
Tonsil
Posterolateral fissure
Ala
Lingula
Central lobule
Culmen
Declive
Folium
Tuber
Pyramid
Uvula
Nodule
Flocculus

Fig. 25.1: Parts of cerebellum

b. Primary fissure
c. Posterolateral fissure.

Each fissure cuts the vermis and both hemisphere

Parts of vermis	*Parts of cerebellar hemisphere*
1. Lingual	1. Ala
2. Central lobule	2. Quadrangular lobule
3. Culmen	3. Simple lobule
4. Decline	4. Superior semilunar lobule
5. Folicum	5. Inferior semilunar lobule
6. Tuber	6. Biventral lobule
7. Pyramid	7. Tonsil
8. Uvula	8. Flocculus
9. Module	

MORPHOLOGICAL AND FUNCTIONAL DIVISIONS OF CEREBELLUM

1. Archicerebellum	Controls axial musculature and bilateral movements used for locomotion and maintenance of equilibrium.
2. Paleocerebellum	Controls tone, posture and crude movements of the limbs.
3. Neocerebellum	Regulate fine movements of body

CONNECTIONS OF CEREBELLUM

Fibers entering or leaving the cerebellum are grouped to form three peduncles, which connect the cerebellum to the midbrain, pons and medulla.

- Superior cerebellar peduncle.
- Middle cerebellar peduncle.
- Inferior cerebellar peduncle.

GRAY MATTER OF CEREBELLUM

- Consist of cerebellar cortex and nuclei
- Four parts of nuclei are (Fig. 25.2):
  a. Nucleus dentatus
  b. Nucleus globosus
  c. Nucleus emboliformis
  d. Nucleus fastigi

FUNCTIONS

- The cerebellum controls the same side of the body, i.e. its influence is ipsilateral.
- The function are:
  - Coordinates voluntary movements so that they are smooth, balanced and accurate.
  - Controls tone, posture and equilibrium

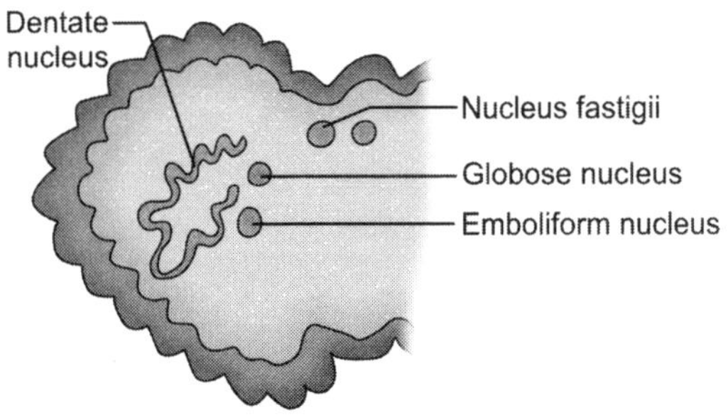
Dentate nucleus
Nucleus fastigii
Globose nucleus
Emboliform nucleus

Fig. 25.2: Nuclei of cerebellum

CLINICAL ANATOMY

Cerebellar Syndrome

Cerebellar lesion give rise to following symptoms and signs:

- Muscular hypotonia
- Intention tremers
- Adiadochokinesia
- Nystagmus
- Scanning speech
- Ataxic gait

PREVIOUS YEAR QUESTIONS

1. Describe briefly anatomy of cerebellum and add a note on cerebellar dysfunction?
2. Write short note on functions of cerebellum.

MULTIPLE CHOICE QUESTIONS

1. Gray matter of cerebellum are the following nuclei:
   a. Nucleus globsus
   b. Nucleus emboliformis
   c. Nucleus dentatus
   d. Nucleus fastigi
   e. All
2. Cerebellar syndrome is characterized by:
   a. Intention tremors
   b. Ataxic gait
   c. Muscular hypotonia
   d. All
3. Two Cerebellar hemisphere are united by each other through:
   a. Median vermis
   b. Fissura Prima
   c. Posterolateral fissure
   d. Superior cerebellar peduncle

Answers

1. (e) 2. (d) 3. (a)

26 Cerebrum

- Cerebrum is made up of two cerebral hemisphere
- Two hemispheres are incompletely separated from each other by **median longitudinal fissure**
- Two hemispheres are connected to each other by **corpus callosum**
- Each hemisphere contains lateral ventricle.

CEREBRAL HEMISPHERE

External Features (Fig. 26.1)

1. **Surfaces**—three
   i. Superolateral surface—convex, related to cranial vault
   ii. Medial surface—flat and vertical
   iii. Inferior surface—Irregular, divided into:
      1. Anterior—orbital surface
      2. Posterior—tentorial surface.
2. **Borders**—four
   i. Superomedial
   ii. Inferolateral
   iii. Medial orbital
   iv. Medial occipital.
3. **Poles**—three
   i. Frontal
   ii. Occipital
   iii. Temporal

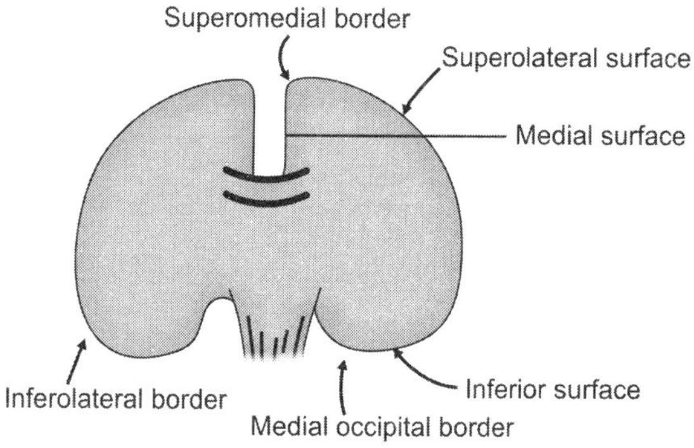

Superomedial border
Superolateral surface
Medial surface
Inferolateral border
Inferior surface
Medial occipital border

Fig. 26.1: External features of cerebral hemisphere

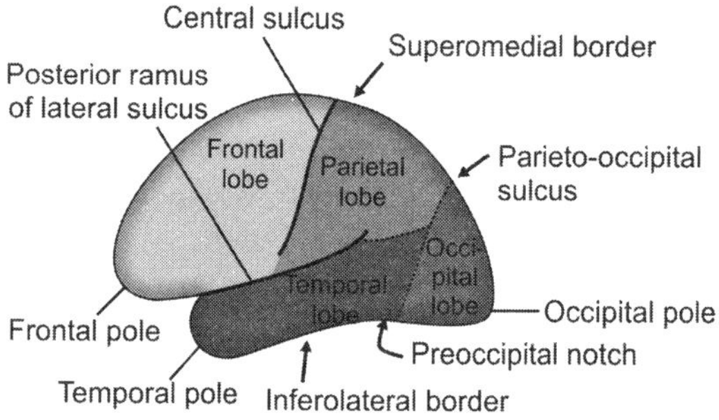

Central sulcus
Superomedial border
Posterior ramus of lateral sulcus
Frontal lobe
Parietal lobe
Parieto-occipital sulcus
Occipital lobe
Temporal lobe
Occipital pole
Frontal pole
Preoccipital notch
Temporal pole
Inferolateral border

Fig. 26.2: Lobes on superolateral surface

Lobes present on superolateral surface of cerebral hemisphere (Figs 26.2 and 26.3)

FRONTAL LOBE

- Lies in front of central sulcus and above the lateral sulcus
- It is bounded by:
  a. Anteriorly: prontal pole
  b. Superiorly: superomedial border.
- It present with three sylci which divide it into four gyri as.

Sulci

- Precentral sulcus:
  – lies in front of central sulcus
- Superior frontal sulcus
- Inferior frontal sulcus.

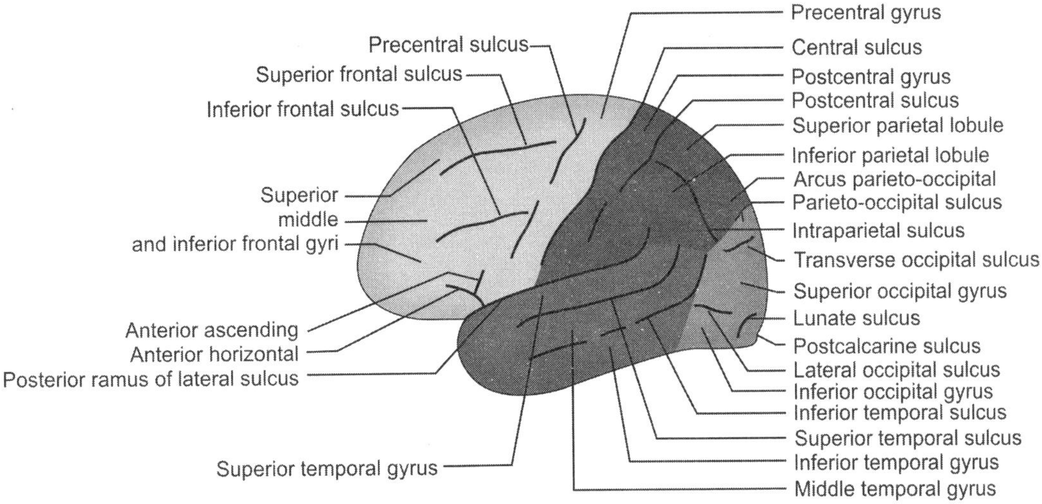

Precentral sulcus
Superior frontal sulcus
Inferior frontal sulcus
Superior
middle
and inferior frontal gyri
Anterior ascending
Anterior horizontal
Posterior ramus of lateral sulcus
Superior temporal gyrus
Precentral gyrus
Central sulcus
Postcentral gyrus
Postcentral sulcus
Superior parietal lobule
Inferior parietal lobule
Arcus parieto-occipital
Parieto-occipital sulcus
Intraparietal sulcus
Transverse occipital sulcus
Superior occipital gyrus
Lunate sulcus
Postcalcarine sulcus
Lateral occipital sulcus
Inferior occipital gyrus
Inferior temporal sulcus
Superior temporal sulcus
Inferior temporal gyrus
Middle temporal gyrus

Fig. 26.3: Sulci and gyri on superolateral surface

Gyri

- Precentral gyrus
  - Lies between central and precentral sulcus
  - It constitute motor area and provide principal origin of corticospinal and cortico bulbar fiber.
- Superior frontal gyrus—lies above superior frontal sulcus.
- Middle frontal gyrus—lies between superior and inferior frontal sulcus.
- Inferior frontal gyrus—lies below inferior frontal sulcus.

PARIETAL LOBE

- Bounded infront by central sulcus, behind by imaginary line extending from preoccipital notch to parieto-occipital sulcus.
- It is bounded by:
  - i. Superiorly—superomedial border
  - ii. Inferiorly—posterior ramus of lateral sulcui is:

It is divided into three gyri by two sulci as:

Sulci

- i. Postcentral sulcus—behind the central sulcus
- ii. Intra parietal sulcus

Gyri

- Postcentral gyrus
  - Lies between central and postcentral Sulci.
  - Receive various somatic and proprioceptive inputs from opposite side of body.
  - Sensory in function.
- Superior parietal lobule—lies between intraparietal sulcus and superomedial border.
- Inferior parietal lobule—lies below intraparietal sulcus and behind postcentral sulcus.

TEMPORAL LOBE

- Lies below lateral sulcus
- The anterior end of temporal lobe is temporal pole.
- It is bounded by:
  - a. Superiorly—posterior ramus of lateral sulcus
  - b. Inferiorly—inferolateral border
- It is divided into three gyri by two sulci as:

Sulci

- Superior temporal sulcus
- Inferior temporal sulcus.

Gyri

- Superior temporal gyrus
- Middle temporal gyrus
- Inferior temporal gyrus

OCCIPITAL LOBE

It is bounded by:

- Superiorly—superomedial border

- Inferiorly—inferolateral border
- Posteriorly—occipital pol.

It is divided into four Gyri by four sulci as:

Sulci

- Transverse occipital sulcus
- Lateral occipital sulcus
- Lunate sulcus
- Superior and inferior polar.

Gyri

- Arcus-parieto-occipitalis
- Superior occipital gyrus
- Inferior occipital gyrus
- Gyrus descendens.

MEDIAL SURFACE OF CEREBRAL HEMISPHERE (TABLE 26.1)

Table 26.1: Cerebral hemisphere of medial surface

Sulci	*Gyri*
• Anterior parolfactory	• Paraterminal
• Posterior parolfactory	• Parolfactory/subcollosal area
• Cingulate	• Medial frontal
• Callosal	• Paracentral lobule
• Suprasplenial or subparietal	• Cingulate
• Parieto-occipital	• Cuneus
• Calcarine	• Precuneus

INFERIOR SURFACE OF CEREBRAL HEMISPHERE (TABLE 26.2)

Table 26.2: Cerebral hemisphere of inferior surface

Sulci	*Gyri*
• Orbital surface – Olfactory – H shaped orbital sulci	• Gyrus rectus • Anterior orbital • Posterior orbital • Medial orbital • Lateral orbital
• Tentorial surface – Collateral – Rhinal – Occipitotemporal	• Lingual • Uncus • Parahippocampal • Medial occipitotemporal • Lateral occipitotemporal

Functions of Cerebral Hemisphere

The left cerebral hemisphere predominates in right handed persons (Table 26.3 and Fig. 26.4).

Table 26.3: Functions of cerebral hemisphere

Right cerebral hemisphere	*Left cerebral hemisphere*
• Nonverbal communications • Musical • Geometrical compre hension • Spatial comprehension • Temporal synthesis	• Verbal communications • Linguistic • Mathematical • Sequential • Analytical • Direct link to conciousness

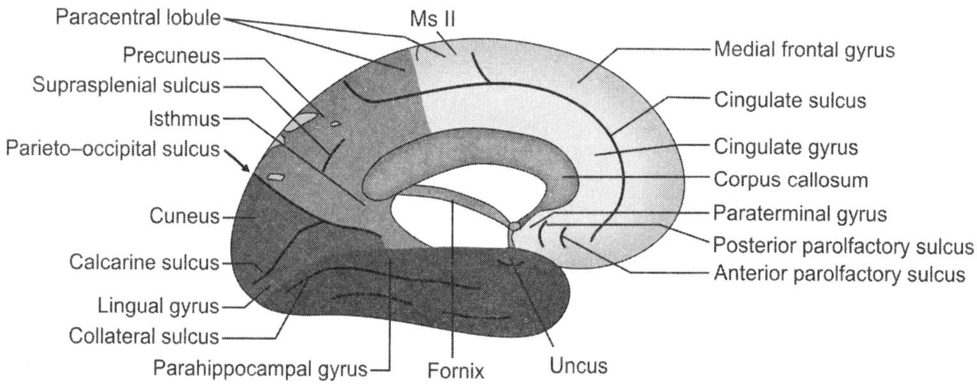
Paracentral lobule
Precuneus
Suprasplenial sulcus
Isthmus
Parieto–occipital sulcus
Cuneus
Calcarine sulcus
Lingual gyrus
Collateral sulcus
Parahippocampal gyrus
Fornix
Uncus
Ms II
Medial frontal gyrus
Cingulate sulcus
Cingulate gyrus
Corpus callosum
Paraterminal gyrus
Posterior parolfactory sulcus
Anterior parolfactory sulcus

Fig. 26.4: Sulci and gyri on medial surface

FUNCTIONAL AREAS OF CEREBRAL CORTEX (FIG. 26.5)

Motor Area

- Located in precentral gyrus on superolateral surface and anterior part of paracentral lobule
- Its stimulation results in movements in the opposite half of the body
- The body is represented upside down in this area.

Premotor Area/Psychomotor Area

- Lies just anterior to motor area
- Occupies posterior parts of superior, middle and inferior frontal gyri
- Patterns of movement are remembered in this area.

Motor Speech Area (of Broca)

- Lies in inferior frontal gyrus
- Injury to this area results in inability to speak (aphasia).

Sensory Area

- Located in postcentral gyrus
- Extends in posterior part of paracentral lobule
- Body is represented upside down.

Visual Area

Located in occipital lobe mainly on medial surface.

Acoustic Area

- Located in temporal lobe
- Lies partly on temporal lobe surface and mainly on part of superior temporal gyrus.

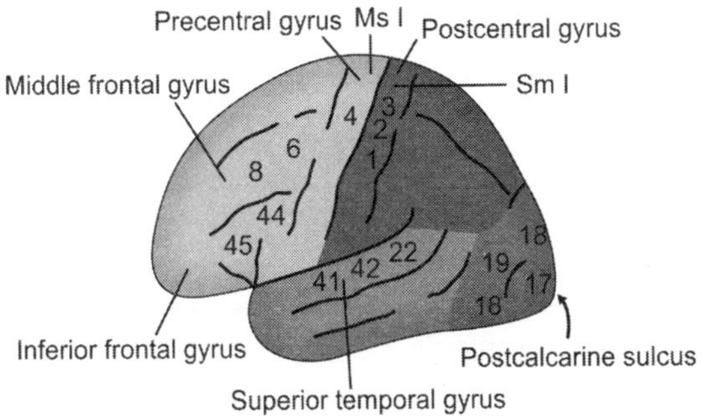
Precentral gyrus
Ms I
Postcentral gyrus
Middle frontal gyrus
Sm I
4
3
2
1
6
8
44
45
22
41
42
18
19
17
18
Inferior frontal gyrus
Postcalcarine sulcus
Superior temporal gyrus

Fig. 26.5: Functional areas of cerebral hemisphere

Clinical and Applied Anatomy

1. The effect of any lesion of motor area:
   a. It causes flaccid paralysis of contralateral side.
2. Injury to acoustic area can lead to loss of hearing.
3. Lesion in area No. 22 leads to sensory aphasia/word deafness.
4. Lesion in area No. 44,45 will lead to loss of fluency of speech or motor aphasia.

White Matter of Cerebrum

Three types of nerve fibers are present in the cerebral hemispheres.

Association Fibers/Arcuate Fibers

a. They connect two functional areas of the same cerebral hemisphere
b. Two types
   i. Long association—connects distant gyri
   ii. Short association—connects two adjacent gyri.

Association fibers are:

- Cingulum
- Superior longitudinal fasiculus
- Inferior longitudinal bundle
- Uncinate fasiculus
- Fronto—occipital fasiculus.

Projection Fibers

Connect cerebral cortex with subcortical gray matter up to the level of spinal cord. They include:

- Fimbria
- Fornix
- Corona radiata
- Internal capsule

Commissural Fibers

- Connects functional area of two cerebral hemisphere
- Two type of fibers
  - Homotopical connect identical functions over
  - Heterotopical—connect different function area
- They include
  - Anterior commissure
  - Posterior commissure

Table 26.4: Parts of internal capsule

Parts	*Extent/Location*	*Fibers prsent*	*Blood supply*
• **Anterior limb**	Lies between head of caudate nucleus and lentiform nucleus	• Frontopontine fibers. • Anterior thalamic radiation • Efferent and afferent fibers from anterior thalamic nucleus to cingulated gyrus • Medial forebrain bundle • Corticostriate fibers	• Anterior cerebral artery • Striate branch of middle cerebral artery (Charcot's artery)
• **Genui**	Lies between anterior and posterior limb	• Corticonuclear fibers from area No. 4, 6, 8 • Corticoreticular fibers.	• Recurrent branch of anterior cerebral artery • Internal carotid artery
• **Posterior limb**	Lies between thalamus and lentiform nucleus	• Corticospinal tract from area No. 4, 6 • Corticorubral tract • Superior thalamic	• Striate branch of middle cerebral artery • Interior choroidal artery • Posterior cerebral artery
• **Sublenticular** part	Extends below the lentiform nucleus	• Medial geniculate body to area No. 41, 42 • Meyer's loop of optic radiation	• Anterior choroidal artery • Posterior cerebral artery
• **Retrolentiform part**	It is backward extension of posterior limb—lies along the posterior horn of lateral ventricle	• Optic radiation • Posterior thalamic radiation • Parietopontine and occipitopontine fibers	• Posterior cerebral artery

- Hippocampal commissure
- Habenular commissure
- Corpus callosum

INTERNAL CAPSULE (FIGS 26.6 AND 26.7)

- It lies in the deep substance of each cerebral hemisphere
- It is a compact bundle of fibers which consists of afferent and efferent fibers of the neocortex.
- It is V shaped on cross-section with concavity diverted laterally, which is occupied by lentiform nucleus
- Small lesion of it produces widespread paralysis because of compact arrangement of fibers in it.
  Parts of internal capsule as given in Table 26.4.

Extent

- Superiorly: Continuous with corona radiata
- Inferiorly: Continuous with crus cerebrum of midbrain
- Medially: Bounded by head of caudate nucleus and thalamus
- Laterally: Bounded by lentiform nucleus.

CORPUS CALLOSUM

It is the largest band of commissural fibers of the neocortex which connects all the functional areas of the cerebral hemisphere except, area No. 17 and hand and foot somaesthetics area of area No. 3, 1, 2.

Shape—arched band of fibers with covexity directed upwards.

Size—10 cm long.

Parts (Fig. 26.8)

1. Rostrum—thin, pointed anterior end of the corpus
2. Genu—lies 4 cm behind the frontal pole
3. Trunk—lies over anterior horn and central part of lateral ventricle
4. Splenium—enlarged posterior end of corpus —lies about 6 cm in front of occipital pole.

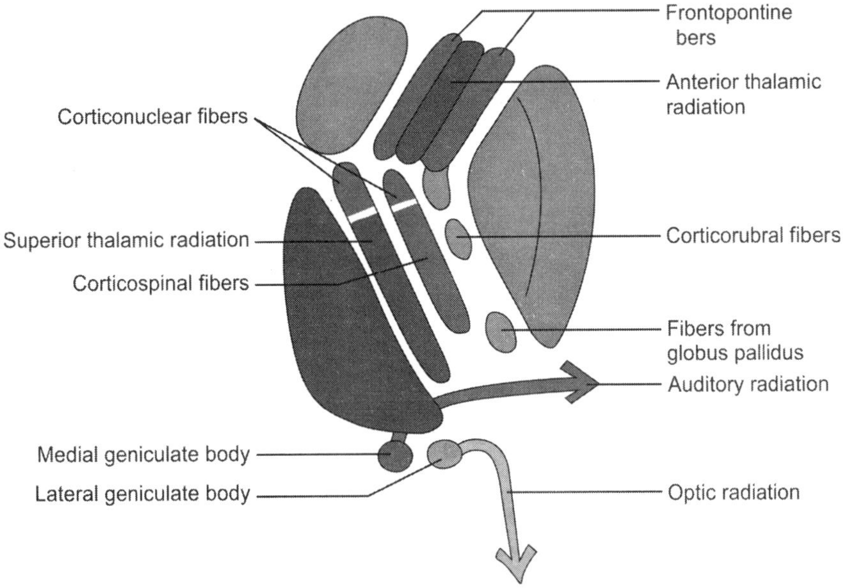
Frontopontine
bers
Anterior thalamic
radiation
Corticonuclear fibers
Superior thalamic radiation
Corticospinal fibers
Corticorubral fibers
Fibers from
globus pallidus
Auditory radiation
Medial geniculate body
Lateral geniculate body
Optic radiation

Fig. 26.6: Relations of internal capsule

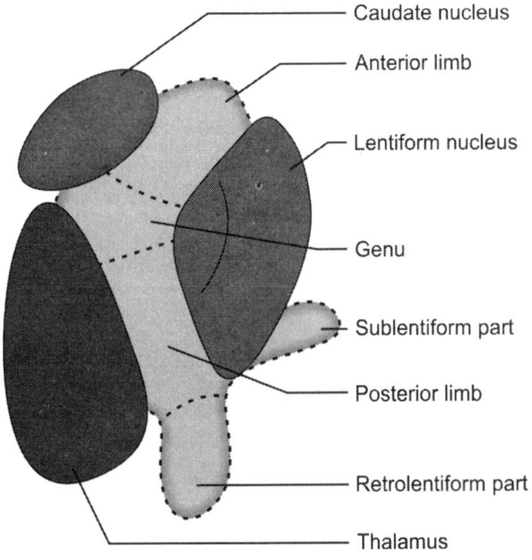
Caudate nucleus
Anterior limb
Lentiform nucleus
Genu
Sublentiform part
Posterior limb
Retrolentiform part
Thalamus

Fig. 26.7: Parts of internal capsule

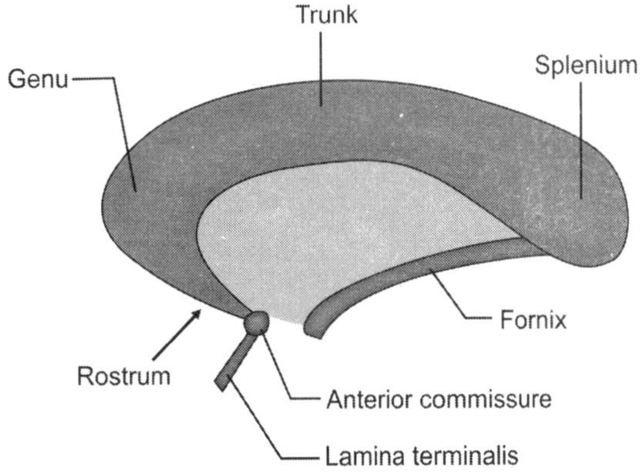
Trunk
Genu
Splenium
Fornix
Rostrum
Anterior commissure
Lamina terminalis

Fig. 26.8: Parts of corpus callosum

Functions

1. Transfer of learning process from one hemisphere to another
2. Transfer of speech function from one hemisphere to another.

Important Relations

Important relations of corpus callosum are described in Table 26.5.

Table 26.5: Relations of corpus callosum

Upper surface	*Lower surface*
• Indusium griseum • Lower free margin of falx cerebri • Inferior saggital sinus • Cynes cinguli	• Fornix • Septum pellucidum • Ependyma of lateral ventricles

BLOOD SUPPLY OF BRAIN

Arterial Supply

Brain is supplied by:
1. Two internal carotid arteries
2. Two vertebral arteries

Internal Carotid Arteries

Following branches supply brain:
- Posterior communicating artery
- Anterior choroidal artery
- Anterior cerebral artery
- Middle cerebral artery
  - Lenticulostriate branches
  - Cortical branches

Vertebral Arteries

- Anterior spinal arteries
- Posterior spinal artery
- Posterior inferior cerebellar artery.

CIRCLE OF WILLIS

It is a polygonal shaped arterial circle that lies in relation to the base of brain at the level of interpeduncular fossa.

Formation (Fig. 26.9)

Circle is formed by branches of the two internal carotid and two vertebral arteries as:

1. Anteriorly - Anterior communicating artery
2. Posterior - Terminal part of basilar artery and proximal part of two posterior cerebral arteries
3. Anterolaterally - 2 anterior cerebral arteries
4. Posterolaterally - 2 posterior communicating arteries
5. Laterally - Proximal part of both internal carotid arteries

Branches of Circle of Willis

See Table 26.6.

Functions

Helps to equalize the blood flow during normal conditions of different parts of brain.

VENOUS DRAINAGE OF BRAIN

Venous Drainage of Cerebral Hemisphere

1. Superficial veins
   i. Superior cerebral vein—from superolateral and medial surface
   ii. Superficial middle cerebral vein—from superolateral surface
   iii. Inferior cerebral veins—from inferior surface and lower part of superolateral surface
2. Deep Veins
   i. Internal cerebral veins
      - Formed by union of thalamostriate and choroid veins
      - Tributaries
        a. Thalamostriate vein
        b. Choroid vein
        c. Septal vein
        d. Lateral ventricular vein

Table 26.6: Branches circle of Willis

Branches	*Territory of distribution*
• Anteromedial branches of anterior communicating and anterior cerebral arteries • Anterolateral branches from Heubner and charcot's artery • Posteromedial branches from posterior communicating and posterior cerebral.	• Preoptic regions of anterior hypothalamus • Supraoptic regions of anterior hypothalamus • Corpus striatum • Internal capsule • Hypothalamus • Medial part of tegmentum and crus cerebri of midbrain • Subthalamus • Pituitary • Mamillary region • Anterior and medial part of thalamus
• Posterolateral branches from posterior cerebral artery	• Pulvinar • Both the geniculate bodies of thalamus

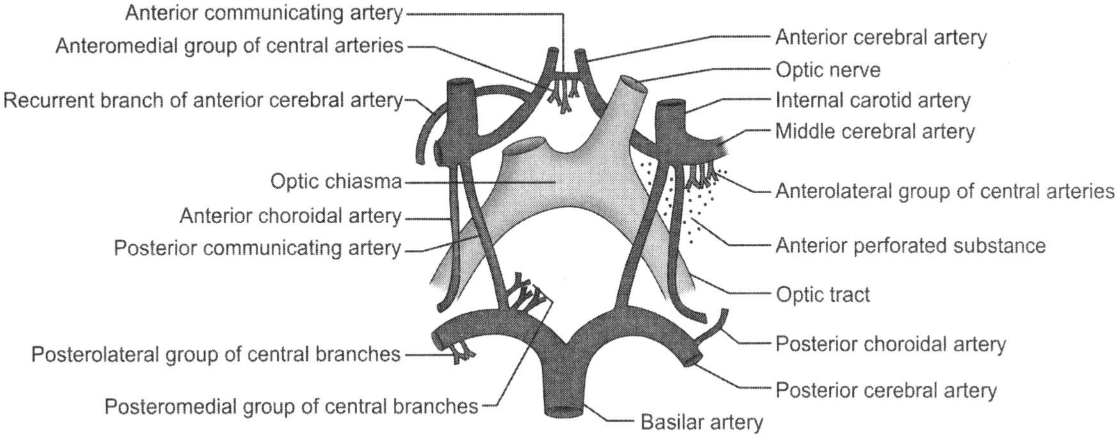
Anterior communicating artery
Anteromedial group of central arteries
Recurrent branch of anterior cerebral artery
Optic chiasma
Anterior choroidal artery
Posterior communicating artery
Posterolateral group of central branches
Posteromedial group of central branches
Basilar artery
Anterior cerebral artery
Optic nerve
Internal carotid artery
Middle cerebral artery
Anterolateral group of central arteries
Anterior perforated substance
Optic tract
Posterior choroidal artery
Posterior cerebral artery

Fig. 26.9: Formation of circle of Willis

ii. Basal vein
- Each basal vein is formed by union of
  a. Anteior cerebral vein
  b. Deep middle cerebral vein
  c. Striate vein

iii. Great cerebral vein of Galen
- Formed by union of two internal cerebral veins
- Tributaries
  a. Internal cerebral veins
  b. Basal veins
  c. Occipital veins
  d. Posterior callosal vein

Venous drainage of cerebellum

1. Superior cerebellar veins
2. Inferior cerebellar veins

Venous drainage of brainstem

1. Midbrain - By basal and great cerebral veins
2. Pons - Terminate into basal, transverse and petrosal sinuses
3. Medulla - By basilar plexus of veins and inferior petrosal sinus

CLINICAL SIGNIFICANCE OF CIRCLE OF WILLIS

1. Acts as principal collateral channel following an occlusion of any one of arterial system, which helps to maintain blood supply and nutrition to the brain of affected side.
2. It is also a common site of berry aneurysms in adults.

PREVIOUS YEAR QUESTIONS

1. Draw a labelled diagram of sagittal section of cerebral hemisphere.
2. Draw a well-labeled diagram of superolateral surface of cerebrum showing functional areas.
3. Enumerate white fibers of brain.
4. Write a short note on corpus callosum with diagram.
5. Give an account of internal capsule with diagram.
6. Enumerate commissures of brains and write about callosum.
7. Draw a labelled diagram of superolateral surface of cerebral hemisphere showing sulci and gyri.
8. Describe the functional areas of cerebral cortex and its clinical anatomy.
9. Name arteries supplying cerebrum and cerebellum.
10. Write short note on circle of Willis with diagram.

MULTIPLE CHOICE QUESTIONS

1. Broca's area is localized in:
   a. Superior temporal gyrus
   b. Parietal lobe
   c. Inferior frontal lobe
   d. Angular gyrus

2. Which cells are not present in cerebral cortex:
   a. Purkinje
   b. Stellate
   c. Cajal
   d. Pyramidal
3. Two cerebral hemisphere are incompletely separated from each other by:
   a. Corpus callosum
   b. Internal capsule
   c. Fornix
   d. Median longitudinal fissure
4. White matter of cerebrum contains:
   a. Association fibers
   b. Projection fibers
   c. Commissural fibers
   d. All
5. Corpus callosum is a/an:
   a. Association fibers
   b. Commissural fibers
   c. Projection fibers
   d. None
6. Widespread paralysis can be produced by lesion in:
   a. Corona radiata
   b. Fimbria
   c. Fornix
   d. Internal capsule
7. Circle of Willis is formed by branches of:
   a. Two internal carotid and two vertebral arteries
   b. Two internal carotid and two vertebral arteries
   c. Two internal carotid arteries
   d. Two vertebral carotid arteries
8. Injury to Broca's area results in
   a. Loss of hearing
   b. Loss of vision
   c. Inability to speak (aphasia)
   d. All of the above

Answers

1. (c) 2. (a) 3. (d) 4. (d) 5. (b) 6. (d) 7. (a) 8. (c)

27 Diencephalons

- Also known as interbrain
- Consists of gray matter which lies b/w two cereberal hemisphere.

PARTS

1. Thalamus (Dorsal thalamus)
2. Epithalamus
3. Metathalamus
4. Subthalamus (Ventral thalamus)
5. Hypothalamus.

THALAMUS

- There are two thalamus
- Each thalamus is an ovoid mass of gray matter
- Both thalami act as highest relay center for all sensations except olfaction.

Presenting Parts

It has two ends → Anterior and posterior end
and four surfaces →
i. Superior
ii. Inferior
iii. Medial
iv. Lateral

Nuclei of Thalamus

Six groups →
i. Anterior
ii. Lateral
iii. Dorsomedial
iv. Midline nuclei
v. Intralaminar
vi. Reticular thalamic

Functions of Thalamus

1. Final relay center for sensory input
2. Significant role in arousal and alertness
3. Regulates the activities of motor pathway
4. Helps in appreciating pain and temperature sense
5. Play a role in an individual's personality and intellect.

Blood Supply

Arterial supply →
i. Posterior cerebral
ii. Posterior choroidal
iii. Posterior communicating
iv. Middle cerebral

Venous drainage →
i. Thalamostriate
ii. Choroid veins of 3rd ventricle

Clinical Anatomy

1. Lesions of thalamus cause impairment of all type of sensibility, joint sense being the most affected.
2. Thalamic syndrome is characterized by disturbances of sensations, hemiplegia or hemiparesis with hyperesthesia and spontaneous pain.

EPITHALAMUS

It consists of following parts:

1. **Pineal Body:** It is neuroendocrine organ in mammals and have antigonadotrophic function.
2. **Habenular Nuclei**
   - Forms part of limbic system
   - Concerned with integration of olfactory impulses.
3. **Habenular Commissure:** Fibers of stria medullaris which connects pineal stalk to habenular nucleus of opposite side form habenuclar commissure.
4. **Posterior Commissure:** These fibers connects pretactal nuclei, interstitial nucleus of cajal and nuclei of posterior commissure.

METATHALAMUS

- It is dorsal part of thalamus
- Consists of two parts.

Medial Geniculate Body

- Oval elevation on inferior aspect of pulvinar
- Contains medial geniculate nucleus which has two parts
  - i. Parva - Cellular
  - ii. Magno - Cellular
- Function : Final relay center for hearing

Lateral Geniculate Body

- Oval elevation an inferolateral aspect of pulvinar
- Larger than medial
- Connects with superior colliculus through superior brachium
- Neurons are arranged in six layers
- Functions final relay center in visual pathway.

SUBTHALAMUS

- It is ventral part of thalamus
- Main nuclei are:
  - i. Zona incerta
  - ii. Subthalmic nucleus
  - iii. Cranial extension of substansia nigra
  - iv. Cranial extension of red nucleus
  - v. Nucleus of ansa lenticularis

HYPOTHALAMUS (FIG. 27.1)

- Lies in the ventral part of diencephalon
- Consists of collection of nerve cells in a matrix of neurological tissue.

Extent

Dorsally	-	Hypothalamic salcus
Ventrally	-	Lamina terminalis
Superiorly	-	Lamina terminalis
Inferiorly	-	Up to the vertical plane
Medially	-	Ependymal lining of 3rd ventricle
Laterally	-	Up to subthalamus and internal capsule

Nuclei of Hypothalamus: nuclei arranged in four regions:

1. Preoptic region
2. Supraoptic region
3. Tuberal infundibular region
4. Mamillary region.

Functions

- Highest Center of autonomic nervous system (ANS) after cerebral cortex
  1. Regulate sympathetic and parasympathetic activity.
  2. Regulate the secretion of pituitary hormones.

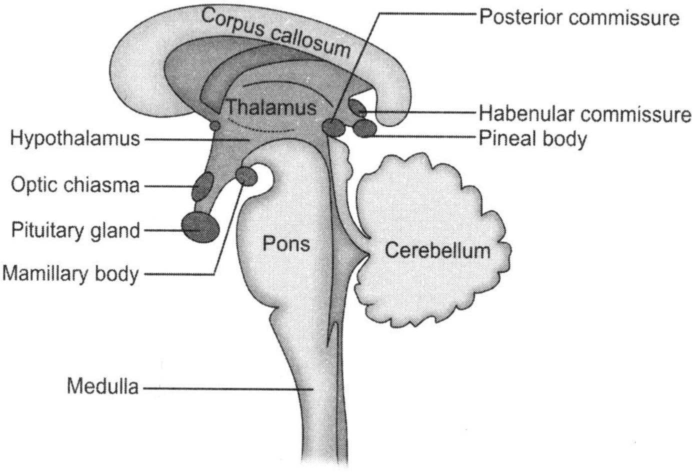

Corpus callosum
Posterior commissure
Thalamus
Habenular commissure
Pineal body
Hypothalamus
Optic chiasma
Pituitary gland
Pons
Cerebellum
Mamillary body
Medulla

Fig. 27.1: Basal ganglia

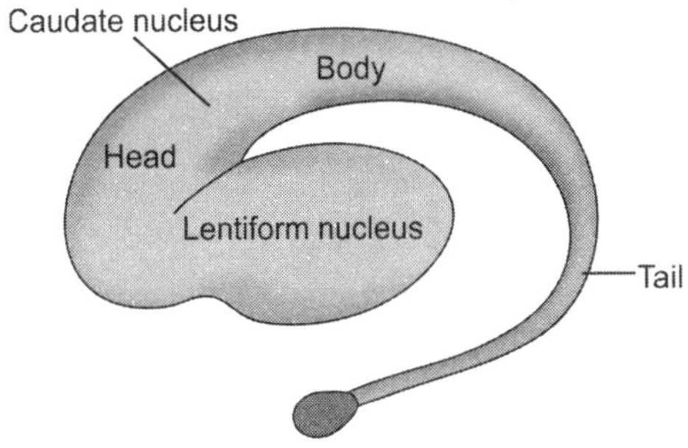
Caudate nucleus
Body
Head
Lentiform nucleus
Tail

Fig. 27.2: Amygdaloid body

3. Temperature regulation.
4. Acts as satiety center and hunger center.
5. Emotional expression is controlled by it.
6. Sex and propogative behavior is controlled by it.
7. Controls the biological clock.

BASAL GANGLIA (FIG. 27.2)

- Primarily masses of gray matter which lie in white core of each cerebral hemisphere.
- Comprise of
  i. Corpus striatum
  ii. Claustrum
  iii. Amygdaloid body

Corpus Striatum

- Divided into two parts by internal capsule.
  i. Caudate nucleus—it is medial band of gray matter divided into:
     (a) Head (b) Body and (c) Tail
  ii. Lentiform nucleus—divided into two part by external medullary lamina
     i. Putamen—dark, outer larger part.
     ii. Globus pallidus—inner pale part.
- It consists of biconvex mass of gray matter that lies lateral to the caudate nucleus.

Claustrum

Thin sheet of gray matter present b/w the putamen and the insular cortex.

Amygdaloid body

- It is continuous with the tail of caudate nucleus
- But structurally and functionally it is related to limbic system.

Functions

- It belong to extra—pyramidal system
  1. Helps in regulation of muscle tone.
  2. Supress abnormal involuntary movements.
  3. Controls the axial and girdle movements of body.

Clinical Anatomy

Lesion in basal ganglia lead to:
  i. Parkinson's
  ii. Chorea
  iii. Athetosis
  iv. Wilson's disease

PREVIOUS YEAR QUESTIONS

1. Write a short note on lateral geniculate body.
2. Write a short note on lentiform nucleus.

MULTIPLE CHOICE QUESTIONS

1. Thalamus is the largest relay center for all sensory input
   a. Touch
   b. Olfaction
   c. Hearing
   d. Pressure
2. Lateral geniculate body is final relay center of
   a. Hearing
   b. Smell
   c. Optic/Visual pathway
   d. Taste pathway
3. Which is the highest center of autonomic nervous system (ANS) after cerebral cortex
   a. Thalamus
   b. Epithalamus
   c. Subthalamus
   d. Hypothalamus

Answers

1. (b) 2. (c) 3. (d)

28 Mandible

- Mandible on lower jaw, is the largest and strongest bone of face.
- It develops from the first pharyngeal arch.

ANATOMICAL FEATURES

1. Body
2. Pair of Rami

Body of Mandible

- Horse-shoe shaped
- Has two surfaces and two borders

External Surface—structures present on external surface (Fig. 28.1)

1. Symphysis menti
2. Mental protuberance
3. Incisive fossa
4. Oblique ridge
5. Mental foramen

Internal Surface—structure present are (Fig. 28.2):

1. Mylohyoid line
2. Mylohyoid groove
3. Genial tubercle/Mental spine

Upper Border/Alveolar Border—bear the sockets for teeth.

Lower Border—base of mandible.

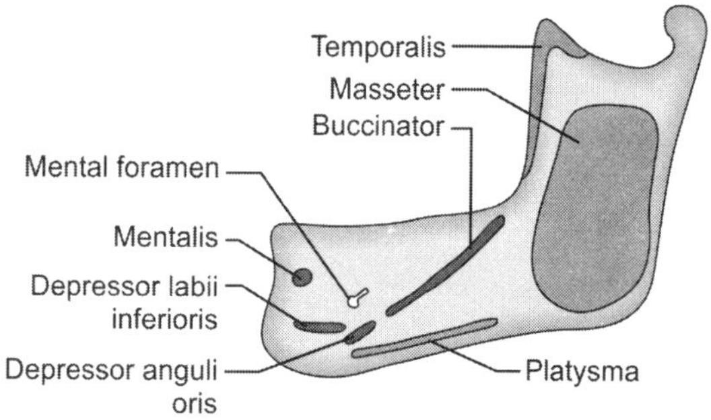

Temporalis
Masseter
Buccinator
Mental foramen
Mentalis
Depressor labii inferioris
Depressor anguli oris
Platysma

Fig. 28.1: Attachment on lateral surface of mandible

Attachments on Body of Mandible

1. Oblique line—origin of buccinator, depressor anguli oris and depressor labii inferioris.
2. Incisive fossa—origin of mentalis.
3. Mylohyoid line—origin of mylohyoid.
4. Superior genial tubercle—origin of genioglossus.

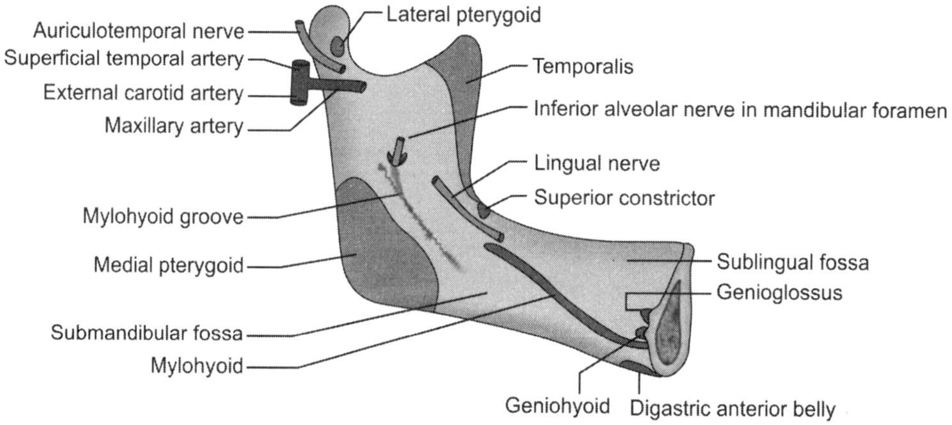

Auriculotemporal nerve
Superficial temporal artery
External carotid artery
Maxillary artery
Lateral pterygoid
Temporalis
Inferior alveolar nerve in mandibular foramen
Lingual nerve
Superior constrictor
Mylohyoid groove
Medial pterygoid
Sublingual fossa
Genioglossus
Submandibular fossa
Mylohyoid
Geniohyoid
Digastric anterior belly

Fig. 28.2: Attachment on medial surface of mandible

5. Inferior genial tubercle—origin of geniohyoid.
6. Base—origin of anterior belly of digastric.
   - Insertion of platysma.

Ramus of Mandible

Ramus is attached on either side of the body.

Two Surfaces

a. Lateral—over lapped posteriorly by the parotid gland.
b. Medial—structures present are:
   i. Mandibular foramen
   ii. Lingula

Four Borders

a. Anterior—superiorly continues with caronoid process.
b. Posterior—thick, overlapped by parotid gland.
c. Superior border:
   It present with anterior and posterior process which are separated by mandibular notch
   i. Coronoid process
   ii. Condylar process
d. Inferior border—base of mandible

Attachment on Ramus of Mandible

i. Masseter—insertion an lateral surface of ramus.
ii. Temporalis—insertion on medial surface of coronoid and anterior borer of ramus.
iii. Medial pterygoid—inserted on medial surface of ramus.
iv. Lateral pterygoid—inserted an pterygoid forea.
v. Sphenomandibular ligament—inserted in lingua.

Angle of Mandible

- It measures 110°-115° in adults.
- In newborn and old people angle is up to 140°

Mandibular Canal—extends from mandibular foramen transmis the inferior alveolar vessels and nerve.

Nerves Related to Mandible

1. Lingual nerve
2. Inferior alveolar nerve
3. Mylohyoid nerve
4. Mental nerve
5. Massetric nerve
6. Auriculotemporal nerve.

PREVIOUS YEAR QUESTIONS

1. Enumerate nerves and vessels related to mandible.
2. Short note on age changes of mandible and general features of mandible.
3. Labeled diagram of attachment relations on internal (medial) surface of mandible.
4. Name the nerves related with mandible. Describe movements of mandible.

MULTIPLE CHOICE QUESTIONS

1. Lingula gives attachment to:
   a. Sphenomandibular ligament
   b. Stylomandibular ligament
   c. Upper medial incisor
   d. Capsular ligament
2. Which of the following structure is not present on the internal surface of mandible:
   a. Genial tubercle
   b. Mylohyoid ridge
   c. Lingula
   d. Mental foramen
3. Which out of the following bones acidify first:
   a. Mandible
   b. Nasal bone
   c. Vomer
   d. Occipital

Answers

1. (a) 2. (d) 3. (a) 4. (a)

29 Embryology

DEVELOPMENT OF FACE

After formation of head fold, the developing brain and pericardium form 2 prominent bulging on the ventral aspect

↓

At 5th week of Intrauterine life
These are separated by buccopharyngeal membrane

↓

Mesoderm covering forebrain proliferates

↓

It forms a downward projection

↓

It is called the **frontonasal process**

Face is derived from:

1. Frontonasal process
2. 1st pharyngeal arch of each side

Mandibular/1st pharyngeal arch form the lateral wall of stomatodeum

↓

Gives off a bud called as **maxillary process**

↓

Growth occurs

↓

Mandibular process developed

↓

Ectoderm of frontonasal process shows bilateral localized thickening called as **Nasal Placodes**

↓

It sinks below the surface

↓

Nasal pits

↓

Edges of each pit raised above the surface

↓

Forms – Median and lateral nasal processes by median and lateral edges respectively

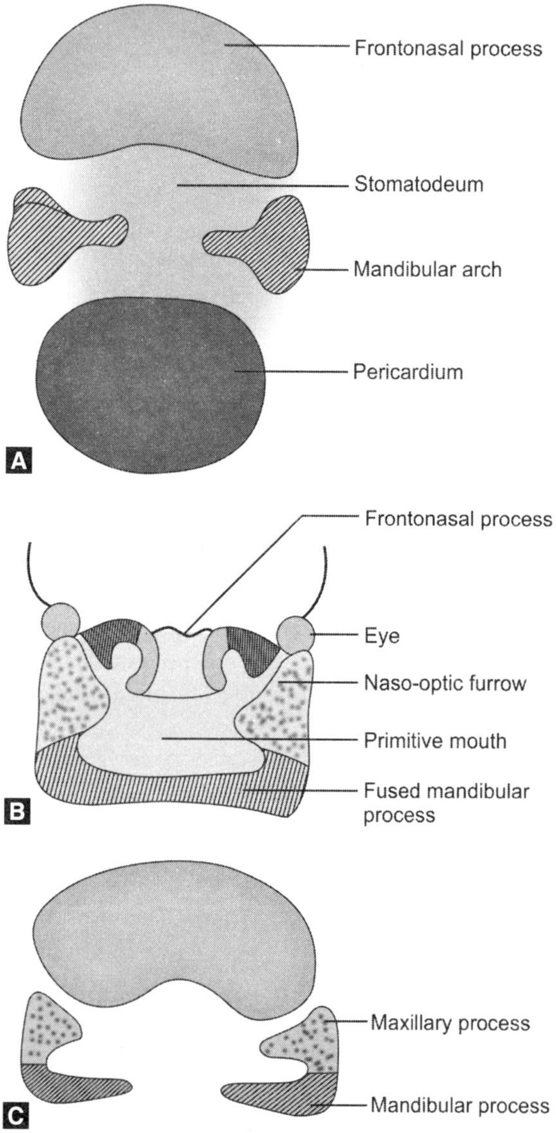
Frontonasal process
Stomatodeum
Mandibular arch
Pericardium
A
Frontonasal process
Eye
Naso-optic furrow
Primitive mouth
Fused mandibular process
B
Maxillary process
Mandibular process
C

Figs 29.1A to C

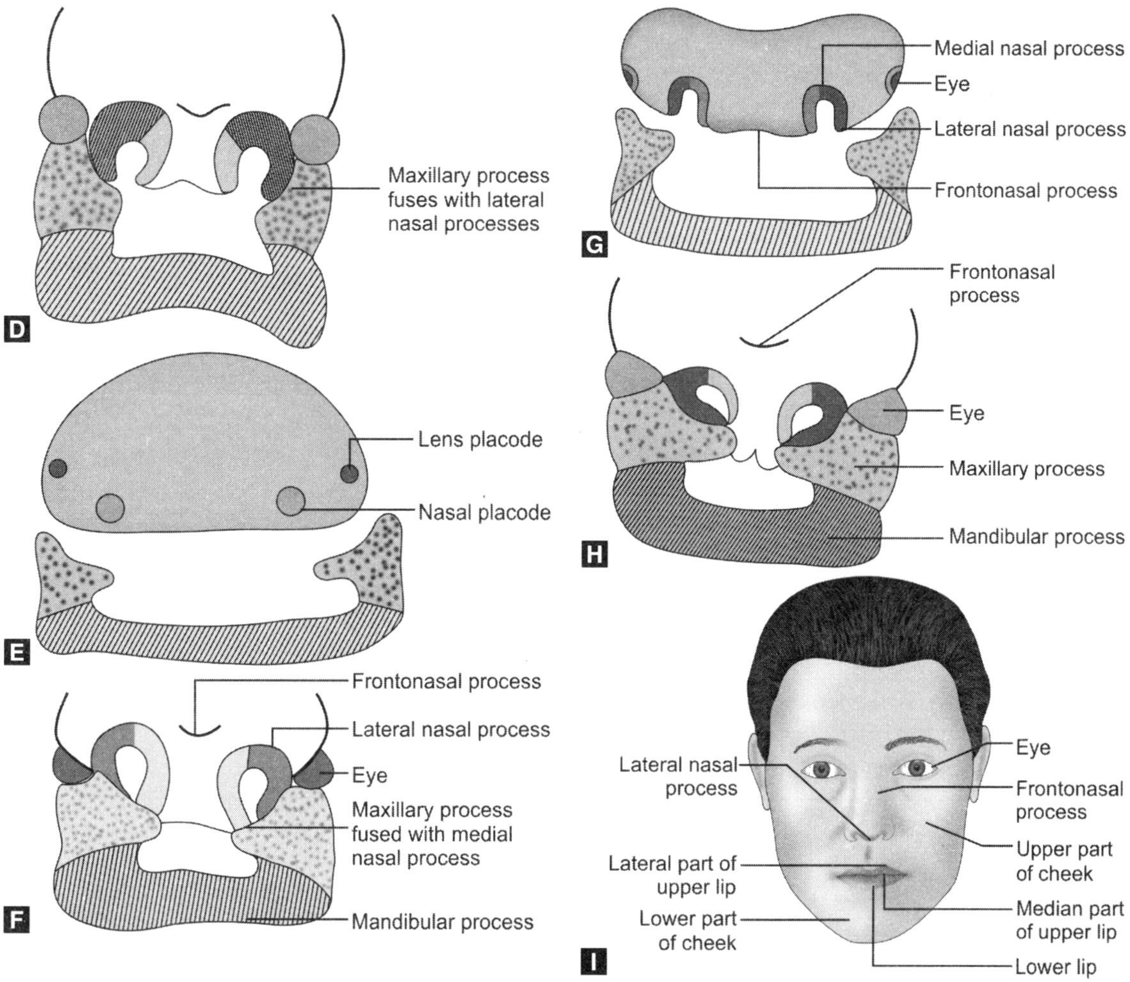

Maxillary process fuses with lateral nasal processes
D
Lens placode
Nasal placode
E
Frontonasal process
Lateral nasal process
Eye
Maxillary process fused with medial nasal process
Mandibular process
F
Medial nasal process
Eye
Lateral nasal process
Frontonasal process
G
Frontonasal process
Eye
Maxillary process
Mandibular process
H
Lateral nasal process
Lateral part of upper lip
Lower part of cheek
Eye
Frontonasal process
Upper part of cheek
Median part of upper lip
Lower lip
I

Figs 29.1D to I
Figs 29.1A to I: Development of face

Development of Different Parts of Face (Table 29.1 and Figs 29.1A to I)

Table 29.1: Development of face

Structure	*Part developed*
• Median process/globular process	• Philtrum of upper lip • Primitive palate • Nasal septum
• Lateral process	Alae of nose
• Maxillary process on each side meets lateral nasal process	• Cheek • Palatine process of maxillae • Upper jaw/maxilla • Lateral part of upper lip • Nasolacrimal duct
• Mandibular processes fuses together	• Lower lip • Lower jaw/mandible

BRANCHIAL APPARATUS/PHARYNGEAL ARCHES

- Made up of following components (Figs 29.2 and 29.3):
  - Pharyngeal/branchial arches
  - Ectodermal clefts
  - Endodermal pouches
- It give rise to the following:
  - Face
  - Neck
  - Definitive mouth
  - Pharynx
  - Larynx

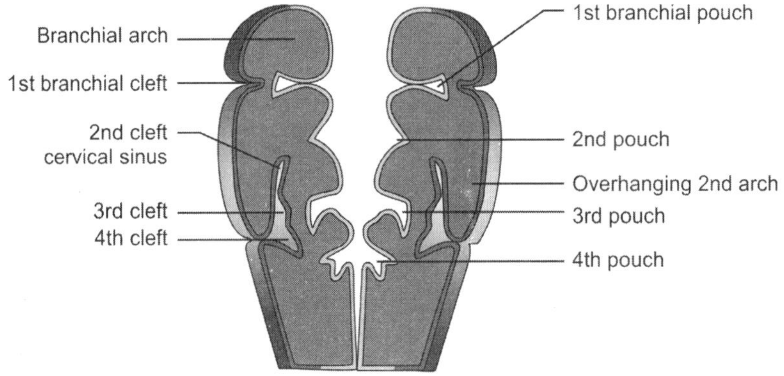

Branchial arch
1st branchial cleft
2nd cleft
cervical sinus
3rd cleft
4th cleft
1st branchial pouch
2nd pouch
Overhanging 2nd arch
3rd pouch
4th pouch

Fig. 29.2: Branchial clefts and pouches

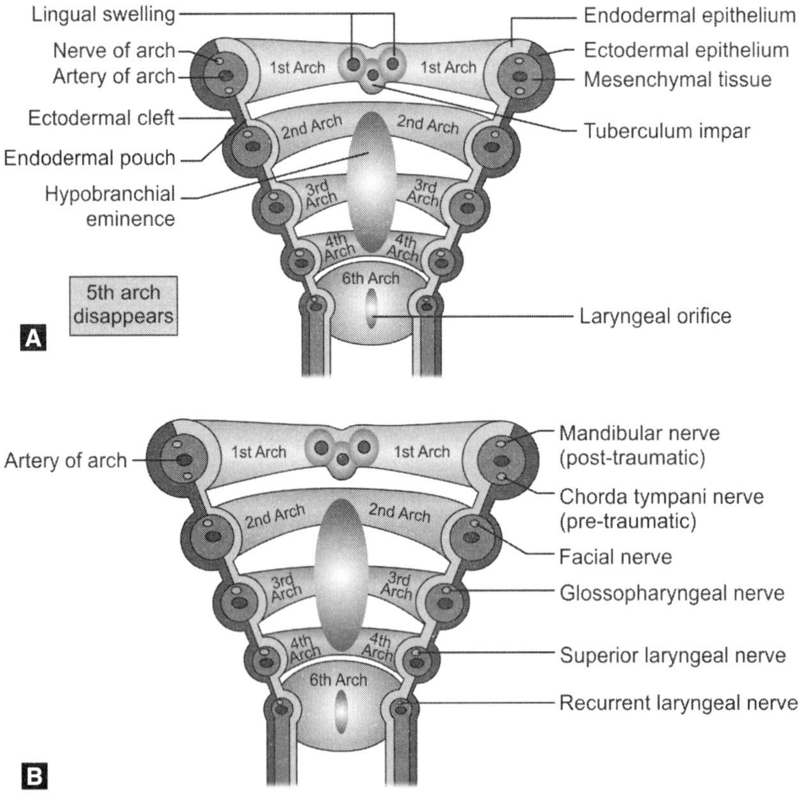

Lingual swelling
Nerve of arch
Artery of arch
Ectodermal cleft
Endodermal pouch
Hypobranchial eminence
5th arch disappears
A
1st Arch
2nd Arch
3rd Arch
4th Arch
6th Arch
Endodermal epithelium
Ectodermal epithelium
Mesenchymal tissue
Tuberculum impar
Laryngeal orifice
Artery of arch
B
Mandibular nerve (post-traumatic)
Chorda tympani nerve (pre-traumatic)
Facial nerve
Glossopharyngeal nerve
Superior laryngeal nerve
Recurrent laryngeal nerve

Figs 29.3A and B: Branchial arches

Derivatives of ectodermal, endodermal and mesodermal are depicted in Tables 29.2 to 29.4.

Table 29.2: Ectodermal derivatives

Arch	*Ectodermal covering*	*Derivatives*
1st	Maxillary process	• Epidermis of upper lip and cheek • Enamel of teeth • Parotid gland
	Mandibular process	• Epidermis of lower lip and jaw • Epithelium of vestibule and palate
	1st Branchial cleft	• Epithelial lining of external auditory meatus • Cuticle of tympanic membrane
2nd	Auricle and neck	Epidermis over the auricle and neck
3rd	Middle of neck	Epidermis over middle of neck

Table 29.3: Mesodermal derivatives

Arch	*Skeleton*	*Muscles*	*Nerves*
1st Arch	**Maxillary process gives** • Upper jaw • Palate • Dentine **Mandibular process** give rise to **Meckel's Cartilage** which forms • Malleus and its anterior ligament • Incus • Sphenomandibular ligament • Body of mandible • Symphysis menti	• Temporalis • Masseter • Lateral pterygoid • Medial pterygoid • Tensor veli palatini • Tensor tympani • Mylohyoid • Anterior belly of digastric	i. Mandibular nerve ii. Chorda tympani
2nd Arch/ Hyoid Arch	Give rise to **Reichert's cartilage** which form: • Stapes • Styloid process • Stylohyoid ligament • Lesser cornua of hyoid • Upper part of hyoid	• Stapedius • Stylohyoid • Posterior belly of digastric • Auricular muscles • Occipitofrontalis • Muscles of facial expression • Platysma	Facial nerve
3rd Arch	Ventral part give rise to: 1. Greater cornu of hyoid 2. Lower part of hyoid	• Stylopharyngeus • Superior constrictor	Glossopharyngeal nerve

Table 29.4: Endodermal derivatives

Pharyngeal	*Derivatives*
1st Pouch	• Auditory tube • Epithelium of tympanic cavity and mastoid antrum • Mastoid air cells • Mucous layer of tympanic membrane • Submandibular and sublingual glands
2nd Pouch	• Tonsillar pits • Tonsillar crypts • Intratonsillar cleft
3rd Pouch	• Inferior parathyroid gland • Reticular fibers and corpuscles of thymus
4th Pouch	• Superior parathyroid gland
4th and 5th Pouch	• Thyrene element • Lateral thyroid • Parafollicular cells of thyroid

DEVELOPMENT OF PALATE

It is derived from two sources (Fig. 29.4):

1. *Primitive palate:* Formed by fusion of globular processes of median nasal process.
2. *Permanent palate:* Formed by fusion of maxillary process.

Process of Development

Maxillary process
↓ At 6th week of intrauterine life (IUL)
Shelf like projection grows medially from each maxillary process
↓
Called as palatine process
↓ At 7th week of IUL
Palatine process assume horizontal position
↓
Fuses with each other and forms **Permanent palate**
↓ At 8th week of IUL
Permanent palate fuses with primitive palate in a Y-shaped manner starts from backward

- Ventral 3/4th of permanent palate is formed by fusion of palatine process with each other and with nasal septum. This part represent **Hard palate**.
- Dorsal 1/4th of permanent palate is formed by fusion of palatine process which fail to fuse with nasal septum. This part persists as **Soft Palate**.

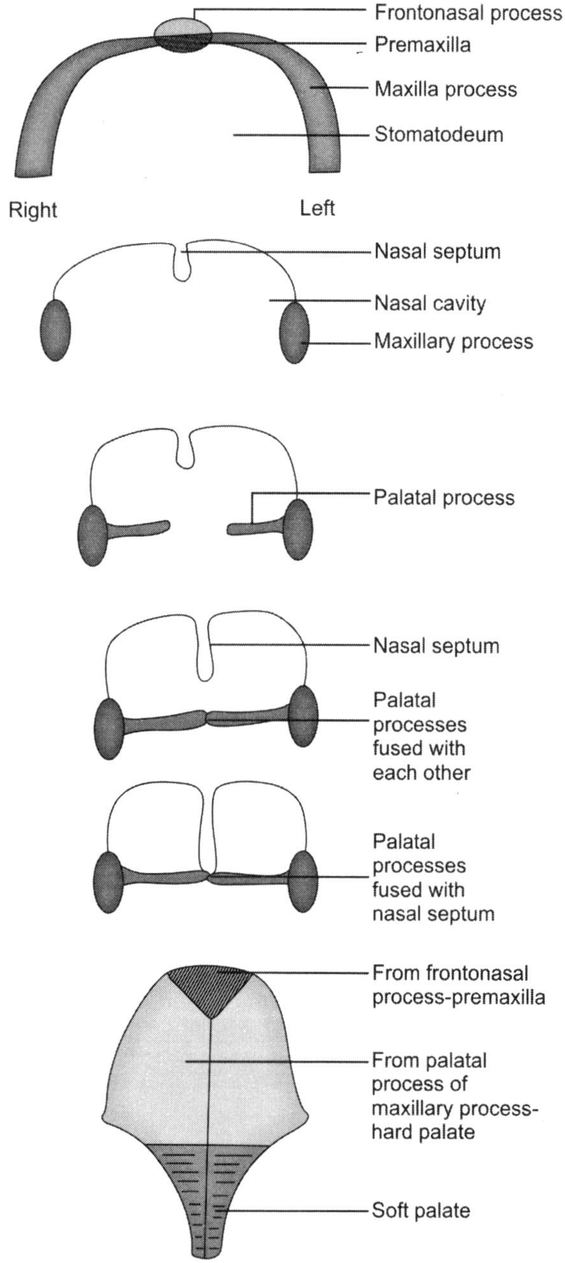
Frontonasal process
Premaxilla
Maxilla process
Stomatodeum
Right
Left
Nasal septum
Nasal cavity
Maxillary process
Palatal process
Nasal septum
Palatal processes fused with each other
Palatal processes fused with nasal septum
From frontonasal process-premaxilla
From palatal process of maxillary process-hard palate
Soft palate

Fig. 29.4: Development of palate

Clinical Anatomy

Cleft Palate

- Defective fusion of various components of palate give rise to cleft in the palate.
- Clefts of the palate result in anomalous communication between mouth and nose.
- May be unilateral or bilateral.
  a. ***Bilateral cleft lip and palate***
  Complete nonfusion: Y-shaped cleft with bilateral harelip.
  b. ***Unilateral cleft lip and palate***
  One palatine process is fused with premaxilla or primitive palate but other is fail to fuse with it. This cleft is accompanied by unilateral harelip.
  c. ***Midline cleft and palate:*** Midline cleft extending into hard palate.
  d. ***Cleft of soft palate***
  e. ***Bifid uvula.***

DEVELOPMENT OF MOUTH

In the region of floor of mouth mandibular process forms (Figs 29.5A to D):

- Lower lip
- Lower jaw/mandible
- Tongue

Process of Development

Floor of developing mouth
↓
Developing tongue forms swelling
↓
Seperated laterally from rest of mandibular process by Linguo-gingival sulcus
↓
Linguo-gingival sulcus is again separated laterally by Labio-gingival sulcus
↓
These sulcus deepens rapidly
↓
Area lying between them becomes raised and called as Alveolar process
↓
It forms jaw and teeth

DEVELOPMENT OF TONGUE

Tongue develops from 3 sources (Figs 29.6A to D):

1. Endoderm
2. Occipital somites
3. Mesoderm of branchial arches.

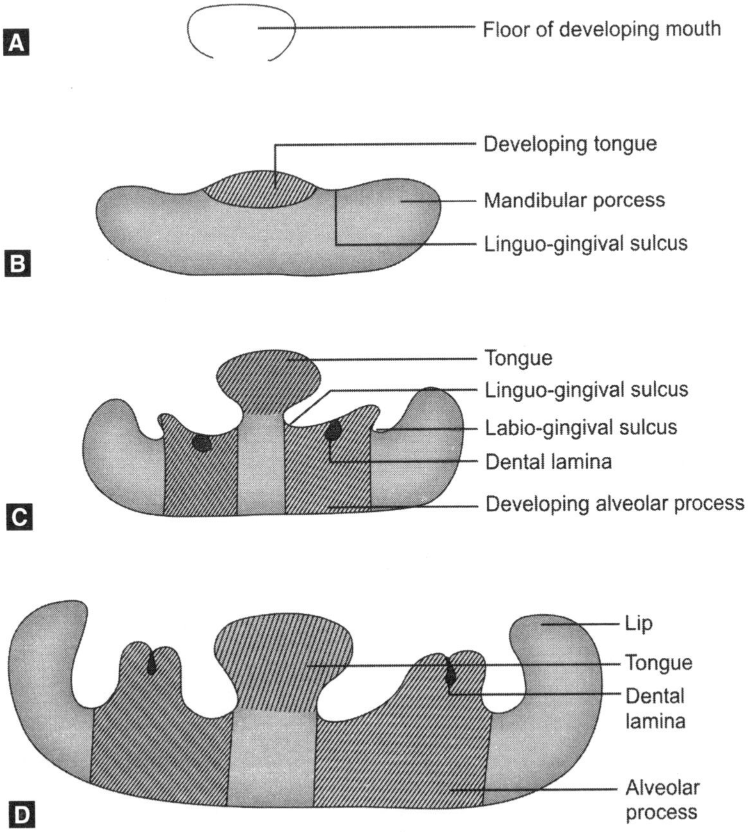
A
Floor of developing mouth
B
Developing tongue
Mandibular porcess
Linguo-gingival sulcus
C
Tongue
Linguo-gingival sulcus
Labio-gingival sulcus
Dental lamina
Developing alveolar process
D
Lip
Tongue
Dental lamina
Alveolar process

Figs 29.5A to D: Development of mouth

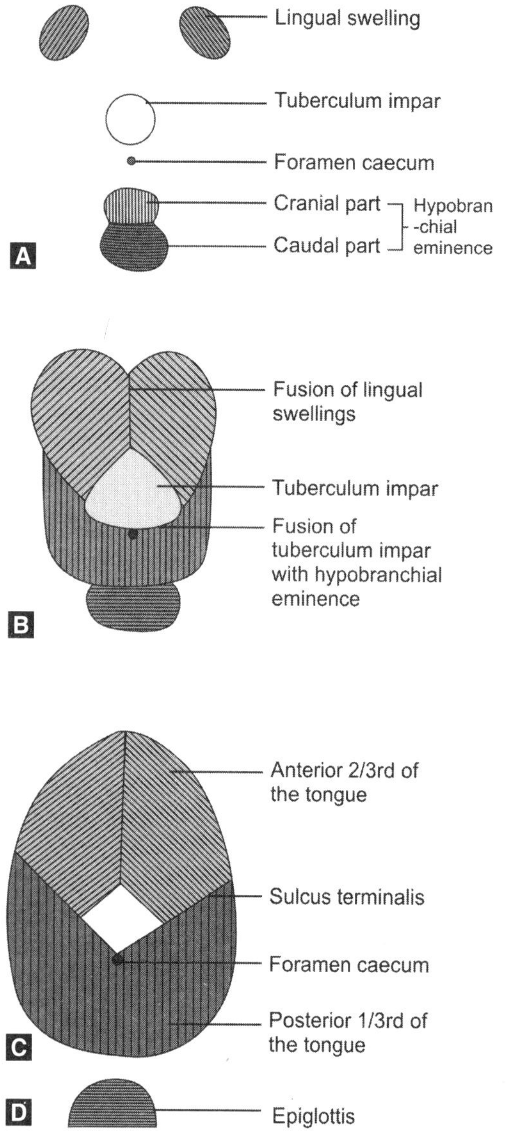
Lingual swelling
Tuberculum impar
Foramen caecum
Cranial part
Caudal part
Hypobran
-chial
eminence
A
Fusion of lingual swellings
Tuberculum impar
Fusion of tuberculum impar with hypobranchial eminence
B
Anterior 2/3rd of the tongue
Sulcus terminalis
Foramen caecum
Posterior 1/3rd of the tongue
C
D
Epiglottis

Figs 29.6A to D: Development of tongue

Process of Development

Development of Mucous Membrane

Derived from endoderm of foregut and arises in 3 parts:

a. *Lingual swelling:* Pair of endodermal elevations which later unite to form a single mass.

b. *Tuberculum impar:* It is single median elevation which appears between 1st and 2nd arches next to lingual swellings.
   Lingual swelling and tuberculum impar give rise to mucous membrane of anterior 2/3rd of tongue.

c. *Hypobranchial eminence:* It is median elevation dorsal to tuberculum impar.
   - It is divided into dorsal and ventral part by a transverse sulcus.
   - Ventral part give rise to mucous membrane of posterior 1/3rd of tongue.
   - It later fuses with anterior 2/3rd of tongue.
   - Line of fusion is known as **sulcus terminalis.**

Development of Masculature of Tongue

It is derived from occipital myotomes.

Development of Fibroareolar Stroma

It is derived from mesenchyme of branchial arches.

Clinical Anatomy

1. Failure of fusion of 2 lingual swellings leads to bifid tongue.
2. Complete agenesis of tongues known as aglossia.

DEVELOPMENT OF THYROID GLAND

Develops form 3 sources (Figs 29.7A to D):

1. **Thyroglossal Duct:** Gives rise to isthmus and lateral lobes of thyroid.
2. **Caudal pharyngeal complex of fourth pouch:**

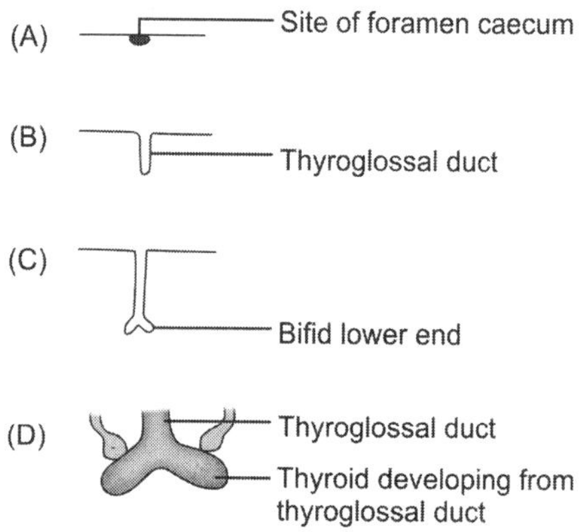
(A)
Site of foramen caecum
(B)
Thyroglossal duct
(C)
Bifid lower end
(D)
Thyroglossal duct
Thyroid developing from thyroglossal duct

Figs 29.7A to D: Development of thyroid gland

This is inducer for the differentiation of lateral lobes.

3. **Ultimobranchial body:** It give rise to parafollicular cells of thyroid gland.

Process of Development

Endodermal cells, dorsal to tuberculum impar proliferate
↓
Form median rediment
↓
These cells invaginate through substance of tongue
↓
Form thyroglossal duct
↓
Duct grows caudally in front of laryngeal cartilages
↓
At the level of prominent part of trachea, duct divides into
↙ ↘
Primordium of isthmus | Lateral lobes of thyroid gland

- Duct disappears and leaves only a trace of its cephallic attachment seen as the foramen cecum of tongue.
- Lateral thyroid rudiments fuse with the bilobed mass.
- Parafollicular cells are derived from the ultimobranchial body and also form part of the thyroid gland.

DEVELOPMENT OF PITUITARY GLAND

Pituitary gland/hypophysis cerebri develops from ectoderm of stomodeum and neuroectoderm of diencephalon in 2 parts (Fig. 29.8).

Development of Anterior Lobe

Diverticulum evaginates from roof of stomodeum
↓
It is known as Rathke's pouch
↓
It extend upto floor of fore brain vesicle
↓
It is separated from stomodeum due to growth of surrounding mesenchyme
↓
It forms following parts

1. Anterior wall of pouch: anterior lobe of pituitary
2. Posterior wall of pouch: pars inter-media
3. Cavity of pouch Intraglandular cleft.
4. Cephalic part of anterior lobe: pars tuberalis.

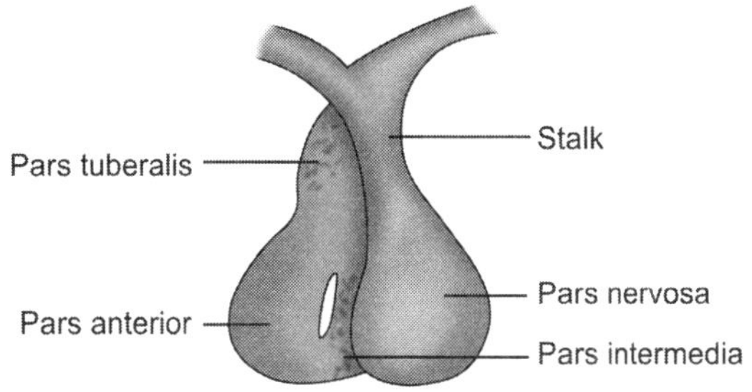
Pars tuberalis
Stalk
Pars anterior
Pars nervosa
Pars intermedia

Fig. 29.8: Development of pituitary gland

Development of Posterior Lobe

Diverticulum from floor of diencephalon
↓
Lower ends proliferates
↓
Forms posterior lobe
↓
Upper ends of diverticulum form infundibulum

DEVELOPMENT OF TONSILS

Palatine tonsils develop in relation to lateral parts of 2nd pharyngeal pouch.

Process of Development

Endodermal lining of pouch
↓
Proliferate
↓
Lymphocytes collected in relation to endodermal cells
↓
Infratonsillar cleft or tonsillar fossa developed

DEVELOPMENT OF TOOTH (FIGS 29.9A TO F)

The teeth are developed from "Stomatodeum"
↓
Epithelium over the alveolar process becomes thickened and projects in underlying mesoderm.
↓

This is called as dental lamina
↓
It shows series of local thickenings, called as **ENAMEL ORGAN**
↓
Cells proliferate
↓
Thus, enamel organ increases in size, changing its shape from **bud** to **cap** and then to **bell**.
↓
Ectomesenchymal cells increase in number forming **Dental Papilla**
↓
Ectomesenchymal cells surround enamel organ and dental papilla, which is called as **Dental Sac/Follicle**

Thus, tooth germ consist of:
1. Ectodermal components: Enamel organ
2. Ectomesenchymal components:
   i. Dental papilla
   ii. Dental follicle

Tooth and its supporting structure are formed from tooth germ as follows:
   a. Enamel: Formed from enamel organ (Ameloblast).
   b. Dentine — Formed from dental
   c. Pulp — papilla (odontoblast)
   d. Cementum
   e. PDL — Formed from dental follicle
   f. Alveolar bone

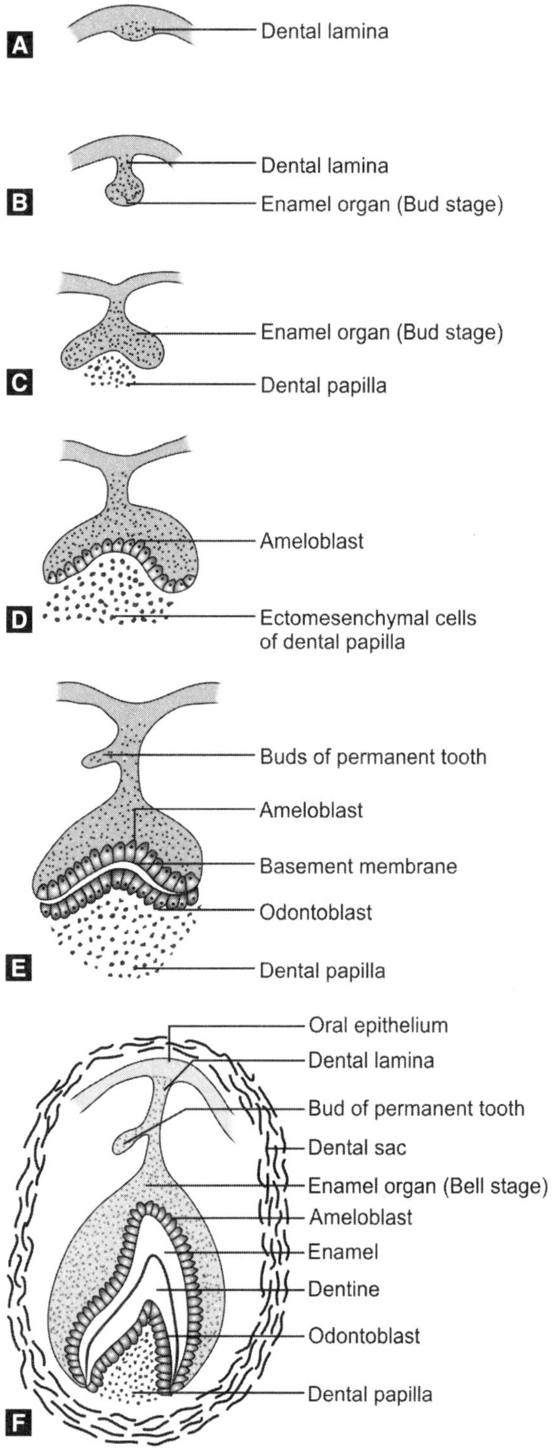
A
Dental lamina
B
Dental lamina
Enamel organ (Bud stage)
C
Enamel organ (Bud stage)
Dental papilla
D
Ameloblast
Ectomesenchymal cells of dental papilla
E
Buds of permanent tooth
Ameloblast
Basement membrane
Odontoblast
Dental papilla
F
Oral epithelium
Dental lamina
Bud of permanent tooth
Dental sac
Enamel organ (Bell stage)
Ameloblast
Enamel
Dentine
Odontoblast
Dental papilla
Fig. 29.9A to F: Development of tooth

PREVIOUS YEAR QUESTIONS

1. Describe the development of face
2. Write short note on:
   a. Development of tongue
   b. Development of thyroid gland
   c. Development of palatine tonsil
   d. Development of tooth
3. Describe the development of tongue and its anomalies.
4. Describe in brief the derivatives of 1st pharyngeal arch.
5. Describe the development of teeth in detail.

MULTIPLE CHOICE QUESTIONS

1. Cleft lip occurs due to failure of:
   a. Fusion of lateral nasal process with maxillary process
   b. Fusion of median nasal process with maxillary process.
   c. Fusion of median and lateral nasal process
   d. None.
2. Philtrum of the upper lip is formed largely by:
   a. Lateral nasal process
   b. Frontonasal process
   c. Maxillary process
   d. Mandibular process
3. Tongue develops from all of the following except:
   a. Tuberculum impar
   b. Hypobranchial eminence
   c. Lingual swelling
   d. Arytenoid swelling.
4. Posterior part of the tongue develops from:
   a. Ist arch
   b. IIIrd arch
   c. IInd arch
   d. All.
5. The tongue as formed from following branchial arches:
   a. Ist, IInd, IIIrd
   b. Ist, IIIrd, Vth
   c. Ist, IIIrd, IVth
   d. Ist, IVth, Vth.
6. The primordial of the craniofacial complex develops from:
   a. Hensen's node
   b. Notochordal process
   c. Cloacal membrane
   d. Blastopore.
7. Which of the following is the nerve of 3rd branchial arch:
   a. Facial
   b. Trigeminal
   c. Vagus
   d. Glossopharyngeal.
8. From which pharyngeal pouches do the parathyroid glands develop:
   a. Ist and IInd
   b. IInd and IIIrd
   c. IIIrd and IVth
   d. IVth and Vth.
9. Thyroid gland develops from
   a. Thyroglossal duct
   b. Rathke's pouch
   c. Notochordal process
   d. Embryonic disc.
10. Hyoid bone is a derivative of which pharyngeal arch:
    a. Ist arch
    b. Ist and IInd
    c. IInd and IIIrd
    d. IVth.
11. Development of palate begins at the age of:
    a. 4 weeks
    b. 6 weeks
    c. 13 weeks
    d. 18 weeks.
12. Derivative of IInd pharyngeal arch is:
    a. Sphenomandibular ligament
    b. Anterior ligament of malleus
    c. Stylomandibular ligament
    d. Stylohyoid ligament

Answers

1. (b) 2. (b) 3. (d) 4. (b) 5. (c) 6. (a) 7. (d) 8. (c) 9. (a) 10. (c)
11. (a) 12. (d)

30 Histology

DEFINITION

Tissue which lines the body cavities and covers the outer surface of the body is known as epithelial tissue.

CLASSIFICATION

Based on number of cell layers, shape of cells:
1. Simple epithelium
2. Pseudostratified epithelium
3. Stratified epithelium.

Simple Epithelium

- Single layer of cells
- Types :
  1. Simple squamous epithelium (Flat cells) – e.g.
     i. Blood vessels
     ii. Alveoli
     iii. Bowman's capsule
  2. Simple cuboidal epithelium (cubical cells) – e.g.
     i. Thyroid
     ii. Respiratory
     iii. Germinal epithelium ovary
  3. Simple columnar epithelium (columnar cells)– e.g.
     i. Uterus
     ii. Gallbladder
     iii. GIT

Pseudostratified Epithelium (Fig. 30.1)

- Single layer of columnar cells with different heights.
- Level of nucleus is different in different cells that give rise to false appearance of stratification.

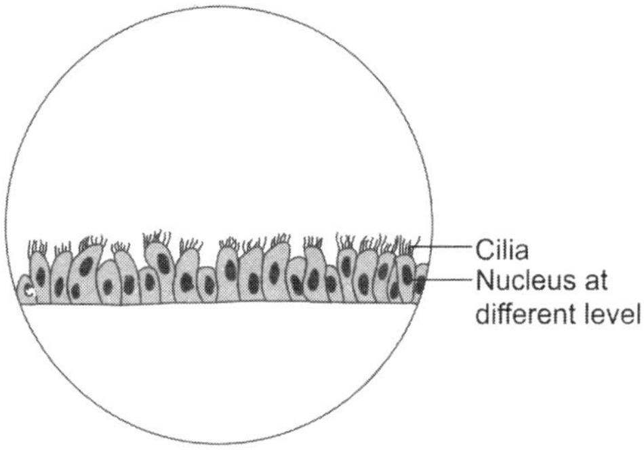

Cilia
Nucleus at different level

Fig. 30.1: Pseudostratified epithelium
(For color version, See Plate 1)

- Present in respiratory tract and male genital system, e.g. Trachea, male urethra, etc.

Stratified Epithelium

- More than one layer of cells are present
- Types:
  - Stratified squamous non-keratinized epithelium
  - Stratified squamous keratinized epithelium
  - Stratified cuboidal epithelium
  - Stratified columnar epithelium
  - Transitional epithelium.

Transitional Epithelium (Fig. 30.2)

- There is transition of cells from basal to superficial layer
- 5-6 layers of cells
- Basal cells are columnar and become polygonal above.
- Superficial cells are umbrella shape
- It lines the urinary tract, e.g. ureter, urethra, urinary bladder (Urothelium).

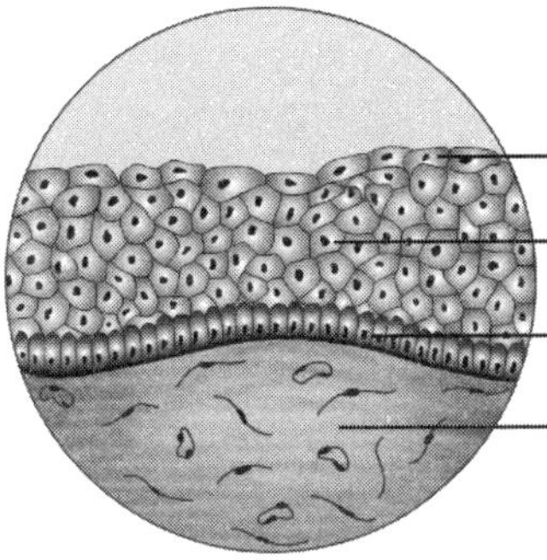
Umbrella shaped cell
Polygonal cell
Columnar basal cell
Connective tissue

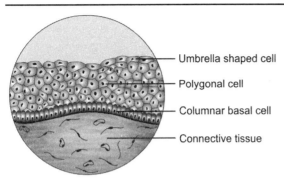

Fig. 30.2: Transitional epithelium
(For color version, See Plate 1)

CONNECTIVE TISSUE

- It connects different tissues
- Facilitates passage of neurovascular bundles in different tissue
- Made up of intercellular material, extracellular matrix and cells.

Components

- Cells
- Fibers
- Matrix.

Classification

Based on relative proportion of cells, fibers and ground substance in connective tissue.

- Irregular connective tissue
  - Loose areolar
  - Dense irregular
  - Adipose tissue
- Regular connective tissue
- Fascia
- Specialized connective tissue, e.g. cartilage, bone, blood, etc.

Functions

- Binds together various structure
- Keeps muscles and tendons in position
- In the form of ligaments, binds the bones
- Attaches muscle to bone with the help of tendons and facilitates a concentrated pull
- Facilitates venous return in lower limb
- Helps in wound repair
- Facilitates passage of neurovascular bundle.

HISTOLOGICAL FEATURES

Salivary Glands

- Three pairs of salivary glands secrete saliva which is poured into the oral cavity (Figs 30.3 to 30.6 and Table 30.1).
- These are:
  a. Parotid gland - Purely serous
  b. Submandibular gland - Predominantly serous
  c. Sublingual gland - Predominantly mucous
- Glands are composed of:
  a. Acini
  b. Intralobular duct
  c. Interlobular duct
  d. Main – duct

Tongue

- Musculature of tongue is covered by stratified squamous non-keratinized epithelium
- Anterior 2/3rd - underlying corium consists of collagen and elastic fibers which project upwards forming **papillae**
- Posterior 1/3rd – Present only irregular bulges due to lymphoid tissue

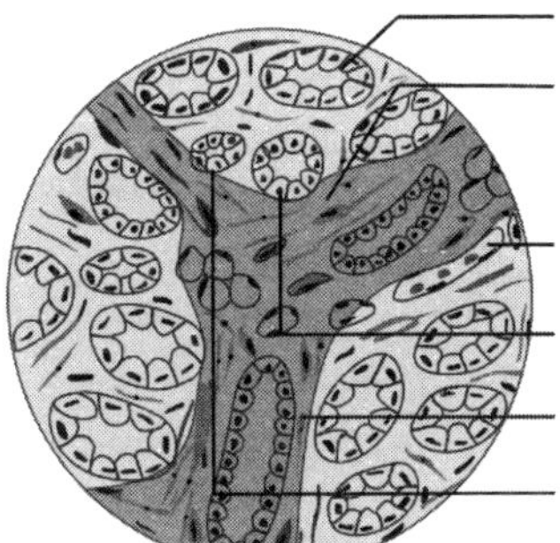
Mucous acini
Connective tissue septa dividing gland into lobes
Blood vessel
Intralobular duct
Interlobular duct
Intercalated duct

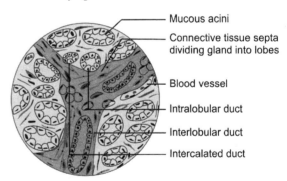

Fig. 30.3: Mucous salivary gland (Sublingual)
(For color version, See Plate 1)

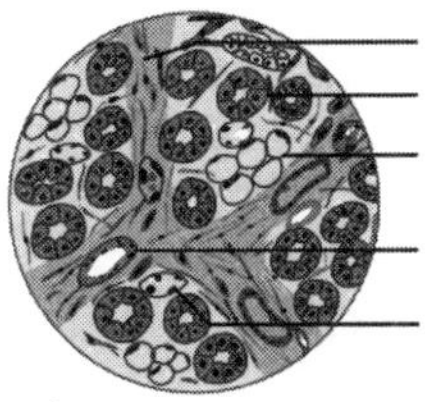
Interlobular connective tissue septa
Serous acini
Adipose tissue
Interlobular duct
Intralobular duct

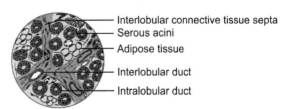

Fig. 30.4: Serous salivary gland (Parotid)
(For color version, See Plate 1)

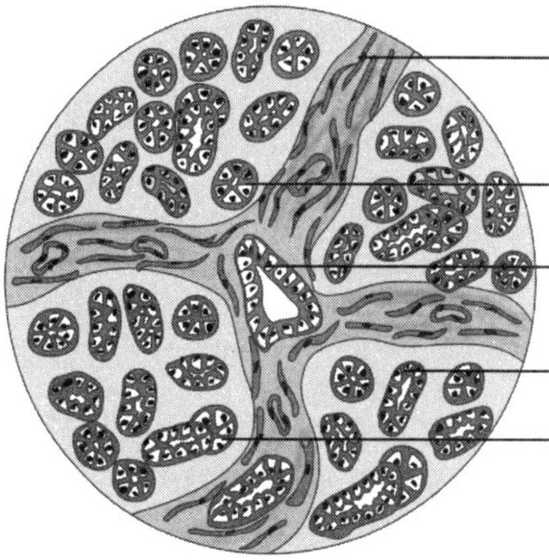
Connective tissue septa dividing gland into lobes
Mucous acini
Interlobular duct
Serous acini
Serous demilunes/demilune of gianuzzi

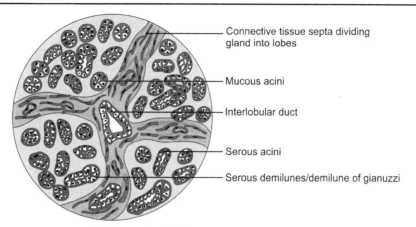

Fig. 30.5: Mixed salivary gland (Submandibular) *(For color version, See Plate 1)*

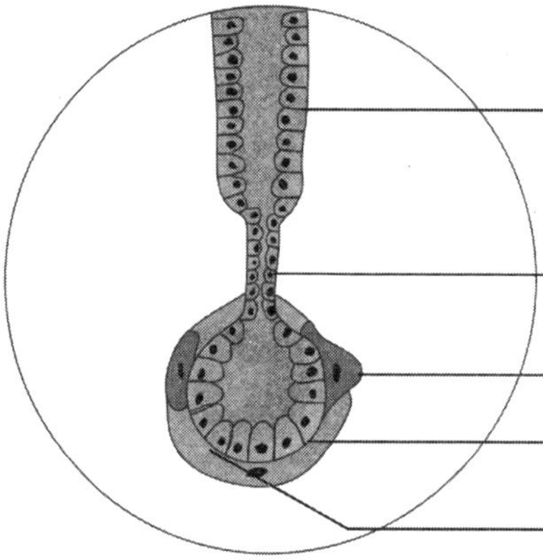
Striated duct
Intercalated duct
Myoepithelial cell
Acinar cell
Basal lamina

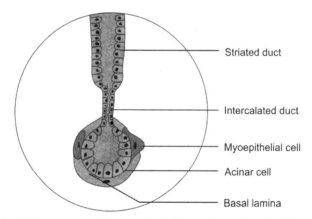

Fig. 30.6: Structure of ducts and acini *(For color version, See Plate 2)*

Table 30.1: Features of serious acini and mucous acini

Serious Acini	*Mucous Acini*
• Smaller in size	Larger
• Rounded in shape	More variable
• Lumen hardly visible	Mostly visible
• Lining cells are pyramidal in shape and more in number	Truncated columnar in shape and cells are fewer in number
• Nuclei are rounded and basal	Flattened and peripheral
• Basophilic cytoplasm	Pale and vacuolated cytoplasm
• Serous acinus may be present as demilunes on one aspect of some mucous acini, known as Demilune of Giannuzzi	Mucous acini only present as complete acini

Papillae

- Three types of papillae are present which contains tastebuds (Figs 30.7 and 30.8)
  - i. Filiform
  - ii. Fungiform
  - iii. Circumvallate

Palatine Tonsil (Fig. 30.9)

- Covered by stratified squamous non-keratinized epithelium which dips into underlying tissue to form crypts.
- No differentiation into cortex and medulla.
- Lymphatic nodules invading the epithelium.

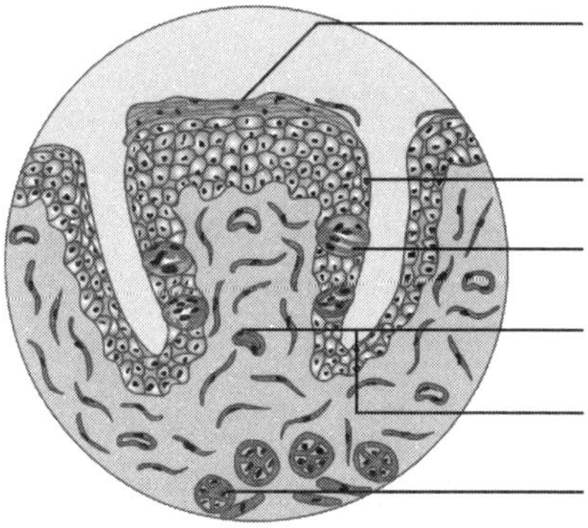
Keratinized stratified squamous epithelium lining superficial surface of papilla
Nonkeratinized epithelium lining lateral surface
Taste buds
Connective tissue core
'V' shaped trough around papilla
Von ebner's salivary gland

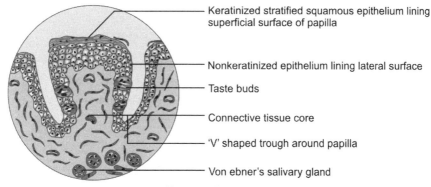

Fig. 30.7: Circumvallate papilla *(For color version, See Plate 2)*

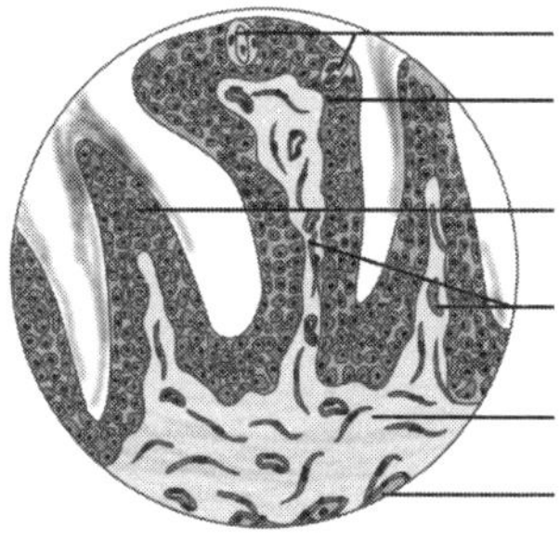
Taste buds
Fungiform papilla lined by nonkeratinized epithelium
Filiform papilla lined by keratinized epithelium
Connective tissue core
Lamina propria
Submucosa containing muscle

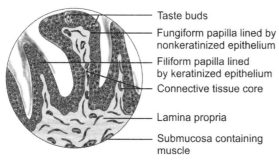

Fig. 30.8: Fungiform and filiform papilla *(For color version, See Plate 2)*

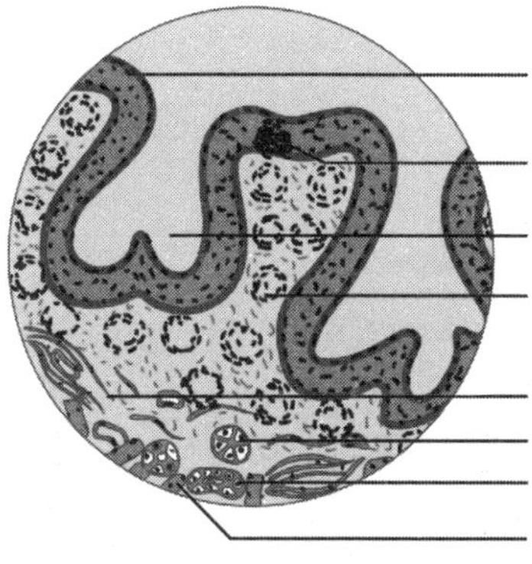
Stratified squamous epithelium
Lymphoid tissue invading epithelium
Crypt
Lymphatic nodules
Connective tissue
Mucous acini
Serous acini
Striated muscle

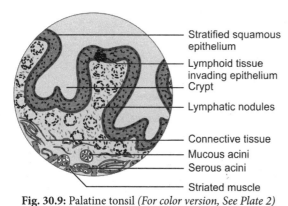

Fig. 30.9: Palatine tonsil *(For color version, See Plate 2)*

- Germinal center may or may not be present.
- Contains large lymphocytes and plasma cells.

Lymph Node (Fig. 30.10)

- Covered by a capsule which consists of dense collagen fiber, fibroblasts and elastic fibers.
- Trabeculae of dense collagenous connective tissue arise from capsule and penetrate the node.
- Medullary card seen and medullary sinus lie in it.

Pituitary Gland/Hypophysis Cerebri (Fig. 30.11)

- It has two major divisions
  - i. Neurohypophysis/Posterior lobe
  - ii. Adenohypophysis
    - → Pars distalis/Anterior lobe
    - → Pars intermedia
    - → Pars tuberalis

1. Pars anterior have lots of cells
   - It contains acidophils, basophils and chromophobe cell
2. Pars intermedia contains vesicles
3. Pars posterior contains nerve fibers

Thyroid Gland (Fig. 30.12)

- It is covered by i. False capsule
  ii. True capsule
- These capsule sends connective tissue septa into gland to form lobes and lobules.
- Thyroid follicles lines by cuboidal to columnar cells containing colloid.
- Scanty connective tissue with capillaries.
- "C" cells in connective tissue or within the follicles.

Pancreas (Fig. 30.13)

- It is a highly cellular gland composed of
  - i. An exocrine part secreting pancreatic juice
  - ii. An endocrine part called islets of Langerhans

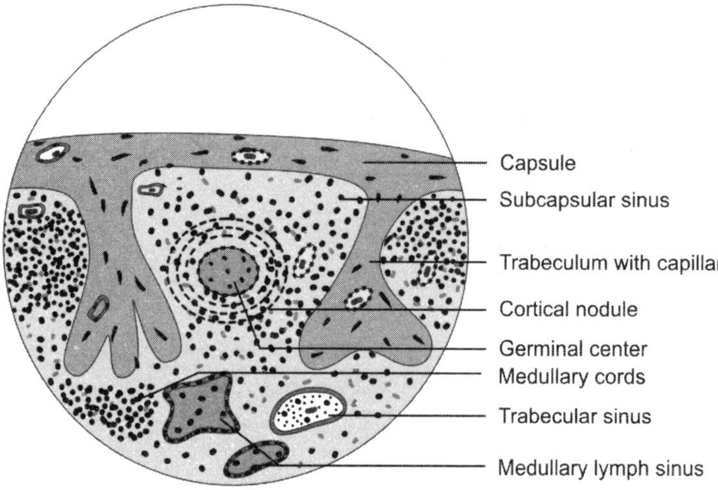
Capsule
Subcapsular sinus
Trabeculum with capillaries
Cortical nodule
Germinal center
Medullary cords
Trabecular sinus
Medullary lymph sinus

Fig. 30.10: Lymph node *(For color version, See Plate 3)*

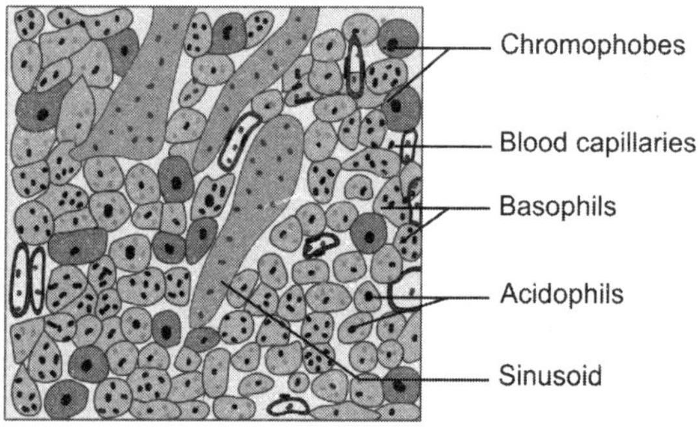
Chromophobes
Blood capillaries
Basophils
Acidophils
Sinusoid

Fig. 30.11: Pituitary gland *(For color version, See Plate 3)*

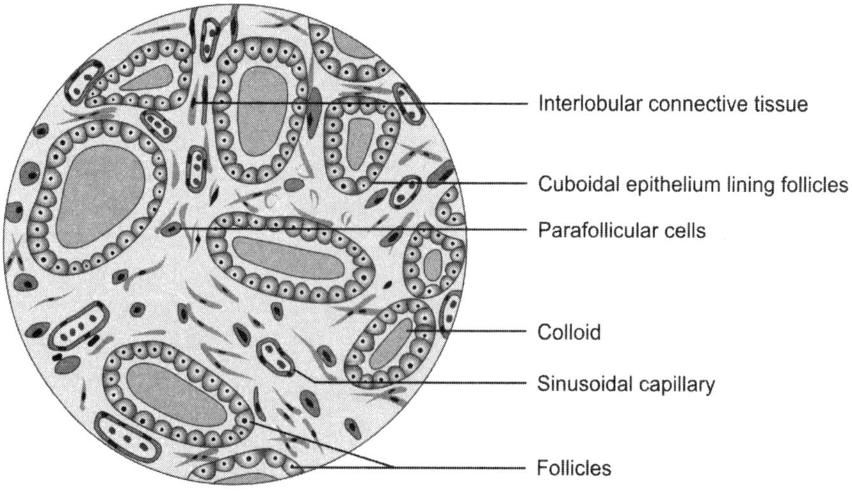
Interlobular connective tissue
Cuboidal epithelium lining follicles
Parafollicular cells
Colloid
Sinusoidal capillary
Follicles

Fig. 30.12: Thyroid gland *(For color version, See Plate 3)*

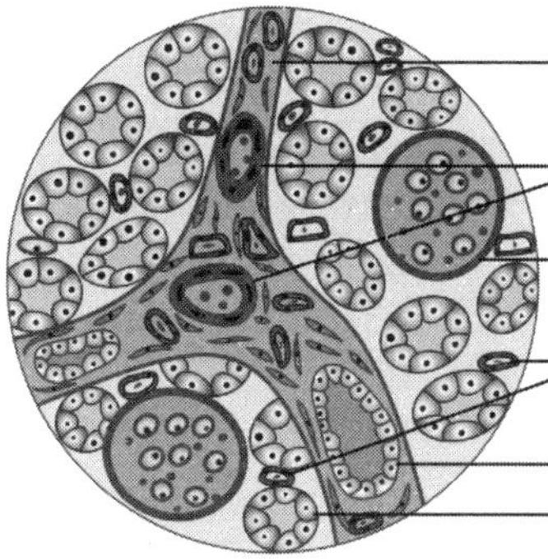
Connective tissue septa
Blood vessels
Islet of Langerhans
Intercalated ducts
Inter lobular ducts
Serous acini

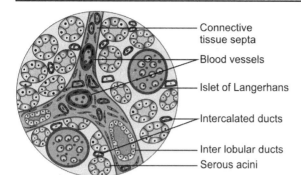

Fig. 30.13: Pancreas *(For color version, See Plate 4)*

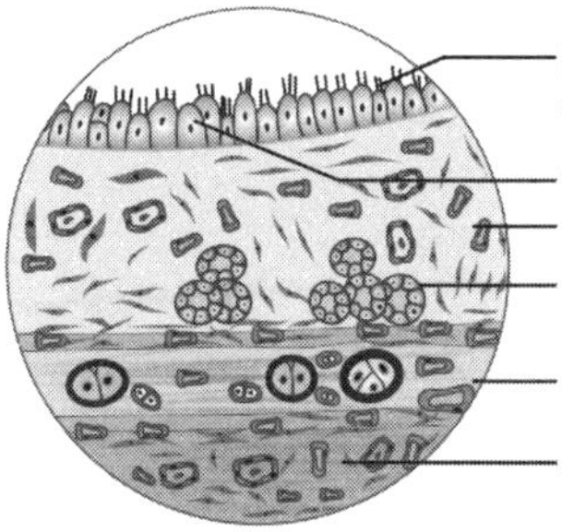
Pseudostratified ciliated columnar epithelium
Goblet cell
Lamina propria
Submucosa with mucous and serous acini
Hyaline cartilage
Adventitia with capillaries

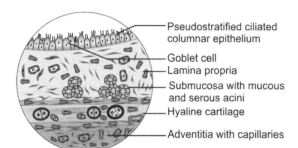

Fig. 30.14: Trachea *(For color version, See Plate 4)*

- Acini lined by pyramidal cells
- Lighter islets of langerhans between acini
- Islet contains number of capillaries

Trachea (Fig. 30.14)

- It is lined by pseudostratified ciliated columnar epithelium.
- Interspersed goblets cells resting on basement membrane.
- Lamina propria consists of
  - i. Elastic fibers
  - ii. Lymphocyte
  - iii. Short ducts
- Deeper part of lamina propria is submucosa which contains both mucous and serous.
- Outermost layer is the adventitia which contains blood vessels and nerves.

Hyaline Cartilage (Fig. 30.15)

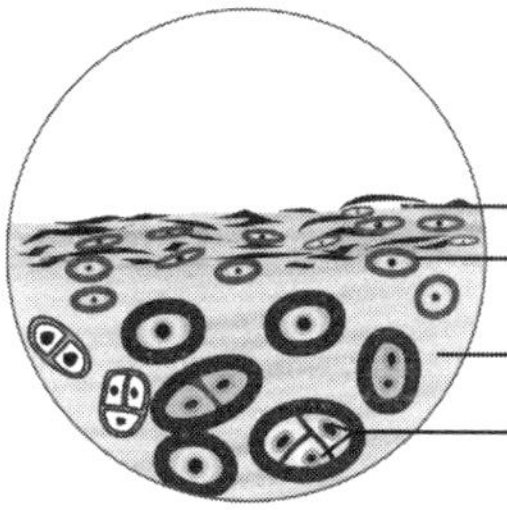
Fibrous layer
Cellular layer
Perichondrium
Matrix
Chondrocytes in lacuna

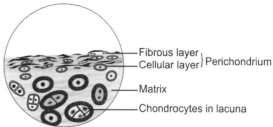

Fig. 30.15: Hyaline cartilage *(For color version, See Plate 4)*

- Subdivided into two types
  - a. Costal cartilage – covered by perichondrium
  - b. Articular cartilage not covered by perichondrium
- Cells are encapsulated in groups of 2-6 "Cell nests"
- Matrix appears homogenous
- Affinity for basic dyes
- Ground substance appears homogenous
- Chondrocytes in lacuna lie in groups of 2-4 cells.

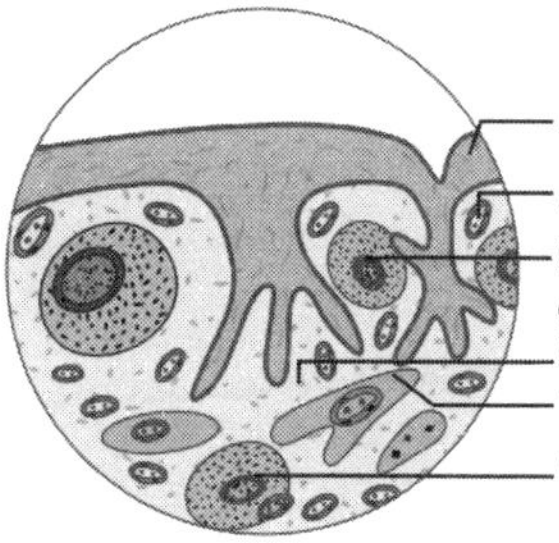
Capsule
Arteriole
Malpighian corpuscle with eccentric arteriole
Red pulp
Trabeculae with arteriole
White pulp

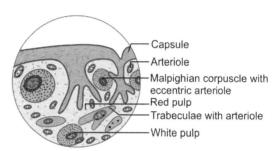

Fig. 30.16: Spleen *(For color version, See Plate 4)*

Spleen (Fig. 30.16)

- Spleen is surrounded by a connective tissue capsule.
- Outer surface of capsule is covered by a layer of flattened mesothelium.
- Trabeculae made up of reticular, elastic and collegenous fibers.
- No differentiation of tissue into cortex and medulla.
- Spleen is comprised of white pulp and red pulp.
- Spleenic corpuscles of malpigian corpuscles.
- Peripheral part contains small lymphocytes.
- Central part/Germinal center has large lymphocytes and plasma cells.

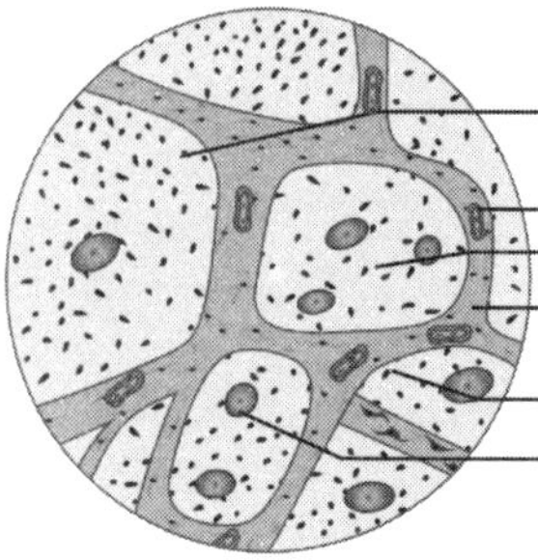
Cortex
Blood vessel
Medulla
Interlobular connective tissue septum
Connective tissue stroma
Hassall's corpuscles

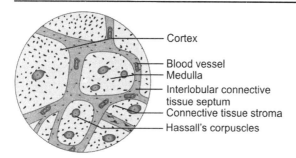

Fig. 30.17: Thymus *(For color version, See Plate 4)*

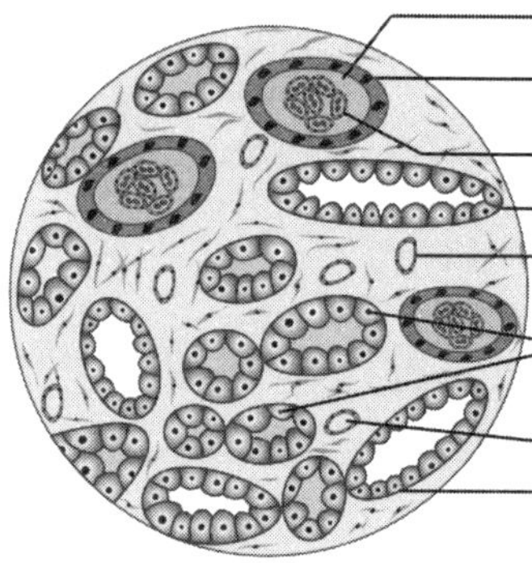
Subcapsular space
Parietal layer of bowman's capsule
Glomerulus
Collecting tubule
Arteriole
Proximal convulated tubule
Blood vessels
Distal convulated tubule

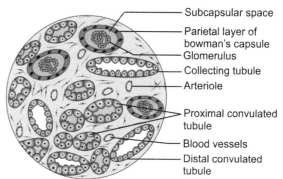

Fig. 30.18: Kidney *(For color version, See Plate 4)*

Thymus (Fig. 30.17)

- It is a lymphoepithelial organ.
- Produces "T-lymphocytes" and lymphocyte stimulating hormone.
- Trabeculae only in cortical part.
- Medulla of adjacent lobules continuous and contains lighter reticular cells.
- Cortex contains dark lymphocytes.
- Hassall's corpuscles made up of concentric lamellae of epithelial cells surrounding a hyaline mass.

Kidney (Fig. 30.18)

- It is covered by a connective tissue capsule and adipose tissue.

Divided into an:

1. Outer cortex – Granular
2. Inner medulla – 8-18 conical masses called renal pyramids.

It contains

- Collecting duct
- Lots of sections of loop of Henle
- Numerous capillaries

PREVIOUS YEAR QUESTIONS

1. Describe various types of connective tissue?
2. Write short notes on:
   a. Urothelium
   b. Microscopic anatomy of pituitary gland.
   c. Histology of thyroid gland
   d. Histology of pancreas.
3. Describe the epithelia under the following heads:
   a. Definition
   b. Classification
   c. Transitional epithelium
4. Describe glands under the following heading:
   a. Definition
   b. Classification with one example each
   c. Differences between serous and mucous gland.
5. Describe histology of palatine tonsil?
6. Draw a well labelled diagram of microscopic anatomy of hyaline cartilage
7. Microscopic structure of salivary glands.
8. Draw the well labelled diagram of
   a. Histology of trachea
   b. Histology of tongue
   c. Histology of lymph node.

MULTIPLE CHOICE QUESTIONS

1. Epithelium in vocal cord is:
   a. Pseudostratified columnar
   b. Stratified squamous
   c. Simple columnar
   d. Cuboidal epithelium
2. Papilla present on margins of tongue:
   a. Fungiform papillae
   b. Filliform papillae
   c. Vallate papillae
   d. Foliate papillae
3. Pseudostratified epithelium is present in:
   a. Respiratory bronchiole
   b. Bowman's capsule

c. Trachea
d. Uterus

4. Transitional epithelium is characteristic of:
   a. Urinary bladder
   b. Blood vessels
   c. Trachea
   d. Gall bladder
5. Purely serous gland is:
   a. Submandibular
   b. Sublingual
   c. Parotid
   d. Minor salivary gland
6. Deep crypts of the epithelium are typical feature of:
   a. Trachea
   b. Lymph node
   c. Palatine tonsil
   d. Spleen
7. 'C' cells are present in:
   a. Parathyroid gland
   b. Thyroid gland
   c. Pituitary gland
   d. Salivary gland
8. Hassall's corpuscles surrounding hyaline mass are seen in:
   a. Thymus
   b. Kidney
   c. Spleen
   d. Pancreas
9. Islets of langerhans are found in:
   a. Thyroid gland
   b. Gall bladder
   c. Pancreas
   d. Liver
10. Spleen is comprised of:
   a. White pulp
   b. Red pulp
   c. White and red pulp both
   d. None

Answers

1. (b) 2. (a) 3. (c) 4. (a) 5. (c) 6. (c) 7. (b) 8. (a) 9. (c) 10. (c)

31 Miscellaneous

FORAMEN (TABLE 31.1)

Table 31.1: Structures passing through foramen

• Foramen Rotundum (ME)	Maxillary nerve Emissary vein
• Foramen Ovale (MALE)	Mandibular nerve Accessory middle meningeal artery Lesser petrosal nerve Emissary vein
• Foramen Spinosum (3 M)	Middle meningeal artery Middle meningeal vein Meningeal branch of mandibular nerve (Nervus Spinosum)
• Foramen Lacerum (MINE)	Meningeal branch of ascending pharyngeal artery Internal carotid artery Nerve of pterygoid canal Emissary vein
• Jugular Foramen	
– Anterior (IM)	Inferior petrosal sinus Meningeal branch of ascending pharyngeal artery
– Middle	IX, X, and XI cranial nerves
– Posterior (IM)	Internal jugular vein Meningeal branch of occipital artery
• Foramen Magnum	
– Anterior Part (MA)	Membrana Tectoria Apical ligament of dens
– Sub-arcanoid Space (VAS)	Vertebral artery Anterior and posterior spinal arteries Spinal accessory nerve
– Posterior Part (LMT)	Lower part of medulla Meninges Tonsil of cerebellum

RED NUCLEUS

- Large ovoid mass of gray matter present on each side of midline.
- It is surrounded by fibers of superior cerebellar peduncle.
- 5 mm in diameter.
- Pink in color.
- Contains iron pigment in its multipolar neuron.
- Situated in tegmentum of the midbrain.
- It consists of two portions.
  1. Caudal part—contains large multipolar neuron.

2. Rostral part—contains small multipolar neuron

Functions

- Acts as an alternative route to pyramidal system.
- Stimulates the flexor tone.
- Inhibits the extensor tone.
- Corticospinal tract helps in learning new movements while rubrospinal tract implement them.

SPINAL CORD

SPINOTHALAMIC SENSORY PATHWAY

- These are ascending and descending tracts (Table 31.2).
- There are two pathways (Fig. 31.1):
  1. Lateral spinothalemic tract
  2. Anterior spinothalemic tract

Lateral Spinothalemic Pathway (Tract)

Origin: Laminae I to IV of spinal gray matter.
Termination: Area 3,1,2 of cerebral cortex.
Crossing over: Fibers cross in the corresponding spinal segment anterior to spinal cord
Sensation carried: Pain and temperature.

Anterior Spinothalamic Pathway (Tract)

Origin: Laminae I to IV of spinal gray meter.
Termination: Joins with medial lemniscus in medulla.
Crossing over: Fibers cross 2 to 3 segment above spinal segment.
Sensation carried: Non-discriminatory touch and pressure.

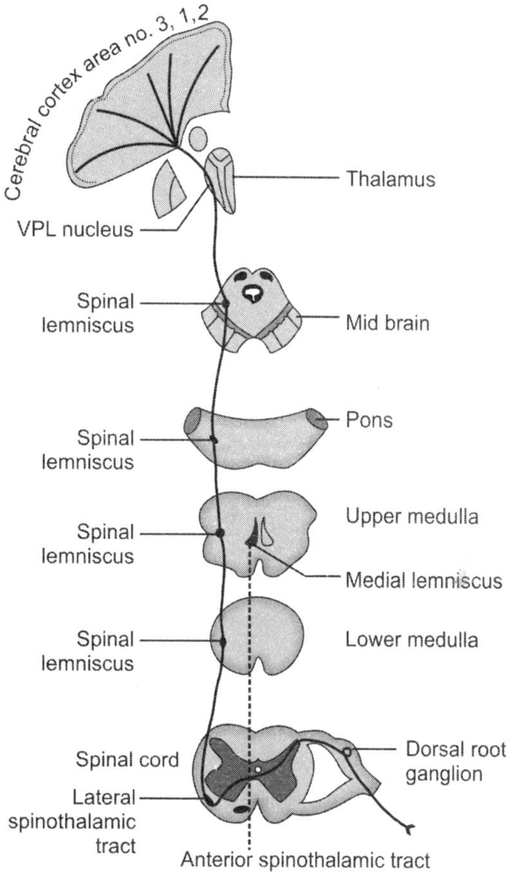
Cerebral cortex area no. 3, 1,2
Thalamus
VPL nucleus
Spinal lemniscus
Mid brain
Spinal lemniscus
Pons
Spinal lemniscus
Upper medulla
Medial lemniscus
Spinal lemniscus
Lower medulla
Spinal cord
Dorsal root ganglion
Lateral spinothalamic tract
Anterior spinothalamic tract

Fig. 31.1: Anterior and lateral spinothalamic tract

Table 31.2: Tracts of spinal cord

Funiculus	*Ascending Tracts (Fig. 31.2)*	*Descending Tracts (Fig. 31.3)*
Anterior	1. Anterior spinothalamic	Anterior corticospinal Tectospinal Vestibulospinal Medial reticulospinal
Lateral	2. Posteior spino-cerebellar 3. Anterior spino-cerebellar 4. Lateral spinothalamic 5. Dorsolateral tract of Lissauer	Lateral corticospinal Rubrospinal Lateral reticulospinal Olivo spinal
Posterior	6. Fasciculus gracilis or tract of gall 9. Fasciculus septomarginalis	Fasciculus cuneatus or tract of Burdach Fasciculus inter fasciculus

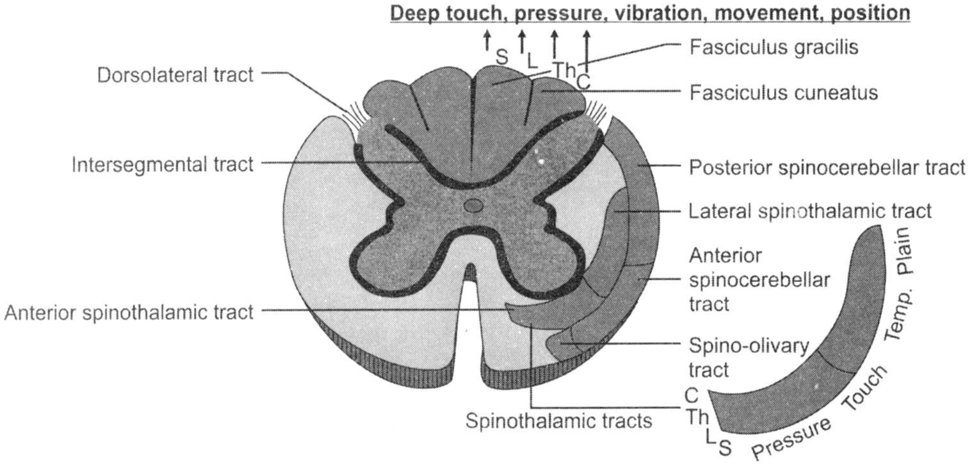
Deep touch, pressure, vibration, movement, position
S L Th C
Dorsolateral tract
Fasciculus gracilis
Fasciculus cuneatus
Intersegmental tract
Posterior spinocerebellar tract
Lateral spinothalamic tract
Anterior spinocerebellar tract
Anterior spinothalamic tract
Spino-olivary tract
Spinothalamic tracts
C Th L S
Pressure Touch Temp. Plain

Fig. 31.2: Ascending tract of spinal cord

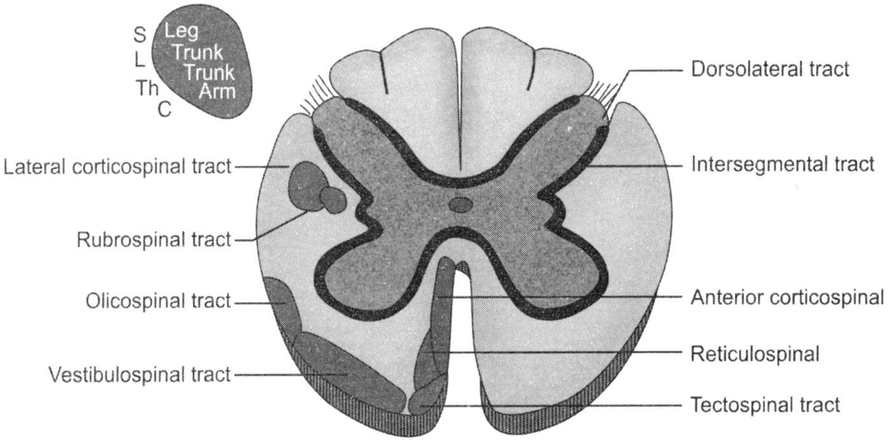
S L Th C
Leg
Trunk
Trunk
Arm
Dorsolateral tract
Lateral corticospinal tract
Intersegmental tract
Rubrospinal tract
Olicospinal tract
Anterior corticospinal
Reticulospinal
Vestibulospinal tract
Tectospinal tract

Fig. 31.3: Descending tract of spinal cord

VARIOUS TYPES OF NEURONS (TABLE 31.3)

Table 31.3: Types of neuron

According to polarity	*According to axon length*	*According to shape of soma*	*Size of soma*
Unipolar: One process arises from the body, e.g. dorsal root ganglion	**Golgi Type-I:** Long axons which forms trads, e.g. fasciculas gracilis	• Stellate shape • Fusiform shape • Basket shape • Flask shape • Pyramidal shape	• Microneurons—7 mm length • Large neuron—12 mm of length
Bipolar: two processes arises from the body, e.g. olfactory mucosa	**Golgi Type-II:** Short axons, e.g. present in gray matter		
Multipolar: More than two processes arise from body, e.g. maximum neuron of body	**Amacrine:** Numerous processes without an axon, e.g. present in retina		

OPTIC PATHWAY

The nervous pathway which carries the retinal impulses to the visual center in cerebral cortex is called optic pathway (Flow chart 31.1).

Flow chart 31.1: Course of Visual/Optic Pathway

Optic nerve leaves eye through optic disc
↓
Medial fibers of each optic nerve cross midline
↓
They join the uncrossed lateral fibers of opposite side
↓
Optic chiasma
↓
Fibers runs towards lateral geniculation body
↓
Fibers pass through internal capsule
↓
Forms optic radiation
↓
Ends in visual cortex

Applied Anatomy

- Lesion of one optic nerve will cause total blindness in corresponding visual field.
- Lesion of optic tract/lateral geniculate body will cause homonymous hemianopia.
- Lesion of visual cortex will causes inferior or superior homonymous hemianopia.

BRACHIAL PLEXUS (FLOW CHART 31.2)

- It is formed by interconnection of ventral primary rami of C5, C6, C7, C8 and T1 spinal nerves which supply upper limb.
- It is made up of roots, trunks and cords which are divided into cervical, supraclavicular and infraclavicular parts respectively.
  - **Roots:** Formed by anterior primary rami of C5, C6, C7, C8 and T1.
  - **Trunks**
    i. *Upper trunk:* Formed by joining of C5 and C6 roots
    ii. *Middle trunk:* Formed by C7 roots
    iii. *Lower trunk:* Formed by joining of C8 and T1 roots
  - **Division:** Each trunk divides into ventral and dorsal divisions
  - **Cords**
    i. *Lateral cord:* Formed by union of ventral division of upper and middle trunks
    ii. *Medial cord:* Formed by ventral division of lower trunk
    iii. *Posterior cord:* Formed by union of dorsal division of all the three trunks.

Branches

From Roots

- Dorsal scapular
- Long thoracic/nerve of bell
- Branches to join phrenic nerve
- Branches to longus coli and scalenus muscles

From Upper Trunk

- Nerve to subclavius
- Suprascapular nerve

From Lateral Cord (LML)

- **L**ateral pectrol nerve
- **M**usculo-cutaneous nerve
- **L**ateral root of median nerve

From Medial Cord (4 MU)

- **M**edial pectoral nerve
- **M**edial cutaneous nerve of forearm
- **M**edial cutaneous nerve of arm
- **M**edial route of median nerve
- **U**lnar nerve

From Posterior Cord (RAT)

- Upper subscapular
- Lower subscapular
- **R**adial nerve
- **A**xillary nerve
- **T**horaco-dorsal nerve

Clinical Anatomy

- Injury to nerve of bell due to sudden pressure on shoulder leads to paralysis of serratus anterior muscle which causes **winging of scapula**.

Flow chart 31.2: Brachial plexus

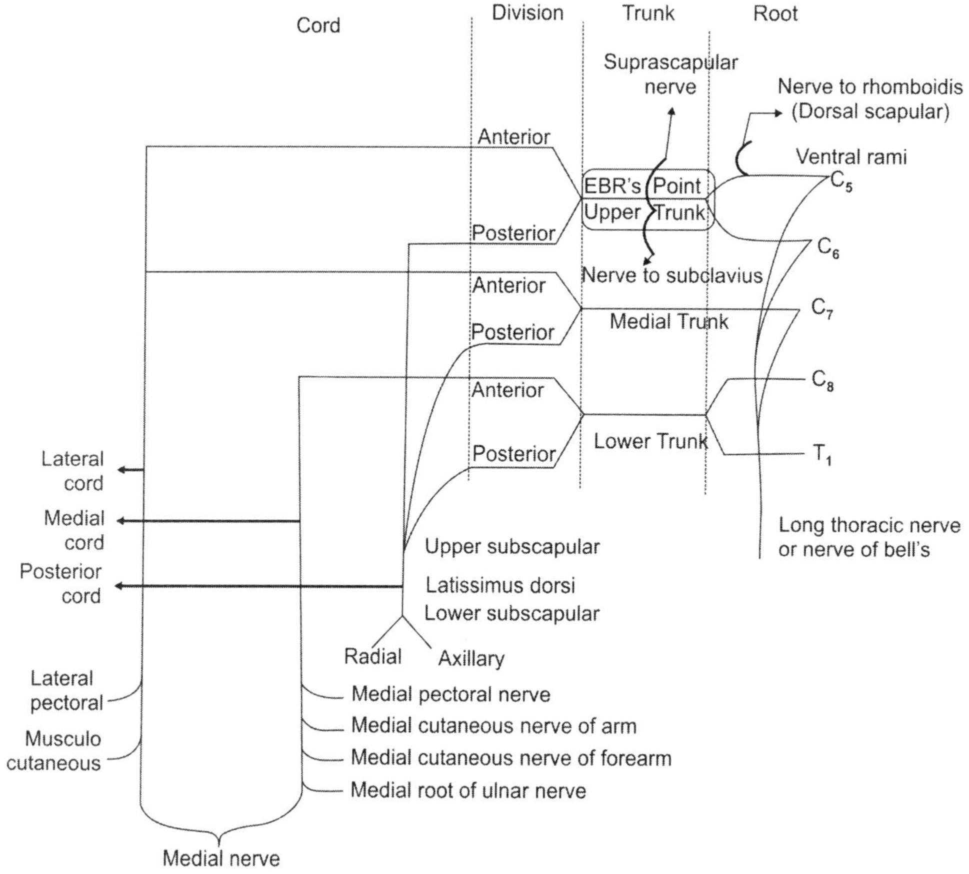
Cord
Division
Trunk
Root
Suprascapular nerve
Nerve to rhomboidis (Dorsal scapular)
Ventral rami
Anterior
EBR's Point
Upper Trunk
Posterior
C5
C6
Nerve to subclavius
Anterior
Medial Trunk
Posterior
C7
Anterior
C8
Lower Trunk
Posterior
T1
Lateral cord
Medial cord
Posterior cord
Long thoracic nerve or nerve of bell's
Upper subscapular
Latissimus dorsi
Lower subscapular
Radial
Axillary
Lateral pectoral
Musculo cutaneous
Medial pectoral nerve
Medial cutaneous nerve of arm
Medial cutaneous nerve of forearm
Medial root of ulnar nerve
Medial nerve

- **Erb's Point:** It is a point in upper trunk which is formed by joining of
  - C5 and C6 roots
  - Suprascapular nerve
  - Nerve to subclavius
  - Anterior and posterior division of upper trunk

Erb's Duchenne Palsy/Paralysis

It occurs due to

- Injury to the upper trunk of brachial plexus where these six nerves meet.
- Breech deliveries of babies.
- Prolonged abnormal posture during surgery.

It leads to sensory and motor loss on lateral side of forearm.

Clinical Signs

- Upper limbs is by the side of body and adducted due to paralysis of deltoid, coracobrachialis and subclavius.
- **Medially rotated** due to paralysis of teres minor and infra spinatus muscle.
- **Pronated** due to paralysis of biceps muscle.
- This is known as **Waiter Tip Hand**.

Klumpke's Paralysis

- It results due to lesion involving the lower trunk (C8 and T1).
- Caused by forceful upwards traction of arm.
  - Motor loss—Hands assumes a characteristic deformity described as Claw hand.

Table 31.4: Classification of joints

Structural	*Functional*	*Region*
• **Fibrous joint** - Suture - Syndesmosis - Gomphosis	• Synarthrosis - Immovable, e.g.- fibrous joint	• Skull type - Immovable
• **Cartilaginous joint** - Primary/synchondrosis - Secondary/symphysis	• Amphiarthrosis - Slightly movable, e.g. - cartilaginous joint	• Vertebral type - Slightly movable
• **Synovial joint** - Ball and socket - Saddle - Condylar - Hinge	• Limb type - Freely movable, e.g. snovial joints	• Diarthrosis

- Sensory loss—along the ulnar side of hand forearm and arm.
- Horner's syndrome.

JOINTS

It is a junction between two or more bones or cartilages (Table 31.4).

Fibrous Joint

- Bones are joined by fibrous tissue.
- Either immovable or permit a slight degree of movement
- Following are the subtypes:

Sutures

- Present in skull
- Immovable
- According to shape of bony margins, it can be plane, serrate, denticulate, squamous, limbous types.

Syndesmosis

- Bones are connected by interosseous ligament.
- For example, inferior tibiofibular joint

Gomphosis (Peg and Socket joint)

- For example, Tooth in its socket.

Synovial Joint (Table 31.5)

- It consist of articular surfaces, which are formed by special variety of hyaline cartilage.
- Articular cartilage is wear resistant, low frictional and consists of fabricated surface and provide easy movement.
- It consists of fibrous capsule which completely encloses the joint.
- It is filled by **synovial fluid.**

Table 31.5: Classification of synovial joints and their movements

	Types of joint	*Movement*
A.	Plane type	Gliding movement
B.	Uniaxial joints - Hinge - Pivot	 Flexion and extension Rotation only
C.	Biaxial joints - Condylar - Ellipsoid	 Flexion, extension, and limited rotation Flexion extension abduction, adduction and circumduction
D.	Multiaxial joints - Saddle - Ball and socket (spheroidal)	 Flexion, extension, abduction, adduction and conjunct rotation Flexion, extension, abduction adduction circumduction and rotation

ARM MUSCLES (TABLE 31.6)

Table 31.6: Muscle of arm

Muscle and nerve supply	*Origin*	*Insertion*	*Actions*
• Deltoids – By axillary nerve	• Upper surface of lateral 1/3rd of clavicle • Lateral border of acromian • Lower lip of spine of scapula	Deltoid tuberosity – V Shape insertion on lateral aspect of humerus	• Abduction • Flexion • Extension - They act as shoulder joint
• Biceps Brachii – Musculocutaneos nerve	• Short head: Tip of coronoid process • Long head: Supraglenoid tubercle	Posterior part of radial tuberosity	• Supination in semiflexed foramen • Flexor of elbow joint • Flexion of shoulder joint • Stabilization of shoulder joint.
• Triceps Brachii – Radial nerve	• Long head – Infraglenoid tubercle of scapula • Lateral head – Oblique ridge of humerus • Medial head – Entire posterior surface of humerus	Posterior part of upper surface of olecranon process of ulna	• Extention of forearm • Acts at elbow joint

FEMORAL TRIANGLE

- It is triangular depression below the inguinal ligament with apex directed below.
- Present in the upper 1/3rd of the front of thigh.

Boundaries

- *Apex:* Meeting point of sartorius and adductor longus muscles
- *Base:* Inguinal ligament
- *Medially:* Adductor longus
- *Laterally:* Sartorius
- *Floor:* Iliacus
  Tendon of Psoas major
  Pectineus
  Adductor lougus
- *Roof:* Fascia lata
  Superficial fascia
  Skin

Contents (6F PD)

- Femoral sheath
- Femoral arteries and its branches
- Femoral vein and its tributaries
- Femoral nerve and its branches
- Fibro fatty tissue
- Femoral branch of genitofemoral nerve
- Part of lateral femoral cutaneous nerve
- Deep inguinal lymph node

BLOOD SUPPLY OF BONE (FIG. 31.4)

Bone is supplied by four sets of blood vessels as

1. Nutrient artery—supplies to bone marrow and inner 2/3rd of cortex.
2. Metaphyseal artery/Juxta epithelia artery—arise from anastomosis around the joint.
3. Epiphyseal artery—derived from periarticular vascular arcades found on non articular bone surface.
4. Periosteal artery—main artery which supplies to short bone. It supplies the harversian system in outer 1/3rd of cortex.

BLOOD SUPPLY OF HEART

1. Arterial Supply—By two coronary arteries from ascending aorta. Both runs in coronary sulcus.

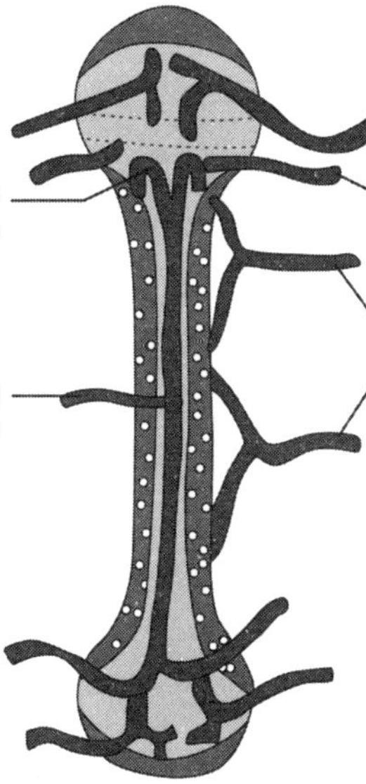
Epiphyseal artery
Pin head artery
Metaphyseal artery
Periosteal artery
Nutrient artery

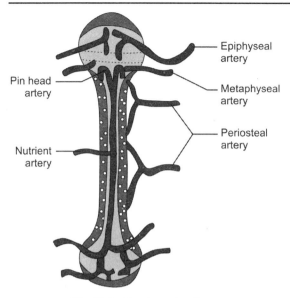

Fig. 31.4: Blood supply of bone

a. *Right Coronary Artery*
   - Smaller than left
   - Arises from anterior aortic sinus
   - Supplies right atrium, ventricle, i.e. major part of right ventricle and smaller part of left ventricle and whole system of heart except left branch of AV bundle.

b. *Left Coronary Artery*
   - Arises from left posterior aortic sinus
   - Supplies to left atrium
   - Ventricle (major part of left and small part of right ventricle)
   - Left branch of AV bundle

2. Venous Supply
   Heart is mainly supplied by 3 veins.
   a. *Coronary Sinus*
      - Longest vein of heart
      - Receive tributaries as
      - Great cardiac vein
      - Middle cardiac vein
      - Small cardiac vein
      - Posterior vein of left ventricle
      - Oblique vein of left atrium of Marshall's
      - Right marginal vein
   b. *Anterior Cardiac Vein*
   c. *Venae Cordis Minimi*

SYNDROMES

1. Turner's Syndrome
   - Monosomy of X chromosome is seen
   - Karyotype 45, X0
   - Patient is female with no Y chromosomes and present with following features
     a. Short stature
     b. Webbing of neck
     c. Underdeveloped breast
     d. Rudimentary ovaries
     e. Majority are infertile
     f. Primary or secretary amenorrhea
2. Down's Syndrome/Mongolism/Triosomy 21
   - It usually follows fertilization of 2 gametes out of which one has two chromosome 21.
   - It can also occur due to translocation.

Clinical Features

- Mental retardation
- Short stature
- Brachy cephaly
- Protruding tongue
- Small ears and flat occiput
- Flat nasal bridge
- Males are inferile and female have reduced fertility.

Risk Factors

- Advancing maternal age.
- Familial history.
- Radiation injuries

3. Klinefelter's Syndrome
   - Trisomy of sex chromosome
   - Karyotype is 47, XXY
   - Patient is male

Clinical Features

- Mild developmental delay
- Behavioral immaturity
- Small testes
- Dysgenesis of seminiferous tubules
- Gynecomastia
- Poor musculature
- Infertile

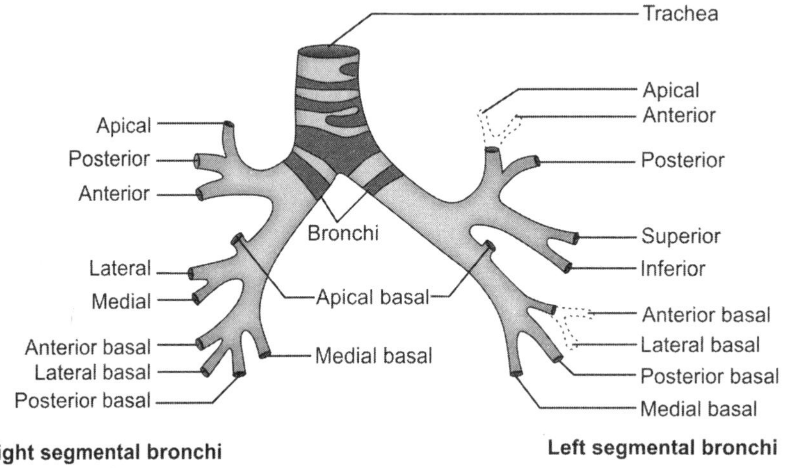
Trachea
Apical
Posterior
Anterior
Bronchi
Lateral
Medial
Apical basal
Anterior basal
Lateral basal
Posterior basal
Medial basal
Apical
Anterior
Posterior
Superior
Inferior
Anterior basal
Lateral basal
Posterior basal
Medial basal
Right segmental bronchi
Left segmental bronchi

Fig. 31.5: Functional unit of lung

BRONCHO-PULMONARY SEGMENTS

- It is the independent functional unit of lung (Fig. 31.5).
- Made up of a tertiary branches with its branchial tree accompanied by an independent branch from pulmonary artery, venous drainage is inter-segmental.
- Each lung has ten broncho-pulmonary segment

Anatomical Features

Shape - Wedge
Apex - Towards tertiary branches
Base - Towards lung surface

Principal branches of lung
↓
Divides into upper and lower end
↓
Subdivides to form 10 segmental bronchi on each side (Table 31.7)

Clinical Anatomy

- Apical segment of lower lobe of right lung is commonest site of aspiration lung abscess and aspiration pneumonia (Mendelson's Syndrome).
- Posterior segment if right upper lobe is commonest site of tuberculosis.

Table 31.7: Ten broncho-pulmonary segments

Lobe	*Right Lung Segments*	*Left Lung Segments*
Upper	Apical Posterior Anterior	Apical Posterior Anterior Upper lingual Lower lingual
Middle	Medial Lateral	
Lower	Apical Medial basal Anterior basal Lateral basal Posterior basal	Apical Medial basal Anterior basal Lateral basal Posterior basal

- Anterior segment of upper lobe is most frequent site of origin of carcinoma.

LMPHATIC DRAINAGE OF BREAST

- Female mammary gland is a modified sweat gland which lies in the superficial fascia in pectoral region.
- Right gland may be larger and lower than left.
- Lymphaytic drainage of breast has a deep and superficial part (Fig. 31.6).

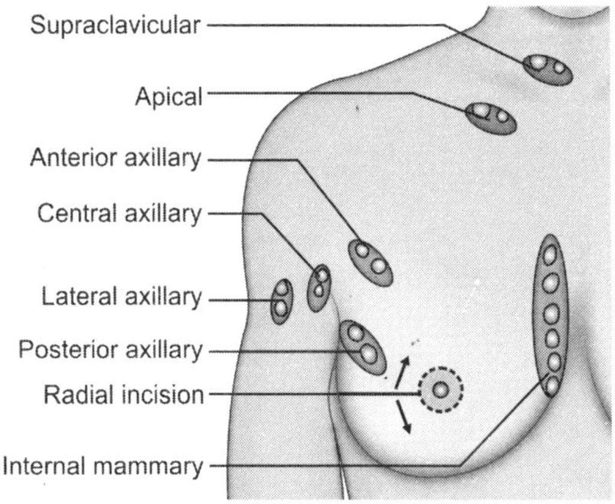
Supraclavicular
Apical
Anterior axillary
Central axillary
Lateral axillary
Posterior axillary
Radial incision
Internal mammary

Fig. 31.6: Lymph nodes draining breast

Deep Part

- Drains parenchyma, nipple and areola.
- Areola and nipple are drained by subreolar plexus of sappey.
- Parenchyma is drained by vessels present in interlobular connective tissue and walls of lactiferous ducts.
  - 75% drain into maxillary nodes
  - 20% drain into parasternal nodes.
  - 5% drain into posterior intercostal nodes.

Superficial Part

- Drains overlying skin except areola and nipple.
- Outer part drains into axillary nodes.
- Inner part drains into parasternal groups of lymph nodes.
- This communicates with the opposite parasternal nodes.
- Upper part drains into supraclavicular group of lymph nodes.
- Lower part drains into subdiaphragmatic nodes.
- They communicates with sub-peritoneal plexus of lymphatic.

Bibliography

1. BD Chaurasia. Handbook of General Anatomy (3rd edn).
2. BD Chaurasia's Human Anatomy (4th edn), volume 1-Upper Limb and Thorax
3. BD Chaurasia's Human Anatomy (4th edn), volume 2-Lower Limb, Abdomen and Pelvis
4. BD Chaurasia's Human Anatomy (4th edn), volume 3-Head, Neck and Brain
5. GP Pal. Textbook of Histology (1st edn).
6. Gowri Shankar. Dentest (2nd edn).
7. Inderbir Singh, GP Pal. Human Embroyology (7th edn).
8. Inderbir Singh. Textbook of Anatomy with Color Atlas (3rd edn) volume 3-Head, Neck and Brain
9. Inderbir Singh. Textbook of Human Histology (4th edn).
10. Krishna Garg, Indira Bahl, Mohini Kaul. Textbook of Histology Color Atlas (4th edn).
11. Mahindra Kumar Anand. Human Anatomy for Dental Student (1st edn).
12. Satheesh Kumar K, Swapna M. Dental Pulse (4th edn).

Index

Page numbers followed by *f* refer to figure and *t* refer to table